OXFORD WORLD'S CLASSICS

KAMASUTRA

THE *Kamasutra* is the oldest extant Hindu textbook of erotic love. It was composed in Sanskrit, the literary language of ancient India, probably in North India and probably sometime in the third century of the common era, most likely in its second half, at the dawn of the Gupta Empire. Virtually nothing is known about the author, Vatsyayana Mallanaga, other than his name and what we learn from this text.

WENDY DONIGER (O'FLAHERTY) is the Mircea Eliade Distinguished Service Professor of the History of Religions at the University of Chicago, and the author of translations of Sanskrit texts, including the *Rig Veda* (1981) and the *Laws of Manu* (1991), as well as books about India—*Splitting the Difference: Gender and Myth in Ancient Greece and India* (1988)—about myth—*Other Peoples' Myths: The Cave of Echoes* (1984)—and about sex—*Siva: The Erotic Ascetic* (1973) and *The Bedtrick: Tales of Sex and Masquerade* (2000).

SUDHIR KAKAR is a psychoanalyst and currently a Senior Fellow at the Center for the Study of World Religions at Harvard University. He is the author of many books on India that cover a wide spectrum from Hindu childhood to India's healing traditions, from male–female relations to Hindu–Muslim violence, from classical love tales to modern mysticism. His most recent books are *The Ascetic of Desire* (1999), a fictionalized account of the life of Vatsyayana, the author of the *Kamasutra*, and the the novel *Ecstasy* (2001).

OXFORD WORLD'S CLASSICS

For over 100 years Oxford World's Classics have brought readers closer to the world's great literature. Now with over 700 titles—from the 4,000-year-old myths of Mesopotamia to the twentieth century's greatest novels—the series makes available lesser-known as well as celebrated writing.

The pocket-sized hardbacks of the early years contained introductions by Virginia Woolf, T. S. Eliot, Graham Greene, and other literary figures which enriched the experience of reading. Today the series is recognized for its fine scholarship and reliability in texts that span world literature, drama and poetry, religion, philosophy and politics. Each edition includes perceptive commentary and essential background information to meet the changing needs of readers.

OXFORD WORLD'S CLASSICS

VATSYAYANA MALLANAGA

Kamasutra

*A new, complete English translation of the
Sanskrit text*

*with excerpts from the
Sanskrit* Jayamangala *commentary of
Yashodhara Indrapada,
the Hindi* Jaya *commentary of
Devadatta Shastri,
and explanatory notes by the translators*

Translated and edited by
WENDY DONIGER *and* SUDHIR KAKAR

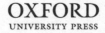

OXFORD
UNIVERSITY PRESS

OXFORD
UNIVERSITY PRESS

Great Clarendon Street, Oxford OX2 6DP

Oxford University Press is a department of the University of Oxford.
It furthers the University's objective of excellence in research, scholarship,
and education by publishing worldwide in

Oxford New York

Auckland Bangkok Buenos Aires Cape Town Chennai
Dar es Salaam Delhi Hong Kong Istanbul Karachi Kolkata
Kuala Lumpur Madrid Melbourne Mexico City Mumbai Nairobi
São Paulo Shanghai Taipei Tokyo Toronto

Oxford is a registered trade mark of Oxford University Press
in the UK and in certain other countries

Published in the United States
by Oxford University Press Inc., New York

British Library Cataloguing in Publication Data

Data available

Library of Congress Cataloging in Publication Data

Data available

ISBN–13: 978–0–19–283982–4
ISBN–10: 0–19–283982–9

6

Typeset in Ehrhardt
by RefineCatch Limited, Bungay, Suffolk
Printed in Great Britain by
Clays Ltd, St Ives plc

For Katha and Kali

This book is specific:

→ It tells what actions to do, speeches to make, etc.

→ Says exactly the steps you need to take. Kind of ridiculous!

→ Ex. Pg 25 → tells what kind of furniture to buy

→ almost like rope. Continues to move forward even if she disagrees. Stupid ex. page 112

CONTENTS

KAMASUTRA

with excerpts from Yashodhara's commentary, the Jayamangala

BOOK TWO · SEX

BOOK THREE · VIRGINS

INTRODUCTION

I. THE TEXT

The Text and its Author(s)

The *Kamasutra* is the oldest extant Hindu textbook of erotic love. It is not, as most people think, a book about the positions in sexual intercourse. It is a book about the art of living—about finding a partner, maintaining power in a marriage, committing adultery, living as or with a courtesan, using drugs—and also about the positions in sexual intercourse. The two words in its title mean 'desire/love/pleasure/sex' (*kama*) and 'a treatise (*sutra*).[1] It was composed in Sanskrit, the literary language of ancient India (related to Latin, in ancient Rome, and ancient Greek, in Greece). The data relevant to a determination of its date are sparse and the arguments complex, but most scholars believe that it was composed sometime in the third century of the common era, most likely in its second half,[2] and probably in North India. Its detailed knowledge of Northwestern India, and its pejorative attitude to other parts of India, particularly the South and the East, suggest that it was written in the Northwest; on the other hand, its reference to Pataliputra alone among cities suggests that it may have been written in Pataliputra (near the present city of Patna, in Bihar), as Yashodhara (who wrote the definitive commentary on this text, in the thirteenth century) believes to be the case. It would be good to have more information about social conditions in India at the time when the *Kamasutra* was written, but the *Kamasutra* itself is one of the main sources that we have for such

[1] Since Kama is also the name of the Hindu god of erotic love, F. F. Arbuthnot referred to the *Kama Shastra* (the *Anangaranga*) as the Scripture of Cupid. See Archer, 'Preface', 24. (Full titles and details for all works cited are given in the Bibliography.)

[2] The *Kamasutra* must have been written after 225 because the western Indian political situation that Vatsyayana describes shows the Abhiras and the Andhras ruling simultaneously over a region that had been ruled by the Andhras alone until 225. Its style seems very close to that of the *Arthashastra*, also of uncertain date, but generally placed in the 3rd century CE; it cites the *Arthashastra* explicitly at 1.2.10, and implicitly elsewhere. The fact that the text does not mention the Guptas, who ruled North India from the beginning of the 4th century CE, suggests that the text predates that period. The *Kamasutra* is mentioned by name in the *Vasavadatta* of Subandhu, composed under Chandragupta Vikramaditya, who reigned at the beginning of the 5th century CE. Chakladar, *Social Life, passim*; Syrkin, *Kamasutra*, 189; Mylius, *Das Kamasutra*, 16–18.

data; the text is, in a sense, its own context. The cultural context is urbane and cosmopolitan, with a real consciousness of the possible regions of 'India', what one scholar has called a 'pre-Imperial consciousness', setting the stage for the Gupta Empire that would dominate North India from the fourth century to the sixth.[3]

Virtually nothing is known about the author, Vatsyayana Mallanaga, other than his name and what we learn from this text; and all that he tells us is that he composed it 'in chastity and in the highest meditation' [7.2.57], about which we may conclude, as he himself remarks about someone else's claim of virtue [5.4.15], that it 'may or may not have happened'. But Vatsyayana tells us something important about his text, namely, that it is a distillation of the works of a number of authors who preceded him, authors whose texts have not come down to us: Auddalaki, Babhravya, Charayana, Dattaka, Ghotakamukha, Gonardiya, Gonikaputra, and Suvarnanabha. These other authors, called 'teachers' or 'scholars', supply what Indian logic called the 'other side' (literally, the 'former wing', *purvapaksha*), the arguments that opponents might raise. In this case, they are 'former' in both the logical and chronological sense of the word; Vatsyayana cites them often, sometimes in agreement, sometimes in disagreement. Always his own voice comes through, as he acts as ringmaster over the many acts that he incorporates in his sexual circus. The *Kamasutra* was therefore certainly not the first of its genre, nor was it the last. The many textbooks of eroticism that follow it, such as Kokkaka's *Ratirahasya* (also called the *Kokashastra*, pre-thirteenth century) and Kalyanamalla's *Anangaranga* (fifteenth century), cite it as a foundational authority. The *Nagarasarvasva* of Bhikshu Padamashri and the *Panchasayaka* of Jyotirishvara (eleventh to thirteenth century) explicitly base themselves on the *Kamasutra*, the first on Books Two, Five, and Seven, and the second on Books Two, Three, Five, and Seven. The *Kamasutra* also made a deep impact on Indian literature; its vocabulary and taxonomies were diffused into later Sanskrit erotic poetry.[4]

The erotic science to which these texts belong, known as *kamashastra* ('the science of *kama*'), is one of the three principal human sciences in ancient India, the other two being religious and social law (*dharma-shastra*, of which the most famous work is attributed to

---

[3] Laura Desmond, personal communication, September 2000.
[4] Hampiholi, *Kamashastra in Classical Sanskrit Literature*.

Manu, the *Manavadharmashastra* or *Manusmriti*, known as the *Laws of Manu*) and the science of political and economic power (*arthashastra*, whose foundational text is attributed to Kautilya, the minister of Chandragupta Maurya). (There were many other sciences, preserved in texts about medicine, astronomy, architecture, the management of horses and elephants, and so forth.[5]) The *Kamasutra* opens with a discussion of *dharma*, *artha*, and *kama*, known collectively as the three aims of human life (*purusharthas*) or the trinity (*trivarga*). For assonance, one might call them piety, profit, and pleasure, or society, success, and sex, or duty, domination, and desire. More precisely, *dharma* includes duty, religion, religious merit, morality, social obligations, the law, justice, and so forth. Vatsyayana's commitment to *dharma* emerges frequently at the end of a chapter. *Artha* is money, political power, and success; it can also be translated as goal or aim (as in the three aims of human life), gain (versus loss), money, the meaning of a word, and the purpose of something. *Kama* represents pleasure and desire (what the Germans call *Lust* and *Wollust*), not merely sexual but more broadly sensual— music, good food, perfume, and so forth.

This basic trinity is one of several important triads in Hinduism, whose role in Hindu intellectual history demonstrates that 'three' became a kind of shorthand for 'lots and lots'; these threes represented the multivalent, multifaceted, multiform, multi-whatever-you-like nature of the real phenomenal world. The world of the triads is the India of fabled elephants encrusted with jewels and temples covered with copulating couples. This paradigm began in the earthy, vibrant text known as the *Rig Veda*, the oldest sacred text in India, composed in about 1000 BCE, and it still prevails in certain sectors of Hindu society and religion today. But it came to share centre stage with another paradigm that might have subverted or destroyed it altogether, but which, instead, simply came to supplement it as an alternative view of human life; this is the ascetic movement. The omphalosceptic yogis who composed the early Upanishads over a period of a few centuries, probably beginning in the seventh century BCE, fled from the sensual world of sex and sacrifice but did not destroy it. The two worlds remain in conversation in the *Kamasutra*. Why, one might ask, does Vatsyayana go to the trouble of

---

[5] Pollock, 'The Theory of Practice and the Practice of Theory'.

inventing fictive pragmatists, straw men who protest against sex [1.2.32], when there were real people there in India, the religious fringe, who thought that sex was terrible? The answer is that there were good reasons for him to avoid picking a fight with them.

For renunciation was an essential part of the system in which Vatsyayana lived, and eroticism, like asceticism, depends upon the technique of control of the body known as yoga.[6] Sometimes the aims of human life are listed not as a triad but as a quartet, in which the fourth goal is release, *moksha*, the goal of the religious renouncer (Yashodhara speaks of four aims at 1.5.8). Vatsyayana gives very short shrift indeed to release [1.2.4], and even applies the term, surely tongue in cheek, to the courtesan's successful jettisoning of an unwanted lover [6.4.44–5]. His discussion about whether you can indulge in *kama* at any stage of life [1.2.1–6] reflects (or perhaps even satirizes?) widespread arguments about whether you can engage in renunciation (*sannyasa*) at any stage.[7] But wandering renunciants meander through the *Kamasutra*; nuns, on the one hand, and courtesans, on the other, were the only women in ancient India who could move freely throughout the entire social system. And there are literary ties, too, between the *Kamasutra* and the literature of asceticism. Shvetaketu Auddalaki, the first human author of the *Kamasutra* [1.1.9], was already famous as a great Upanishadic sage.[8] The title of the seventh book of the *Kamasutra*, which we have translated as 'Erotic Esoterica', is actually the 'Upanishadic Book', perhaps because it is secret, like those texts, but perhaps because the extreme realms of sensuality and the control of sensuality have much in common. Perhaps Vatsyayana really did remain chaste while he composed this book.

---

[6] Doniger, *Siva: The Erotic Ascetic*.

[7] Doniger, 'Three (or More) Forms'.

[8] Shvetaketu introduces several key passages (in the *Brihadaranyaka Upanishad* 6.2 and *Chandogya Upanishad* 5.3–10) about the doctrine of five fires, of which one passage [6.2.13] goes: 'A fire—that's what a woman is, Gautama. Her firewood is the vulva; her smoke is the pubic hair; her flame is the vagina; when one penetrates her, that is her embers; and her sparks are the climax. In that very fire the gods offer semen, and from that offering springs a man.' Olivelle, *Upanishads*, 83. S. K. De cites Shvetaketu Auddalaki as one of several indications that the *Kamasutra* began within the genre of religious literature (*Ancient Indian Erotics*, 89–90).

The Genre of the Kamasutra

Michel Foucault, in *The History of Sexuality* (1990), made a distinction between 'two procedures for producing the truth of sex'. The first consists of texts of the *ars erotica* type, characteristic of 'China, Japan, India, Rome, the Arabo-Moslem societies'.[9] The choice of a Latin terminology suggests that Foucault has taken Ovid's *Ars Amatoria* as his paradigm for texts of this sort, and lest there be any question of their otherness he adds: 'On the face of it at least, our civilization possesses no *ars erotica*.'[10] These esoteric texts, technical treatises, remain secret and may be learned only from a master. 'Our civilization', by contrast, is the only one to have the *scientia sexualis*, which Foucault limits, with characteristic Euro-centrism, to Europe, taking as his criterion the element of confession. But if we set confession aside, the subsidiary criteria of the *scientia sexualis*, such as 'the testimony of witnesses, and the learned methods of observation and demonstration', place the *Kamasutra* in this camp. For Vatsyayana cites witnesses in the form of previous scholars, and his arguments are based on close observation and experience. In fact, however, the *Kamasutra* has characteristics of both 'procedures', thus posing a challenge to Foucault's taxonomy.

The very style in which most of the text is composed, aphoristic prose passages, or *sutras*, has associations with both religion and science. A *sutra* is literally a thread (cognate with the English words 'sew' and 'suture'), on which pages (generally palm leaves) and thoughts are strung like beads to form a kind of atomic string of meanings. The text is so intensely condensed, so starkly cryptic, that the task of understanding it frequently seems more like deciphering than translating. A *sutra* that states literally, in its totality, 'Because of the close connection with it' [1.1.4] requires the reader to understand what is being connected with what, most of which, but not always all, may be deduced from the context. (It probably means, 'Because those subjects are integral to the text [scholars made known their mutual agreement].') This renders the text ambiguous in many places, and, to that extent, unclear; it cries out for the help of a commentary to unpack it, just as the cryptic nature of the early religious texts, the Vedas, required the help of a guru. (Yashodhara fulfilled that role in the thirteenth century, as did Devadatta Shastri

[9] Foucault, *The History of Sexuality*, 57.   [10] Ibid. 58.

and several other modern commentators in the twentieth century.) That method of transmission lends the *Kamasutra* a mantle of religious authority; the 'scholars' that Vatsyayana cites are called *ach-aryas*, the word for a spiritual guide or guru. It also lends it an archaic tone, since, by and large, *sutras* precede *shastras* in Indian history. These aspects of the text assimilate it to Foucault's *ars erotica*.[11]

On the other hand, that very same aphoristic form gives this text the veneer of science, the aura of a grammatical treatise (the basis of all sciences, in ancient India) or a logical discourse, each syllogism boiled down to the most concise form possible, each word an indicator for a complex and previously established concept. Logical syllogisms appear at some length in the first two books and in abbreviated form in Vatsyayana's arguments with his opponents in the rest of the work. Alexander Syrkin argues that, in contrast with Ovid's *Ars Amatoria*, 'which is the model of artistic didacticism, the *Kama Sutra* is primarily a scientific-didactic work, reflecting in both expression and content specific features of Ancient Hindu scientific description'.[12] Those features would include not only syllogisms but encyclopedic lists and logical debates. The prose form of the *Kamasutra* also makes it possible for the author to cite other authors by names that might not have fitted into a poetic metre and to quote their texts within his own, taking up the views of several opponents and disposing of them one by one. It allows him to cite observed evidence in each case and to cap it with the assertion: 'This is evident.' This is the procedure of the *scientia sexualis*, and places Vatsyayana, if not in the company of Newton and Einstein, at least closer to Freud and Kinsey than to D. H. Lawrence or Henry Miller. By contrast, Manu, the author of the text that does for *dharma* what Vatsyayana does for *kama*, claims direct descent from the Creator, has a mythical name (equivalent to Adam), and cites at the start of his text only mythical predecessors, whose voices he incorporates into his text without attribution, so that he often seems to be saying contradictory things in two different places.[13]

[11] Burton and Arbuthnot called the *Anangaranga* the Ars Amoris Indica. Archer, 'Preface', 32.

[12] Syrkin, 'Notes on the *Kama Sutra*', 34. In ancient Greece, by contrast, the medical-scientific tradition of aphorisms, starting with Hippocrates, is used for forms of knowledge that cannot be formalized, that have a practical dimension (as in medicine and ethics, but also experimental science). For that tradition, the elliptical, compact form is more a mnemonic than an instruction book.

[13] See Doniger, *The Laws of Manu*, liv–lvii.

As a scientific *shastra*, the *Kamasutra* is both a model of and a model for (to use Clifford Geertz's terms), both descriptive and prescriptive (as well as occasionally proscriptive). More precisely, by claiming to be merely descriptive it is able to position its prescriptions and proscriptions as if they were facts rather than suggestions. It situates itself in the no man's land between the world of possibilities and the world of observations, between 'should' and 'is'. For the *shastric* 'should' functions both in the sense of, 'The sun should rise in the east at 8 a.m. tomorrow', and in the sense of, 'A servant should never look at a Brahmin woman.' These two mutually enforcing goals are supported by two different literary forms, prose and verse. For the *Kamasutra* is not entirely in prose. A few verses are cited at the end of every chapter, usually without explicit attribution, and through them some other voices may enter the text; in all, these verses constitute about a tenth of the text. They are in the form of *shlokas*, not a complex poetic form but the normal improvisational form of poetry, rather like blank verse in English, with a loose rhythm and no rhyme. This is the verse form in which the great Sanskrit epics and the *Laws of Manu* are composed. The prose, by and large, describes what people do; only in the verses does Vatsyayana explicitly suggest what people should do. He may be quoting some of these verses from earlier texts, though if so it is odd that he does not name the authors, as he does in his prose arguments (and as Yashodhara does in several notes). He himself may have invented some of the verses. The Sanskrit commentator says from time to time that Vatsyayana is quoting someone else because the act in question is not actually forbidden, implying that this is a way of allowing it without actually taking responsibility for it; the verses at the end of a chapter may also serve this function. In any case, the voice of these verses is one of moderation and reason, a voice that speaks not only in Manu's *shloka* form but, often, with Manu's moralizing tone, 'reeling *kama* in and contextualizing it within the larger framework of moral and social ideals', functioning like verbal 'speed-bumps' to remind the reader to proceed with caution.[14] Some of these verses offer advice on ways to use the text, either by limiting it (specifying that certain acts should be done only in the right time

---

[14] These two phrases, and the broader idea of the conservative nature of the verses at the end of each chapter, are taken from William Bradford Hunt's essay, 'Sex for Dharma: Framing the *Kamasutra* in Manu's World'.

and place, and only by certain people, and so forth) or, on the other hand, by extending it (suggesting that anything that both partners find acceptable can be done, even if the text has not mentioned it).

A blatant example of the first function of these verses, the limiting function, occurs near the end of the whole text, at the end of the book about drugs:

> The unusual techniques employed to increase passion,
> which have been described as this particular book required,
> are strongly restricted right here in this verse,
> right after it. [7.2.54]

A more complex example occurs at the end of the long, Machiavellian discussion of ways to seduce other men's wives [5.6.46–8]. Vatsyayana appends here a few verses insisting that he intends his work not as a handbook for adulterers but, rather, to help husbands detect the clues of *other people's* adulteries in order to confound them. Is this the author's paper-thin attempt to avoid being accused of teaching people to commit adultery? Or a warning that says, in effect, 'Kids, don't try this at home'? Or is it a deeper warning, encouraging the reader to imagine himself not as the cuckolder but as the cuckold, to recall that eternal vigilance is the price of fidelity? Or the voice of religion, long silent, returning at a crucial moment?

The verses that function in the second way, extending the possibilities, seem to have the very opposite effect, opening up the text. For instance, after describing many embraces, some of which 'can only be learned with practice', Vatsyayana concludes with these verses:

> Some sexual embraces, not in this text,
> also intensify passion;
> these, too, may be used for love-making,
> but only with care.
> The territory of the texts extends
> only so far as men have dull appetites;
> but when the wheel of sexual ecstasy is in full motion,
> there is no textbook at all, and no order. [2.2.30–31]

Often Vatsyayana seems to invoke an ancient Indian cultural relativism: certain acts are permitted only in certain regions. This opens up the text until, in some instances, he qualifies it, as he does in the case of violent blows called 'wedges': 'This is a particular local custom.

But Vatsyayana says: It is a painful and barbarous thing to do, and not to be sanctioned. So, too, one should not take any other custom used in one particular region and use it in another. One should also avoid, even in the region where it is used, anything that is dangerous' [2.7.24–7].

Whether these capping verses limit or extend the preceding chapter, they seem to increase the options by arguing for the particularity of individuals who may use the text. In the context of ancient Hindu social theory, however, they may have precisely the opposite effect, of constraining the possibilities. For they return the reader to another conservative framework that is conspicuously absent from the text: the framework of caste, of the belief that each individual has his (or, in relatively few cases, her) own *dharma* and therefore his own limited range of actual options appropriate to him, out of the totality of ideal human options. Do these verses express Vatsyayana's true voice, what he wants the reader to remember and take away? (It is always easier to remember poetry than prose, and the last lines rather than earlier lines.) Does he really believe that the reader should be able to have a choice of all possibilities, and then add the verses at the end merely as a safety net, a disclaimer?[15] Or does his dedication to the scientific goal of the totalizing project of the encyclopedia force him to include options that he in fact deplores, and wishes to take back at the end?

Devadatta Shastri, at the end of the chapter on unusual sexual acts [2.6], argues for this last option:

In writing his treatise, Vatsyayana was always vigilant in paying due attention to the character and the inherent principles of a treatise. He has also made it clear in this section that unusual sexual acts are base. Even when the author of a treatise considers something as base, he gives it a place in his treatise because there are all sorts of people in this world with different characters and inclinations. Some have an animal nature; they get enjoyment from unusual sexual acts. The *Bhagavata Purana* [11.5–11] says that it is necessary to be free from such tendencies: 'At the times of marriage, sacrifice and other such occasions, we may need to engage ourselves with

---

[15] In our day the author of a text like this might like to protect himself against possible lawsuits: 'I got a whiplash from practising position 15.' In fact, *The Pillow Book Kama Sutra* has a warning on the ISBN page: 'WARNING: With the prevalence of AIDS and other sexually transmitted diseases, if you do not practice safe sex you are risking your life and your partner's life.' Compare Vatsyayana's concern about 'the Wedge' at 2.7.24–7.

these inclinations. But our goal should be freedom. Sexual intercourse, drinking, and eating meat do not need an impetus because people are naturally inclined towards them. Because of this natural bent, these inclinations cannot be destroyed. That is why they are regulated and why rules are made governing an engagement with them on special occasions.' The *Rig Veda* has openly elaborated on this intention, in verses 10.86.16–17, in which Indrani berates Indra. There is some embarrassment in translating these mantras. Griffith did not translate them into English,[16] writing, in a footnote: 'I pass over stanzas 16 and 17, which I cannot translate into decent English.'[17] In his *Manusmriti* [5.56], Manu has also written that there is no sin or fault in eating meat, drinking alcohol, and having sex because they are natural inclinations of all embodied beings. But one attains happiness in becoming free of them.

Shastri renews his defence of Vatsyayana again at the end of the first chapter in the book devoted to adultery [5.1], identifying this conservative moment as the true voice of Vatsyayana:

The treatises on religion require a man to look at another man's wife as if she were his own mother. The *Kamasutra*, however, tells us how to seduce another man's wife. It will not do to maintain that the latter is a treatise on a particular kind of behaviour and has no link to religion. Actually, religion, power, and pleasure are interconnected. The goal of pleasure is related to the other world as much as it is to this one. A treatise never turns its gaze away from reality. The *Kamasutra* is not a religious text but it does not transgress social and ethical boundaries.

Based on human psychology, the *Kamasutra* is a way of looking at the world. After analysing the inclinations of men, good and bad, its conclusions are guided by a concern for human welfare. A treatise incorporates a discussion of both the good and the bad, but one should act only on the good. In the eyes of the author of the *Kamasutra*, adultery is a great sin. But how could he deny its pervasive reality? How could he not discuss this human tendency which has manifested itself throughout the whole of human history? That is why Vatsyayana gives a place to adultery in the *Kamasutra*. The Upanishads, too, view the satisfaction of 'left-handed' desires as the purpose of sex with other men's wives. The *Ayurveda* prescribes adultery as a remedy for erotic fever.

Vatsyayana was not only a scholar but a reformer and builder of society.

[16] Griffith, *The Hymns of the RgVeda*, 597.
[17] Verse 16 (of which 17 is a mirror image) may be translated into indecent English thus: 'That one is not powerful, whose penis hangs between his thighs; that one is powerful, for whom the hairy organ opens as it swells and sets to work. Indra supreme above all!' Translation from O'Flaherty, *The Rig Veda*, 260.

He clearly states that a treatise demands the inclusion of everything, good or bad. Using their discrimination, reflective people should accept only the good. Just because the *Ayurveda* prescribes dog's flesh for a particular disease, it does not mean that dog meat should be consumed for every disease. Similarly, if a person must sleep with another man's wife because of the exigencies of a specific situation, then it is not bad— if he does so after a study of the *Kamasutra* and after employing a mature judgment. But if everyone believes that adulterous sex is a prescription to be followed, then society will lose all its moorings, children will lose their caste. Humanity will become a laughing-stock, religion lose its pre-eminence, and nation and society take on attributes of the animal kingdom.

Perhaps all of these voices are Vatsyayana's, both in prose and in verse, expressing the view of a man dedicated both to the encyclo-pedic goals of science and the often repressive moral concerns of religion, or a man who tempers his goal of including everything that could be relevant (the view of totality) by admitting that one cannot corral all of the possibilities (the view of infinity).[18]

The Science and Magic of Numbers

One quasi-scientific feature, typical of other ancient Hindu *shastric* works besides the *Kamasutra*, appears here in such an exaggerated form that it has become (particularly in Western receptions) a point of satire: the enumerations, particularly of the sexual positions. (Most editions of the Burton translation exacerbate this quasi-scientific appearance by numbering lists that Vatsyayana does not number, or even count, in the Sanskrit original, such as the reasons for women to commit, or not to commit, adultery [5.1].) The num-bers alone would not qualify a text as scientific, though they do serve to bolster two more significant characteristics of that genre, the appeal to empirical evidence and the logical syllogism. Numbers are useful in a literature of this genre, as they serve as mnemonic devices and help scribes to check to see if they have left something out. The numbers in the *Kamasutra* are used in the service of both mystical and scientific agendas.

A telltale sign of the scientific genre of ancient Hindu texts is the list, particularly the numbered list ('the sixty-four arts'), which con-veys an aura of totality here as it does in the *shastras* composed in

[18] Levinas, in *Totality and Infinity*, develops the implications of these two views.

verse, such as Manu's.[19] In the *Kamasutra*, no longer corseted by the *shloka* metre, the lists blossom in even greater profusion. The *Kamasutra* lists consist of strings of aphorisms, each of which often takes the form of a long compound noun that could be unpacked into a sentence. Thus, the list of married women likely to commit adultery includes a woman who hangs about the house of the young man who is her neighbour, a woman who has been supplanted by a co-wife for no cause, a woman whose husband travels a lot, and so forth [5.1.52–4]. Each item hints at a soap-opera story redolent with messy human implications, but herded together in a list, they give the impression of scholarly tidiness.[20]

The *Kamasutra* begins with a myth about numbers: the original text had a hundred thousand chapters, and it was then boiled down to a thousand chapters, then a hundred and fifty chapters, and finally reached its present form of what it declares to be 'thirty-six chapters, in sixty-four sections, in seven books, consisting of 1,250 passages' [1.1.4–23]. This claim to have boiled down a divine original to a human digest is standard operating procedure for an ancient Hindu sacred text; similar declarations are made at the start of the *Mahabharata*, the *Bhagavata Purana*, the *Kathasaritsagara*, and other works of that genre.[21] But the *Kamasutra* goes on to play number games of a different sort. Vatsyayana claims that his text has sixty-four sections.[22] Now, sixty-four is not merely a nice round number

[19] Doniger, *The Laws of Manu*, lvii–lviii.

[20] Gian Biagio Conte notes that such a list is a rhetorical affective figure called *enumeratio caotica*, which consists 'precisely in emphatic accumulation and designating such an abundance of these referents that they cannot be clearly organized by distinguishing what counts more from what counts little . . . by distinguishing the true from the false, the plausible from the incredible, the documented from the fanciful, the useful from the useless', 'The Inventory of the World', 72. Thanks to Lorraine Daston for this citation.

[21] See Doniger, 'Echoes of the *Mahabharata*'. The woman who prepared milk-rice for the Buddha when he ended his long meditation after achieving enlightenment is said to have milked a thousand cows, and fed the milk to five hundred cows; then she milked those five hundred cows and fed the milk to two hundred and fifty, and so on, until she fed the milk of sixteen cows to eight, and used the milk of those eight cows to prepare the milk-rice for the Buddha. See *Introduction to the Jataka* 1.68; trans. Warren, *Buddhism in Translation*, 71–2. The Roman historian Pliny cited a similar myth, about 20,000 facts digested from 2000 volumes written by 100 authors, condensed in 36 books (*Historia Naturalis*, Prefatio, 17). Thanks to Lorraine Daston for this reference.

[22] The total number of sections is actually sixty-seven, according to Vatsyayana's own list of sections in 1.1.15–22. Vatsyayana does not allude to the sections anywhere in the text except once in Book Seven, but Yashodhara identifies them all. He makes it

(more precisely, a squared number, in fact the square of a square, or 2 to the 6th power) but a sacred number in India, indeed a 'natural' number. Ayurvedic medical texts list sixty-four main diseases of the body, a number that also occurs in the ancient law books. The *Laws of Manu*, pronouncing on the weight of transgressions committed by the four different classes, says that the guilt of a thief who belongs to the lowest class is eight times the value of the stolen object, of the third class sixteen times, of the second class thirty-two times, and of a Brahmin sixty-four times [8.337–8]. In the initiation rites the circle symbolizing the universal spirit is divided into four quarters, every quarter again into four parts, to indicate that the initiate is to receive sixteen branches of knowledge. If each of these sixteen branches is again divided into four, we get the sixty-four arts, which cover the whole circle.

Vatsyayana's lists of the sixty-four arts, and his discussion of the traditional lists of the sixty-four positions of intercourse and the elements of foreplay, seem to be efforts to include all that is even remotely possible in the realm of sexual love, even when some of the items on a list appear improbable. Vatsyayana, however, expresses his scorn for this sort of number-crunching: 'But Vatsyayana says: Since the division into eight theoretical varieties is too few for some categories and too many for others, and since sex involves other categories, too, such as slapping, screaming, the sexual strokes of a man, and unusual sexual acts, this is merely a manner of speaking, just as we speak of the "seven-leaf" devil tree or the "five-colour" offering of rice' [2.2.5].[23] He has already expressed similar misgivings: 'Since

come out at sixty-four by failing to number two sections in Book Six ('Reasons for Taking a Lover', which he appends to the first section, and 'Types of Courtesans') and one section in Book Four ('A Man's Management of Many Women'). In addition, one section in Book One, 'Reasons for Taking Another Man's Wife', is referred to as such a section at the start of Book Five but is not mentioned in the list at 1.1.15–22. Yashodhara balances this out by numbering the extra section in Book Five (in which the introduction lists eleven sections but counts only ten). If we add this section to the sixty-four numbered sections and the other four unnumbered sections, we end up with the one number [sixty-four + five = sixty-nine] that has strong sexual associations in English, sixty-nine, which is what Vatsyayana calls 'sex in the style of a crow' [2.9.38]. For our culture, too, has its number mysticism. It is possible that the list of sections in the introduction was added by a redactor of the text at some period after the time of Vatsyayana and before that of Yashodhara.

[23] This sort of casual enumeration continues to the present day. Sanjeev Bhaskar, interviewed about his documentary on the *Kamasutra*, admitted to lying for years about the text when people assumed, wrongly, that he knew it. Sometimes he would say that there were three positions, sometimes that there were 237; sometimes he said it was written in 1932, sometimes in 1847. Lane, 'A Book at Bedtime'.

there are nine kinds of sex according to each of the criteria of size, time, and temperament, when they are combined it is not possible to enumerate all the forms of sex. There are just too many' [2.1.33]. At this, Yashodhara remarks, rather flat-footedly, that they are not innumerable at all: 'There are nine forms of each of the three categories, making twenty-seven possibilities for each man and the same number for each woman. If these mate in all possible combinations, the total comes to 729 (27 × 27).' But this is a path down which Vatsyayana disdains to tread. As he remarks [at 2.7.31]:

> This is no matter for numerical lists
> or textbook tables of contents.
> For people joined in sexual ecstasy,
> passion is what makes things happen.

Enumeration may be a way of taming a subject that always threatens to break out of its *shastric* cage. Some of the most sensitive issues in the *Kamasutra* are domesticated by being enumerated; this is particularly true of Book Two, about the sexual act. In addition to the sixty-four that summarizes the text of that book, as we have just seen, and the 729 combinations of sexual types, many other aspects of sexuality stand up to be counted. There are 4 types of love [2.1.39–45], and some 105 other techniques: 12 embraces, 17 kisses, 16 bites and scratches, 17 positions, 6 unusual acts, 16 slaps and screams, 10 sexual strokes of a man, and 3 more movements for a woman acting the role of a man, 8 acts in oral sex, and, finally, 7 kinds of sex. But other tabulations prove more slippery, such as the reasons for sleeping with another man's wife, which number 3, or 4, or 5, or 6, or 7, or 8, depending on whose system you follow [1.5.3–26]. The very fact that there is such disagreement about the precise number of reasons for adultery, and that the so-called fourth reason is basically a catch-all for any convoluted justification, with numerous separate items (thirteen or seventeen, depending on how you divide it), shows that the constraining net of numbers quickly stretches rather thin. The scientific and mystical aspects of numbers work in tandem. Although they may give the illusion of controlling and 'demystifying' sex, they may, at the same time, be mystifying it, by suggesting that the possible types of a particular sexual phenomenon coincide with a 'natural' number that is believed to represent something given in the cosmos.[24]

Vatsyayana's recurrent attempts to break out of the numerical forms express his hope of moving beyond totality toward infinity in love. He seems at first to be guaranteeing totality, by assuring the reader that there are just sixteen ways of biting, not fifteen, not seventeen.[25] But then, on the one hand, he limits the totality by remarking that some of these sixteen may not always work well, and, on the other hand, he extends the totality into an infinity by suggesting that there may be other ways than the sixteen, that the text is in fact incomplete, its lists merely suggestive, not definitive—in effect, that there are different strokes for different folks. (Manu, too, formulates totalities in this way and then pulls back to qualify them. He constructs a network of rules so tight as to make life virtually impossible, and then offers the escape clause of *apad*, the emergency situation in which no rules apply at all.[26]) At these points, the *Kamasutra* is moving out of its scientific body into a non-scientific frame with a religious or moral viewpoint.

The Kamasutra *as a Play in Seven Acts*

Beneath the veneer of a sexual textbook, the *Kamasutra* resembles a work of dramatic fiction more than anything else. The man and woman whose sex lives are described here are called the *nayaka* and the *nayika* (male and female protagonists), and the men who assist the *nayaka* are called the *pitamarda*, *vita*, and *vidushaka* (the libertine, pander, and clown). All of these are terms for stock characters in Sanskrit dramas—the hero and heroine, sidekick, supporting player, and jester—according to yet another textbook, the one attributed to Bharata and dealing with dramatic writing, acting, and dancing, the *Natyashastra*. The very last line of the *Kamasutra* speaks of a man playing the part of a lover, as if on the stage. Is the *Kamasutra* a play about sex? Certainly it has a dramatic sequence, and, like most

---

[24] Personal communication from Laura Desmond, January 2001.

[25] 2.5.1–18. This method is reminiscent of the scene in John Frankenheimer's 1962 film *The Manchurian Candidate*, where the gaze of the McCarthyite senator, who is struggling to lend an air of authority and precision to his anti-Communist witch-hunts by answering the demand for a precise number of infiltrators, lights upon a bottle of Heinz Tomato Catsup ('57 Varieties'), and we next see him, in the Senate, declaiming, 'There are precisely FIFTY-SEVEN known Communists . . .'.

[26] Doniger, *The Laws of Manu*, lii–liv.

classical Indian dramas, it has seven acts. In Act One, which literally sets the stage for the drama, the bachelor sets up his pad; in Act Two, he perfects his sexual technique. Then he seduces a virgin (Act Three), gets married, and lives with a wife or wives (Act Four); tiring of her (or them), he seduces other men's wives (Act Five); and when he tires of that, he frequents courtesans (Act Six). Finally, when he is too old to manage it at all, he resorts to the ancient Indian equivalent of Viagra: aphrodisiacs and magic spells (Act Seven).[27]

In the course of this plot, the text, like a play, unfolds through a series of dialogues that take place on several levels. In the outermost frame, Pirandello-like, the author is a character in constant conversation with other authors who are characters. Inside this outer frame,[28] there are numerous dialogues between men and women and between women and women, as well as a number of soliloquies, such as the passage alluded to above, in which men justify to themselves their reasons for committing adultery [1.5.3–26], and others in which courtesans justify to themselves their methods for jettisoning, or taking back, ex-lovers [6.4.1–34]. Even the lists in the text sometimes become dialogues in the commentary, when Yashodhara expands upon a single noun by imagining a dialogue around it. Thus, for example, Yashodhara glosses one of the reasons for a courtesan to take a lover, 'compassion': 'Taking pity on someone who says, "I will die if you will not make love with me"' [6.1.17]. Or, glossing the phrase 'she is suspicious of love-magic done with roots': 'When he says, "You are always using root-magic to put me in your power, so that I will be totally submissive to you", she replies, "No! I would never do anything like that!"' [6.2.56].

And, finally, the text is like a drama because it is a fantasy. More precisely, it combines a survey of actual sources of pleasure in ancient India ('is') with imaginative suggestions for other sources of pleasure ('should', or perhaps, 'could'). For example, the passage

---

[27] In keeping with the text's character as a dramatization, it might have been more appropriate to translate the terms for the major divisions (what the *Kamasutra* calls *adhikaranas*) as Acts, the subdivisions (*adhyayas*) as Scenes, and the sub-sub-divisions (*prakaranas*) as Episodes. We decided not to do this, but there is support for it in the Sanskrit tradition, in which major works give distinct names to their subdivisions: the *Mahabharata*, for instance, calls its sections *parvans* (bamboo segments), the *Ramayana* calls its *kandas* (segments of any plant), the *Ocean of Stories* calls its *tarangas* (waves), and the *Rig Veda* calls its *mandalas* (circles).

[28] For the framing technique, see O'Flaherty, *Dreams, Illusion*.

about sneaking into the harem [5.6] is pure fairy-tale, including ways
to become invisible and the trick of wearing woman's clothing,
straight out of the romances of the *Ocean of Story* ('could'); but it is
also laced with some rather closely observed psychological tips on
ways to break into a house ('is'). On the one hand, the *Kamasutra*
abounds in realia, in details about foods and clothing and games and
drugs and the most banal aspects of housekeeping ('is'). On the other
hand, it imagines a world not only of total sexual freedom but of total
social freedom altogether ('could'). The male protagonist may be of
any class, as we learn from Vatsyayana [at 3.2.1], Yashodhara [on
1.4.1] and Shastri [on 1.4.35]: 'This classification of rich and poor
citizens acquaints us with the social order that prevailed in Vatsyayana's times. Here, it is nowhere mentioned that only persons of high
caste were rich and of low castes, poor. It appears that after becoming
rich one rose high in the social order; the low caste disappeared.' But
the man-about-town has no caste, no social ties.

Moreover, he has, as we say of a certain type of man today, no
visible source of income. Vatsyayana tells us, at the start of the section headed 'The Lifestyle of the Man-about-Town', that the playboy may have to live 'wherever he has to stay to make a living' and
that he finances his lifestyle by 'using the money that he has obtained
from gifts, conquest, trade, or wages, or from inheritance, or from
both'. His sidekicks, too, have quite realistic present money prob-
lems [1.4.31–3], his wife is entrusted with all the household management, including the finances, and his mistresses work hard to
make and keep their money. But we never see the man-about-town at
work. Busy teaching his birds to talk, he never drops in to check
things at the shop. Throughout the text, his one concern is the
pursuit of pleasure. Well, there were undoubtedly men in ancient
India who had that sort of money, and the privilege that came with
it; Sanskrit literature tells us, in particular, of wealthy merchants
whose sons engaged in the sorts of adventures, erotic and otherwise,
that other literatures often reserve for princes.[29] Vatsyayana insists
that anyone, not just the man-about-town, can live the life of
pleasure—if he or she has money [1.4.29–30]. But were there also
other sorts of implied readers, less privileged readers, of this text?
And if there were, was this, for them, a world that merely snapped

---

[29] These stories were collected in *The Ocean of Story* [*Kathasaritsagara*] in about the
tenth century.

into place on holidays? Was it real for the rich, and for city-dwellers, and mere fantasy for the poor, and for villagers? Or was it, for all readers, a world of ideal sex like Erica Jong's 'zipless fuck',[30] or the capitalist fantasies of Hugh Hefner's glossy *Playboy* empire?

The text is an instrument of desire, as its title proclaims. It may even have been intended as a sourcebook for other fantasies, for poets composing erotic works.[31] N. N. Bhattacharya argues that not only the social circumstances but the sex itself is fantastic: 'Vatsyayana's attempt to write a scientific treatise is indeed praiseworthy, but the difficulty was that . . . he had no practical knowledge of the subject. We must say that it is a pedantic and superficial production of scholasticism.' In Bhattacharya's view, the sexual positions are 'acrobatic techniques, most of which are impossible to follow in the practical field. The drugs he prescribes are mostly imaginative and superstitious, and they do not correspond to those found in the standard Ayurvedic texts.'[32] The sexual fantasy in the *Kamasutra* is the culmination of centuries of erotic meditations every bit as complex as the parallel ascetic meditations of the literature of the Upanishads and their commentaries.

The Genders of the Kamasutra

If the ideal reader of this text, like its protagonist, is a person with no social ties or economic responsibilities, could that reader be a woman?[33] It is difficult to assess how broad a spectrum of ancient Indian society knew the text first-hand. The production of manuscripts, especially illuminated manuscripts, was necessarily an élite matter; men of wealth and power, kings and merchants, would commission texts to be copied out for their private use. It is often said that only upper-class men were allowed to read Sanskrit, particularly the sacred texts, but the very fact that the texts prescribe punishments for women and lower-class men who read these texts suggests that some of them might do so.[34] In some, but not all, Sanskrit

---

[30] Erica Jong, *Fear of Flying*.

[31] Personal communication from Sheldon Pollock, January 2001.

[32] Bhattacharya, *History*, 90–1.

[33] The assumption that the intended reader is male persists even in popular culture today, where Vinod Verma, apparently hoping to rectify this imbalance, published (in 1997) *The Kamasutra for Women: The Modern Woman's Way to Sensual Fulfillment and Health* (Tokyo: Kodansha International), applying Ayurvedic techniques to female heterosexual relationships.

[34] See e.g. Manu 11.36–7.

dramas, the women speak dialects, Prakrit or Apabhramsha, while the men speak Sanskrit.[35] But women and people of the lower classes may well have read non-religious Sanskrit of various kinds, including the scientific literature, which was circulated by specialists, called *shastris*, who knew the *shastra*s and explained them.

Large portions of the *Kamasutra* are clearly written for men, yet the women in the *Kamasutra* speak in Sanskrit, and Vatsyayana argues at some length that some women, at least, should read this text, and that others should learn its contents in other ways [1.3.1–14]. Book Three devotes one section to advice to virgins trying to get husbands [3.4.36–47], and these women certainly have agency. Book Four consists of instructions for wives; and Book Six is said to have been commissioned by the courtesans de luxe of Pataliputra, presumably for their own use. Their powers may have been extensive but fragile; the devious devices that the courtesan uses to make her lover leave her, rather than simply kicking him out [6.3.39–44], are an example of what the anthropologist James Scott has taught us to recognize as the 'weapons of the weak.' Yet Shastri [on 1.5.3] suggests that these women were very privileged indeed:

The difference between the courtesan [*veshya*] and the courtesan de luxe [*ganika*] is the difference between the earth and the sky. The most beautiful, talented and virtuous among the courtesans was given the title of courtesan de luxe. The *Lalitavistara* calls a princess versed in the texts a courtesan de luxe. In the *Kavyamimamsa*, Rajashekhara writes that in ancient times many courtesans de luxe and princesses were excellent poets. The daughters of these courtesans de luxe had the right to study together with the sons of men-about-town. In fact, a courtesan de luxe was regarded as the wealth and glory of the entire kingdom. The whole society was proud of her. On hearing the name 'courtesan', one should not imagine that this was a woman who had had discarded all social conventions and customary modes of conduct. The courtesan is an uncommon woman whose upbringing and education is also extraordinary. She is educated in a way that facilitates physical and mental development, an education of which ordinary women are deprived. Courtesans have been educated and skilled since ancient times. Well-born maidens profited from their abilities. They were regarded as a special part of the society. Courtesans are often mentioned in Tantric treatises. Buddhist literature is also

[35] For a discussion of the ways in which being forbidden to speak Sanskrit enables one woman, Ahalya, to commit adultery with relative impunity, see Doniger, *Splitting the Difference*.

full of praise for courtesans. They are described in detail in the Puranas, the Kavyas and in Jaina literature. All courtesans were proud of their beauty. The works of Bhasa, Kalidasa, Vishakhadatta, Magha, Dandin, Shudraka, Bana and other poets provide interesting descriptions of courtesans.

Some women, and not only courtesans, may well have had both the economic power to obtain a copy of the *Kamasutra* and the power to learn to read Sanskrit.

If parts of the text are directed toward women, is it also the case that they reflect women's voices? The women in the *Kamasutra* are not only less idealized than the men, but more differentiated. The men are briefly and occasionally dichotomized,[36] but the number of the types of women is debated at some length, some authors counting as many as eight, while Vatsyayana limits them to four (with an ambiguous addition of the third nature) [1.51–27].[37] Both men and women are objects of desire; and, within the basic categories, Vatsyayana on numerous occasions reminds us that both men and women are individuals, and that the rules must be modified for individual tastes. But are both men and women subjects in the *Kamasutra*?

The text not only assumes an official male voice (the voice of Vatsyayana) but presents methods that deny that women's words truly represent their feelings; women's shouts of 'Stop!' or 'Mother!' are taken not as indications of their wish to escape the pain being inflicted on them, but merely as part of a ploy designed to excite their male partners [2.7.1–21]. These passages inculcate what we now recognize as the rape mentality—'her mouth says no, but her eyes say yes'—a dangerous line of thought that leads ultimately to places where we now no longer want to be: disregarding a woman's protests against rape. Indeed, at 3.5.26–7 Vatsyayana lists rape as one of the worst, but still acceptable, wedding devices, and Shastri comments: 'If one has intercourse with a girl who is sleeping or has been made unconscious by the administration of a drug and who is then forced to marry the villain because of the loss of her virginity, this is

---

[36] There are open or concealed lovers [1.5.27–8], or men that a courtesan takes up with for love or for money [6.1.2], and there are six sorts of ex-lovers [6.4.3–9].

[37] Underlying these behavioural differences, both men and women are divided into nine basic physical types according to the size of the organs, the time it takes to reach the climax, and the temperament of the partners, each of these three factors divided into three levels [2.1.1–31].

the ghoulish form of marriage. The scriptures call such men ghouls and prescribe the death penalty for them.'[38] The type of rape that we now call sexual harassment is taken for granted by Vatsyayana, who describes men in power who can take whatever women they want: 'the man in charge of threads may take widows, women who have no man to protect them, and wandering women ascetics; the city police-chief may take the women who roam about begging, for he knows where they are vulnerable, because of his own night-roamings' [5.5.7–9].

The *Kamasutra*, however, often quotes women in direct speech, expressing views that men are advised to take seriously, and it is surprisingly sympathetic to women, particularly to what they suffer from inadequate husbands. Of course, male texts may merely engage in a ventriloquism that attributes to women viewpoints that in fact serve male goals. But in numerous places, the *Kamasutra* expresses points of view clearly favourable to women,[39] particularly in comparison with other texts of the same era. The discussion of the reasons why women commit adultery, for instance, rejects the traditional patriarchal party line that one finds in most Sanskrit texts such as the *Laws of Manu*: 'Good looks do not matter to women, nor do they care about youth; "A man!" they say, and enjoy sex with him, whether he is good-looking or ugly' [9.15]. The *Kamasutra* begins its discussion of adultery with a far more egalitarian, if equally cynical, formulation: 'A woman desires any attractive man she sees, and, in the same way, a man desires a woman. But, after some consideration, the matter goes no farther' [5.1.8]. The text does argue that women have less concern for morality than men have, and does assume that women don't think about anything but men. And it is written in the service of the hero, the would-be adulterer, who reasons, if all women are keen to give it away, why shouldn't one of them give it to him? But the author empathetically imagines various women's reasons *not* to commit adultery [5.1.17–42]; and the would-be seducer takes the woman's misgivings seriously, even if only to disarm her. This discussion is ostensibly intended to teach the male reader of the text to manipulate and exploit such women, but,

---

[38] Not so. Manu [8.364] prescribes death or corporal punishment for a man who rapes an unwilling virgin, but does not inflict even that punishment on a man who rapes a woman who is not a virgin; and a Brahmin who rapes a Brahmin woman is merely fined [8.378].

[39] Doniger, *The Implied Spider*, ch. 5. Frances Zimmermann agrees that there is a woman's voice in the *Kamasutra*; personal communication, April 1994.

perhaps inadvertently, it provides a compassionate exposition of the reasons why inadequate husbands drive away their wives [5.1.51–4].

Vatsyayana tells us that a woman who does not experience the pleasures of love may hate her man and leave him for another [3.2.35 and 4.2.31–5]. If, as the context suggests, this woman is married, the casual manner in which Vatsyayana suggests that she leave her husband is in sharp contrast to such *shastras* as Manu's: 'A virtuous wife should constantly serve her husband like a god, even if he behaves badly, freely indulges his lust, and is devoid of any good qualities' [5.154]. But the belief that she might hate him was hardly unique to the *Kamasutra*. 'Hated by her husband' or 'hating her husband' (the compound can be tantalizingly ambiguous in Sanskrit, as it is in *Kamasutra* 3.2.35) is an established taxonomic category in ancient Hindu texts; a woman in the *Rig Veda* is 'hated by/hating her husband',[40] and other Vedic texts contrast the 'favourite' wife with the 'avoided' wife.[41] 'Hated' in the first sense in this context usually means that the husband prefers, and sleeps with, the other wives; it serves as a synonym for 'unlucky in love'. A husband could not be 'hated' in this way, but there were other ways. Even Manu grants that 'A husband should wait for one year for a wife who hates him. . . . If she hates him because he is insane, fallen, impotent, without seed, or suffering from a disease caused by his evil, she should not be deserted or deprived of her inheritance' [9.77 and 9.79]. Vatsyayana incorporated this tradition even as he incorporated an argument in favour of female orgasm far more subtle than views that prevailed in Europe until very recently indeed [2.1.10–31].

In addition to his general representations of women's voices and needs, Vatsyayana tells us that an entire work, the basis of Book Six of his own work, was commissioned by women, courtesans [1.1.11]. And Yashodhara tells us how this happened: Dattaka happened to be cursed to be a woman for a while, and so knew how to write about courtesans from both sides of the bed, as it were. It is an inspired move on the part of Yashodhara to make the author of this text a bisexual, who 'tastes both flavours', or, as we would say, swings both ways.[42] Yet this is also a move that greatly mitigates the strong female

---

[40] *Rig Veda* 8.91.4, the song of Apala; O'Flaherty, *The Rig Veda*, 256–7.

[41] The *parivrikta*. See Jamison, *Sacrificed Wife*, 99 ff.

[42] The Arabic expression is 'he eats both pomegranates and figs', and the British, '. . . oysters and snails'.

agency in the text: where Vatsyayana tells us that women had this text made, Yashodhara tells us that an extraordinary man knew more about the courtesans' art than they knew themselves. In a culture in which men and women speak to one another (which is to say, in most cultures), we might do best to regard the authors of most texts as androgynes, and the *Kamasutra* is no exception.[43] Yet we must admit that we find these voices, carrying meanings that have value for us, only by transcending, if not totally disregarding, the original context. Were we to remain within the strict bounds of the historical situation, we could not notice the women's voices speaking against their moment in history, perhaps even against their author. Only by asking our own questions, which the author may not have considered at all, can we see that his text does contain many answers to them, fortuitously embedded in other questions and answers that were more meaningful to him.

We may search in this way for the voices not only of women but of people who engage in homosexual acts. Classical Hinduism is in general significantly silent on the subject of homoeroticism, but Hindu mythology does drop hints from which we can excavate a pretty virulent homophobia.[44] The *dharma* textbooks either ignore or stigmatize homosexual activity. Male homoerotic activity was punished, albeit mildly: a ritual bath [Manu 11.174] or the payment of a small fine [*Arthashastra* 3.18.4] was often a sufficient atonement. In contrast to the modern notion of homosexuality, which is defined by a preference for a partner of the same sex, queerness in ancient India was determined by atypical sexual or gender behaviour.[45] The Sanskrit word *kliba* (which has traditionally been translated as 'eunuch', but almost certainly did not mean 'eunuch') includes a wide range of meanings under the general rubric of 'a man who does not act the way a man should act', a man who fails to be a man, a defective male, a male suffering from failure, distortion, and lack. It is a catch-all term that traditional Hindus coined to indicate a man who is in their terms sexually dysfunctional (or in ours, sexually challenged), including someone who was sterile, impotent, castrated, a transvestite, a man who had oral sex with other men, who had anal sex, a man with mutilated

[43] Doniger, *The Implied Spider*.
[44] Doniger, *Splitting the Difference*.
[45] Sweet and Zwilling, 'The First Medicalization'.

or defective sexual organs, a man who produced only female children, or, finally, a hermaphrodite.

But the *Kamasutra* departs from this view in significant ways. It does not use the term *kliba* at all. It mentions sodomy in only one passage, and in the context of heterosexual sex: 'The people in the South indulge in "sex below", even anally' [2.6.49]. (Southerners have a pretty poor reputation in this book composed in the North, and it may be that their geographical position suggested their sexual position in this passage: down under.) Fellatio is regarded as the defining male homosexual act, and Shastri argues that Vatsyayana discusses even this only because his totalizing project forces him to do so:

It is clear that this act [fellatio] is extremely base and that it is not a new but an old and wicked deed in our tradition, since *Dharmashastras* condemn it. One might ask if this act is so reprehensible then why does it find a supporter in Vatsyayana? A treatise (*shastra*) is a reference book. Fellatio is a sexual act; it is related to sexual desire and it has a tradition. How, then, can a treatise ignore it? Giving primacy to human inclinations and local customs, Vatsyayana says that a *shastra* has no meaning for the dissolute, nor does acting against the *shastra* bring sin to the wicked. Fellatio is an act which is proper if permitted by local custom or if it suits a person's particular taste. [At the end of 2.9]

In fact, though the *Kamasutra* quickly dismisses the cross-dressing male, it discusses the fellatio technique of the closeted man of the third nature in considerable sensual detail, in the longest consecutive passage in the text describing a physical act, and with what might even be called gusto [2.9.6–24]. Moreover, as in several other cultures, the active partner in a homoerotic encounter was not stigmatized as the passive partner was. The *Kamasutra*'s man-about-town who uses the masseur's mouth for sexual pleasure is thus not considered 'queer'; the masseur is. (Elsewhere the text quotes scholars who warn the bridegroom that if he is too shy, his bride 'will be discouraged and will despise him, as if he were someone of the third nature' [3.2.3].) Two verses that immediately follow this section describe (in striking contrast with men of the third nature, always designated by the pronoun 'she') men who seem bound to one another by discriminating affection rather than promiscuous passion, and although these men, too, engage in oral sex, they are designated with nouns and pronouns that unambiguously designate males [2.9.35–6]. The female messenger, praising the man's charm, says, according to Yashodhara, 'He has such luck in love that he was desired even by a man' [5.4.15]. Colin Spencer's *The Gay Kamasutra* (1996), which does not pretend to be a translation, mines the parts of the text ostensibly designed for heterosexuals and finds in them possible readings of sexual relationships between men. Yashodhara, as we have seen, even makes Dattaka a bisexual [Y1.1.11].

Lesbian activity is described at the beginning of the chapter about the harem, in a brief passage about what Vatsyayana calls 'Oriental customs' [5.6.2–4].[46] These women use dildos, as well as bulbs, roots, or fruits that have the form of the male organ, and statues of men that have distinct sexual characteristics. But they do this only in the absence of men, not through the kind of personal choice that drives someone of the third nature. As for other sorts of lesbians, Manu says that a woman who corrupts a virgin will be punished by having two of her fingers cut off [8.369–70]—a hint of what Manu thinks lesbians do in bed; Yashodhara specifies that that is how a woman deflowers another woman [7.1.20]. Shastri comments on lesbians [at the end of 2.9 and 5.5]:

In passage 2.9.36, Vatsyayana hints at homosexuality. The commentator Yashodhara has explicated Vatsyayana's opinion by mentioning homosexuality in men and also in women. These days, the act of women rubbing their vulvas together is called a *chapati*. [A *chapati* is an Indian bread shaped somewhat like a pita bread.] Vatsyayana has discussed all kinds of natural and unnatural means for the satisfaction of unslaked sexual desires. But it is surprising that he does not talk of '*chapati*' [lesbian] intercourse among unsatisfied queens. Perhaps '*chapati*' intercourse had not yet appeared at Vatsyayana's time; otherwise, it could not have remained hidden from his penetrating gaze. Today, when the emphasis on virginity has increased, the playing of '*chapati*' and the employment of artificial means for sexual satisfaction among girls are also increasing.

The commentators, therefore, seem more troubled by the topic than Vatsyayana is.

And so, despite the caution with which this topic is broached,

---

[46] The use of the term 'Oriental'—or 'Eastern'—for what Vatsyayana regards as a disreputable lesbian practice in what was soon to be a colonized part of the Gupta Empire suggests that what Edward Said has taught us to call 'Orientalism' began not with the British but with the Orientals themselves.

there are ways in which some parts of the *Kamasutra* might be read as a text for homoeroticism. More precisely, it is possible to excavate several alternative sexualities latent in the text's somewhat fuzzy boundaries between homoeroticism and heteroeroticism. At the end of the discussion of the third nature, Vatsyayana grants that some women, too, perform oral sex, though he strongly disapproves of it and attributes it largely to women from distant parts of India [2.9.25–41]. (He says that this is one of the ways that a group of men can pleasure one woman [2.6.46–7], and even that it is what makes women prefer otherwise useless men to good men [2.9.39], and he clearly disapproves of both of these types of women.) Fellatio, therefore, is permitted for (some) men, and not for (our) women. But the fact that the word 'nature' is feminine in Sanskrit (as it, and most abstract nouns, are also in Latin and Greek), leads Vatsyayana to use the feminine rather than the male pronoun throughout the description of the masseur seducing his male client. (He also lists the third nature among women who can be lovers [at 1.5.27].) This passage, therefore, can be read heterosexually, instructing a woman how to seduce a man through oral sex.

By the same token, one might argue that the female pronoun used for the active partner in the section on 'the woman playing the role of the man' (the woman on top) might refer to a male of the third nature and represent homoerotic rather than heteroerotic sex. The belief that the children produced when the woman is on top might be 'a little boy and a little girl with reversed natures' [Yashodhara on 2.8.41] supports this view: the 'reverse' intercourse of parents was thought to wreak embryonic damage, resulting in the reversed gender behaviour of the third nature—significantly, for a boy as well as a girl.[47] (Here, as in his treatment of the third nature, Vatsyayana is far more relaxed than other texts of the period, which generally stigmatize the 'reversed' position; the bloodthirsty goddess Kali, for instance, is depicted 'on top', straddling the corpse of her husband Shiva.) Though Vatsyayana never uses the verb 'to play the man's role' (*purushayitva*) when he describes lesbian activities [5.6.1–4], Yashodhara cites one text in which that verb is used of a woman with

---

[47] Manu [at 3.49] tells us that a male child is born when the semen of the man is greater than that of the woman, and a female child when the semen of the woman is greater than that of the man; if both are equal, a hermaphrodite is born, or a boy and a girl.

another woman [2.1.18]. Alain Daniélou's translation takes this possibility to two extremes, reading this passage first as the sodomization of a man by a woman using a dildo and then as an encounter between two women, one of whom sodomizes the other with a dildo. This is an ingenious and suggestive reading, but at the cost of ignoring the gender of the pronouns and the meaning of several key Sanskrit words in the text. Daniélou makes the woman the subject and the man the object ('she unties his undergarment'), reversing the genders expressed in the text [2.8.8]; he translates *svairini*, designating an independent and presumably promiscuous woman (which we translate as a 'loose' woman), as 'lesbian'. When the text uses the phrase that always describes the man's sexual organ inside the woman's (*yukta-yantra*, literally 'when the instrument has been attached'), Daniélou interprets this as meaning that the woman inserts a dildo in her partner's anus. But Vatsyayana always uses *apadravya*, not *yantra*, to designate a dildo that women use. Even this often cryptic text is not infinitely elastic; it simply will not stretch to accommodate these readings. Our suggestion that the pronouns in the passage about the third nature might *also* be read with reference to a man and a woman, as an alternative, or perhaps even a subversive, subtext, is a far cry from suggesting, against the pronouns and much else, that the passage about the woman on top is *only* about two women.[48] Yet, without going so far as to distort the text with sodomizing dildos, that passage could be read in lesbian terms.

Yashodhara's commentary on the woman in the man's role [2.8.6] suggests other ways in which the *Kamasutra* does not simply dichotomize gender:

All of this activity is said to be done with a woman's natural talent [2.7.22]. The acts he demonstrated before are acts that he executed with roughness and ferocity, the man's natural talent; she now does these acts against the current of her own natural talent. She hits him hard, with the back of her hand and so forth, demonstrating her ferocity. And so, in order to express the woman's natural talent, even though she is not embarrassed, nor exhausted, and does not wish to stop, she indicates that she is embarrassed and exhausted and wishes to stop.

Vatsyayana has already defined the 'woman's natural talent' [2.7.22]

---

[48] Daniélou's error here is much like Burton's error in putting the commentary into the text instead of offering it as an alternative reading.

as 'suffering, self-denial, and weakness', in contrast with the man's natural talent, his roughness and ferocity, just as he has defined the woman's nature as passive, the man's as active [2.1.26]. He has also listed the female traits that one sort of man of the third nature imitates: 'chatter, grace, emotions, delicacy, timidity, innocence, frailty, and bashfulness' [2.9.2]. Now, since he has maintained [at 2.8.39] that the woman 'unveils her own feelings completely when her passion drives her to get on top', the feelings of the woman when she plays the man's role seem to be both male and female. Or, rather, when she acts like a man, she pretends to be a man and then pretends to be a woman.

The poet Amaru wrote a verse about a girl who forgets herself, and forgets her womanly modesty, as she makes love on top of her male partner, but then, as her memory returns, and with it her sense of shame, she suddenly becomes aware of her own body and releases [*mukta*] first her male nature and then her lover.[49] The thirteenth-century commentator Arjunavarmadeva glosses the verse, in part, like this:

An impassioned woman in the woman-on-top position abandons, first, maleness, and, right after that, her lover. What happened? She perceived her own body, which she had not recognized at all while she was impassioned. Only later is there any mention of the distinction between being male or female. She is described as becoming modest only at the onset of memory.[50]

The sequence here seems to be that she takes on a male nature, loses her natural female modesty, suddenly regains her memory, regains her modesty, recognizes her female body, lets go of her male nature, and lets go (physically) of the man. The interrelationship between gendered actions (male on top, female on the bottom), gendered natures (males rough, females modest), and gendered bodies, together with the loss and recovery of a sense of one's own body balanced against the holding and releasing of the body of a sexual partner, is complex indeed. (It becomes even more complex when we recall that 'release' is the same word that, on the one hand, Vatsyayana uses for the courtesan's technique of getting rid of an unwanted

---

[49] *Amarushataka*, verse 89.
[50] Thanks to Blake Wentworth for bringing this commentary to our attention and translating it.

lover [at 6.3.44] and that, on the other hand, in a religious context, signifies ultimate liberation from the wheel of rebirth.) Altogether, these readings of homo- and heteroerotic passages, some closer to the text than others, suggest various ways in which the *Kamasutra*'s implicit claim to sexual totality might be opened out into a vision of gender infinity.

Psychology and Culture in the Kamasutra

The *Kamasutra* can be viewed as an account of a psychological war of independence that took place in India some two thousand years ago. The first aim of this struggle was the rescue of erotic pleasure from the crude purposefulness of sexual desire, from its biological function of reproduction alone. The first European translators of the *Kamasutra* in the late nineteenth century, clearly on the side of sexual pleasure in a society where the reigning Christian morality sought to subordinate, if not altogether eradicate it in service of a divinely ordained reproductive goal, regarded the ancient Sanskrit text, devoted to the god of love without even a nod to the divinities who preside over fertility and birth, as a welcome ally. To them, the *Kamasutra* was the product of a place and people who had raised the search for sexual pleasure to the status of a religious quest. Lamairesse, the French translator, even called it a 'Théologie Hindoue' that revealed vital truths regarding man's fundamental, sexual nature. Richard Schmidt, the German translator, would wax lyrical: 'The burning heat of the Indian sun, the fabulous luxuriance of the vegetation, the enchanted poetry of moonlit nights permeated by the perfume of lotus flowers and, not least, the distinctive role the Indian people have always played, the role of unworldly dreamers, philosophers, impractical romantics—all combine to make the Indian a real virtuoso in love.'[51]

Vatsyayana and other ancient Indian sexologists can certainly be viewed as flag bearers for sexual pleasure in an era where the sombre Buddhist view of life which equated the god of love with Mara or Death was still influential. But they were also inheritors of another world-view, that of the Sanskrit epics, the *Mahabharata* and *Ramayana*, in which sexual love is usually a straightforward matter of desire and its gratification. This was especially so for the man, for

---

[51] Richard Schmidt, *Beiträge zur Indischen Erotik*, 1. Translation by Sudhir Kakar.

whom a woman was an instrument of pleasure and an object of the senses (*indriyartha*), one physical need among many others. There is an idealization of marriage in the epics, yes, but chiefly as a social and religious act. The obligation of conjugal love and the virtue of chastity within marriage were primarily demanded of the wife, while few limits were set on a husband who lived under and looked up at a licentious heaven teeming with lusty gods and heavenly whores, otherworldly and utterly desirable at once, and most eager to give and take pleasure. The Hindu pantheon of the epics was not unlike the Greek Olympus where gods and goddesses sport and politic with a welcome absence of moralistic subterfuge.

Vatsyayana and the early sexologists were thus also heirs to a patrimony where sexual desire ran rampant, unchecked by moral constraints. Indeed, Shvetaketu Auddalaki, one of the legendary composers of the first textbooks on sex, was credited with trying to put an end to unbridled sexual coupling and a certain profligacy in relation to intercourse with married women which is so prominent in the *Mahabharata*. Prior to Shvetaketu's treatise, both married and unmarried women were viewed as items for indiscriminate consumption, 'like cooked rice', Yashodhara tells us [1.1.9]. Shvetaketu was the first to make the novel suggestion that men should not generally sleep with the wives of other men.

In addition to rescuing erotic pleasure from the confining morality of fertility and reproduction, the *Kamasutra*'s 'freedom struggle' also had a second aim. This was to find a haven for the erotic from the ferocity of unchecked sexual desire. For desire has an open, lustful intent, imperiously and precipitously seeking satisfaction for its own sake, a tidal rush of gut instinct. Human beings have always sensed that sexual desire may also have other aims besides the keen pleasure of genital intercourse and orgasm. For instance, the sexual fantasies of men and women are often coloured with the darker purposes of destructive aggression.[52] Without an imagined violence, however minimal, attenuated, and distant from awareness, many men fail to be gripped by powerful sexual excitement; aggressiveness towards the woman is as much a factor in their potency as are their loving feelings. One of the major fantasies of such men is of taking by force that which is not easily given; some imagine the woman not

---

[52] Jean-Paul Sartre, *Being and Nothingness*, part iii.

wishing to participate in the sexual experience but then being carried away by the man's forcefulness despite herself. We find a variant of this 'possession fantasy' in classical Sanskrit love poetry composed about the time of the *Kamasutra*, with its predilection for love scenes where the woman trembles in a state of diffuse but nongenital bodily excitement as if timorously anticipating an attack, her terror a source of excitement for both herself and her would-be assailant. In the eighth canto of Kalidasa's *Kumarasambhava*, a masterpiece of erotic poetry also roughly contemporaneous with the *Kamasutra*, Shiva's excitement reached a crescendo when Parvati 'in the beginning felt both fear and love'.[53]

In women, the counterpart of violent possession, encompassing the woman's urge to attract, entrap, and control the male, is rarely expressed in the same way as in men, namely in conscious or unconscious fantasies of conquest, ravishment and mastery. Whereas one of men's violent fantasies is of penetrating the woman, in women's imagination the insertion of the penis into the vagina may become not only a loving acceptance but a seizure, for some even a wrenching off of the lover's organ, to be retained inside her as a victor's trophy.[54] The male version of this fantasy appears in an attenuated form in the *Kamasutra*'s warning that certain positions 'must allow a way for the man to slide back' [2.6.9], because, as the commentator cautions, 'If he moves inside her too roughly, she can be injured, and the man's foreskin can be torn off, which physicians call "ruptured foreskin".' It is more strongly expressed in the description of the position known as the 'mare's trap', in which she grasps him, like a mare, so tightly that he cannot move [2.6.21].

To fulfil its aim as an authentic textbook of eroticism, the *Kamasutra* could not gloss over the possessive violence of sexual desire. In its chapters on biting, scratching, and slapping, we again encounter the darker purposes of sexual desire, which, Vatsyayana admits, is combative by its very nature. His effort, though, is to civilize the violence of sex, ritualize the cruelty of intercourse. By giving examples of serious injury caused to women, he warns against the danger of playful violence in sex slipping into murderous cruelty. Sexual desire, then, in which the body's wanting and violence, the excitement of orgasm and the exultation of possession, all flow

---

[53] Kalidasa, *Kumarasambhava*, 8.1.
[54] Kakar and Ross, *Tales of Love, Sex and Danger*, 198–9.

together, can easily overwhelm erotic pleasure. Today, when what were once called 'perversions' are the normal fare of television channels, video films and internet sites, where small but specialized professions exist for the satisfaction of every sexual excess, the *Kamasutra*'s second project of rescuing the erotic from raw sexuality would find many supporters. In today's post-moral world, the danger to erotic pleasure is less from the icy frost of morality than from the fierce heat of instinctual desire. The *Kamasutra*'s most valuable insight, then, is that pleasure needs to be cultivated, that in the realm of sex, nature requires culture.

Culture, in the *Kamasutra*'s sense, the sixty-four arts that need to be learned and so on, requires leisure and means, time and money, none of which was in short supply for the text's primary intended audience, an urban (and urbane) élite consisting of princes and barons, high state officials, and wealthy merchants. Vatsyayana, who disapproves of sexual relations with rural and tribal women because they could have adverse effects on the erotic refinement and sensibility of his reader, the cultivated man-about-town, would have been baffled by Lady Chatterley's sexual transports with a gamekeeper.[55] Erotic pleasure, then, partakes of the moral order and of instinctual desire at the same time as it seeks to emancipate itself from both. As a flag bearer of the erotic, the *Kamasutra* is a champion of *sensible* pleasure.

Despite its awareness of the role of violence in sexuality, the feeling-tone of the *Kamasutra*'s eroticism is primarily one of lightness. In its pages, we meet leisured gallants who spend hours in personal grooming and teaching their mynah birds and parrots to speak. Their afternoons and evenings are devoted to drinking, music and dance; that is, when they are not busy in talking poetry and engaging in sexual banter with artful courtesans. In its light-hearted eroticism, the *Kamasutra* is part of a literary climate during the first six centuries of the common era when the erotic was associated with all that was bright, shining, and beautiful in the ordinary world. The Sanskrit poems and dramas of this period are also characterized by this lightness, an eroticism more hedonist than impassioned. The mood is a playful enjoyment of love's ambiguities, a delighted savouring of its pleasures, and a consummately refined suffering of

---

[55] Vatsyayana does, however, admit that the man-about-town may on occasion stoop to have a low-class servant-girl [2.10.22].

its sorrows. The poems are cameos yielding glimpses into arresting erotic moments, their intensity enhanced by the accumulation of sensuous detail. The aesthetic theory of this period could confidently proclaim that certain emotions such as laziness, violence and disgust do not belong to a depiction of the erotic. The *rasa*, 'flavour' or 'essence', of sexual love today knows no such limits.

Another aspect of the *Kamasutra*'s eroticism is the discovery of the woman as a subject and full participant in sexual life, very much a subject in the erotic realm, not a passive recipient of the man's lust. Women are no longer 'cooked rice'. The text both reflects and fosters the woman's enjoyment of her sexuality. Of the four kinds of preliminary love-play Vatsyayana describes, the woman takes the active part in two. In one she encircles her lover as a vine encircles a tree, offering and withdrawing her lips for a kiss, driving the man wild with excitement. In the other, familiar from its sculpted representation in the temple friezes of Khajuraho, she rests one of her feet on the man's feet and the other against his thigh. One arm is across his back, and with the other clinging to his shoulder and neck she makes the motion of climbing him as if he was a tree [2.2.15–16]. In the final analysis, though, given the fact that the text was composed by a man primarily for the education of other men, the fostering of a woman's sexual subjectivity is ultimately in the service of an increase in the man's pleasure. The *Kamasutra* recognizes that a woman who actively enjoys sex will make it much more enjoyable for him. One might speculate that this more active role of the woman in sex was enhanced, if not inspired, by the more active nature of the Goddess in the religious sphere, since the Glorification of the Goddess (*Devi-Mahatmya*), the earliest Sanskrit text in praise of the Goddess, was composed during this same period.

Women in the *Kamasutra* are thus presented not only as erotic subjects but as sexual beings with feelings and emotions that a man needs to understand for the full enjoyment of erotic pleasure. Book Three instructs the man on a young girl's need for gentleness in removing her virginal fears and inhibitions. Erotic pleasure demands that the man be pleasing to his partner. In recommending that the man not approach the woman sexually for the first three nights after marriage, using this time to understand her feelings, win her trust, and arouse her love, Vatsyayana takes a momentous step in the history of Indian sexuality by introducing the notion of love in sex. He even goes so far as to advance the radical notion that the ultimate goal of marriage is to develop love between the couple and thus considers the love-marriage (which the religious texts regarded as ritually 'low' and disapproved of, and which is still a rarity in contemporary Indian society) to be the pre-eminent form of marriage.

The erotic love of the *Kamasutra* is not of the romantic variety as we know it today, from a tradition born in the twelfth century, in Bedier's *Tristan and Isolde* in Europe and Nizami's *Laila and Majnun* in the Islamic world. Its tenderness and affection for the partner is still, largely, in the service of sexual desire. Thus Vatsyayana's detailed instructions to the man on the tender gestures required of him at the end of sex, 'when their passion has ebbed', end with the words, 'Through these and other feelings, the young couple's passion grows again' [2.10.6–13]. What distinguishes romantic love from the erotic love of the *Kamasutra* is the pervasive presence in the former of what may be called longing, a willing surrender, adoration and cherishing of the person for whom one lusts. Longing requires an idealization that makes a lover experience the loved one as an infinitely superior being to whom he (in the case of the man) willingly subordinates his desire, to whom he can surrender and obey and thus reverse the accents of the master–servant metaphor of possessive desire. This is no part of the erotic love we find in the *Kamasutra* or, for that matter, in the classical literature of that period. In the Sanskrit and Tamil love poems, as in the textbook of erotics, the beloved is a partner who is a source of excitement and delight, enlivening the senses. A lover is to be explored thoroughly, in enormous detail, and therefore is not quickly abandoned. Yet the inner life or the past and future of a lover are not subjects of entrancement; the impulse is not of fierce monogamy.

For most modern readers who have an affinity for the personal and the subjective, this emphasis on love as a depersonalized voluptuous state, while delighting the senses, does not touch the heart. For those whose sensibility has been moulded by romanticism and individualism it is difficult to identify with the impersonal protagonists of the poems. These are not a particular man or woman but man and woman as such—provided he is handsome, she beautiful, and both young. The face of the heroine, for instance, is always like a moon or lotus flower, eyes like water lilies or those of a fawn. She always stoops slightly from the weight of her full breasts, improbable fleshy flowers of rounded perfection that do not admit even a blade of grass between them. The waist is slim, with three folds, the thighs round and plump, like the trunk of an elephant or a banyan tree. The navel is deep, the hips heavy. These lyrical yet conventional descriptions of body parts seem to operate like collective fetishes, culturally approved cues for the individual to allow himself to indulge erotic excitement without the risk of surrender so longed for in romantic love.

The erotic love of the *Kamasutra* and the classical Sanskrit literature of the period is bright and shiny; romantic love, by contrast, in spite of its exquisite transports of feeling, is often experienced by the lovers as dark and heavy. In the full flowering of romantic love, sexual desire loses its primacy as the lover strives to disappear in the contours of another, a person whose gender fits the mould but whose flesh is almost incidental to the quest for wholeness.[56] The suffering of erotic love, on the other hand, the dark spot on its brightness, has less to do with the soul's elemental longing to end separation than with the bodily nature of sexual desire. Sexual desire does not subside with seeming satiation. Memory as well as the deliciousness of pleasure's ache gnaw further, making for the distress that marks the separation of lovers in erotic love. This sentiment casts only a small shadow on the *Kamasutra*, where it takes the rather different form of the sufferings of the rejected wife and the anxiety of the not-yet-successful suitor. The erotic love of the *Kamasutra* is then a precarious balancing act between the possessiveness of sexual desire and the tenderness of romantic longing, between the disorder of instinctuality and the moral forces of order, between the imperatives of nature and the civilizing attempts of culture. It is a search for harmony in all the opposing forces that constitute human sexuality, a quest often destined to be futile by the very nature of the undertaking. As Vatsyayana remarks: 'When the wheel of sexual ecstasy is in full motion, there is no textbook at all, and no order' [2.2.31].

II. THE COMMENTARIES

In our translation we have drawn upon the earliest Sanskrit commentary, by Yashodhara Indrapada, and the most recent Hindi

[56] Kakar and Ross, *Tales of Love*, 202

commentary, by Devadatta Shastri. These commentaries elucidate
obscure or difficult parts of the texts, but they also introduce their
own points of view. By comparing and contrasting a modern commentator's interpretations with those made centuries ago it is possible to see what kind of attitudes, social mores, moral responses and
so on, influence their glosses.

Yashodhara's Jayamangala

A few Sanskrit commentaries on the *Kamasutra* are known to exist in
manuscript form in libraries, such as the commentary called *Prau-*
dhapriya composed in Varanasi in 1788 by Bhaskara Nrisimha, and
another by Malladeva. But only one has been published, the one
composed by Yashodhara Indrapada, almost certainly in the thirteenth century of the present era.[57] Yashodhara gives us an
unusually intimate insight into his own motives, which he repeats as
a colophon at the end of the first chapter of each of the first six
books: 'Yashodhara, whose guru gave him the name of Indrapada,
made this commentary, called the *Jayamangala*, in one piece,
because he was terrified of suffering a lover's separation from
sophisticated women.' This erotic motivation stands in striking contrast to Vatsyayana's claim that his own work was composed in
chastity. Moreover, since Yashodhara lived about a millennium after
Vatsyayana, he may not always know what was in Vatsyayana's
mind, and we have not always taken his advice, though we have
always been glad to have it. But Yashodhara usually makes good
sense of the text and is, in any case, also an original source, now
some seven centuries old. It is fascinating both to know what someone thought about sex then, too, and to contrast what the two
authors say, to see how ideas changed over that millennium. Since
the commentary is many times the size of the text, and often tedi-
ously technical, we have appended to the translation of Vatsyayana
only those portions of Yashodhara that shed light on specific
obscurities in the text or that expand that text in interesting ways.
But some of Yashodhara's longer glosses break away from the text to

---

[57] One of the *Jayamangala* manuscripts says it was written under King Vishaladeva
(1243–61), and it is quoted in 1307 by Jinaprabha in his commentary on the *Kalpasutra*.
Yashodhara's detailed knowledge of South India has led some scholars to suggest that he
might have come from the South, the place that Vatsyayana so despised, but there is far
too little evidence to judge this.

present his basic approach and thus may alert the reader to the general bias of his interpretations.

Yashodhara loves to divide Vatsyayana's already somewhat taxonomic text into further taxonomies. Thus, at 1.1.5: 'Creatures exist in three conditions: creation, sustenance, and dissolution. And sustenance is of two sorts: good and bad. The three aims of human life, too, are of two sorts: acceptable and unacceptable. The acceptable forms are *dharma*, *artha*, and *kama*; the unacceptable, the violation of *dharma*, loss, and hatred.' And at 2.1.30 he divides a woman's pleasure into two ('the scratching of an itch and the pleasure of melting') and then divides the melting into two ('the flowing and the ejaculation of the seed'). He taxonomizes at some length in his discussion of the nature of *kama* (at 1.2.11–12). Here is the gist of it:

Kama takes two forms, general and particular. It is the general form that operates under the control of the mind and heart joined with the self, which governs the senses, each in its own appropriate sensation: the ear engages in sound, the skin in touch, the eye in form, the tongue in taste, and the nose in smell. The consciousness of sound and so forth is undergirded by a wish to enjoy the appropriate sensation; that wish is *kama*. And when the self enjoys a sensation through that wish and experiences pleasure, that pleasure is *kama* of the general kind.

Particular *kama* has two forms, primary and secondary. The speech organs, hands, feet, anus, and genitals are organs of action, which perform the acts of speaking, taking, moving about, defecating, and experiencing bliss. Now, a man and a women have an organ in their lower parts, the vagina and so forth, which is actually a part of the sense organ of skin, for touch is the essence of skin, and a certain place on the skin, called the sense organ of the genitals, causes the experience of bliss on the occasion of ejaculation. Touching a man on the thigh or calf and so forth, or a woman on the thigh or navel and so forth, is also a particular sensation of touch, but that is not what is meant here, because it is secondary. In fact, this sort of experience is an example of general *kama*.

What, then, makes the experience described here an example of particular *kama*? To answer this, Vatsyayana says: 'It bears fruit.' When this experience goes on uninterrupted, there is an ejaculation of semen and a simultaneous pleasure and fruit, namely bliss. The pleasure of erotic arousal is the pleasure that comes when kissing, scratching, biting, and so forth are applied to this place and that, arousing the perception of pleasure in a man and a woman through the power of the imagination of passion. This is primary *kama*. By this definition, even the fruitful experience of the object is not primary *kama* if it is done in something other than a vagina or in the wrong kind of vagina, or between a man and woman who are not attracted to one another, because it lacks the pleasure of erotic arousal and is therefore secondary.

Here Yashodhara distinguishes between general *kama* (pleasure) and particular *kama* (sexual pleasure) and then divides particular *kama* (sexual pleasure) into two types: primary (involving the sexual organs) and secondary (involving other parts of the body). His assumption that the 'fruit' of *kama* is pleasure may not be what Vatsyayana has in mind; at 1.5.1, for instance, and elsewhere, Vatsyayana mentions sons as one of the fruits of the right sort of *kama*. Shastri, too, comments on this discrepancy:

The words 'a direct experience of an object of the senses, which bears fruit' in this *sutra* express a serious mood. Yashodhara has taken the word 'fruit' to mean the pleasure of kissing, embracing and ejaculation. But it appears to us that Vatsyayana's viewpoint differs from that of Yashodhara. Here it would be proper to understand the birth of able offspring as Vatsyayana's chief goal. The Vedas and the Upanishads also express the same intention. [See *Atharva Veda* 14.2.31, 14.2.32, 14.2.38, 14.1.58, 14.2.36, 14.2.66 and *Chandogya Upanishad* 2.13.1.] It is thus clear that for the creator of the *Kamasutra*, the meaning of the fruit of kissing and embracing is the birth of offspring.

Shastri seems to speak here with the full weight of morality and social mores behind him. Where Yashodhara was in many ways apparently freer from social constraints/responsibility, emphasizing the erotic over the reproductive function, Shastri insists on it and finds support in the text. Vatsyayana can be called in to testify on behalf of either of these commentators because he is ambiguous; his text can bear many interpretations, and commentators, as well as other readers, may well interpret it in a way that best suits their personal circumstances

Yashodhara then goes on to make further distinctions between basic sex (centred on the woman) and subsidiary sex (centred on things like gardens and garlands); and between public sex (the meeting) and private sex (the act):

Both general and particular *kama* depend upon sex. There are two sorts of sex, basic and subsidiary. The base of *kama* is the woman, and the subsidiary limbs are garlands and such things. And so it is said:

> *Kama* is pleasure, and its limbs are
> jewellery, perfumed oils, and garlands.
> as well as forest groves, roof-top gardens,
> the playing of lutes, and wine.
> Its base is women—
> unrestrained, beautiful, young,
> amorous, flirtatious, clever at flattery,
> drawing to themselves the minds and hearts of men.

Basic sex is of two sorts: public and private. The private sort is a sexual act done in secret; it is the occasion for a kind of particular *kama*. The public sort of sex is characterized by getting together for the sexual act. Subsidiary sex takes place when each of the sense organs, beginning with the mind, is intimately united with the appropriate subsidiary attribute; it is characterized by the close contact between the sense organs and their objects, and is the occasion for a kind of general *kama*. Public sex requires a method if one or the other, the man or the woman, has no desire or is closely guarded, or ashamed, or afraid, because he or she is dependent on someone else, so that nothing is happening. And how could private sex, the sexual act, happen without the knowledge of the sixty-four arts of love? The text is the method. Even private sex requires a method, for it does not happen without the constant, daily efforts of the man-about-town [1.2.18].

Erotic arousal, for Yashodhara, is therefore primary *kama* even when it does not involve genital contact, because it *imagines* genital contact. On the other hand, sex 'in something other than a vagina or in the wrong kind of vagina' (i.e. self-masturbation, oral sex, anal sex, or bestiality) is not primary *kama*, not just because it lacks (human) genital contact but because the pleasure does not involve true erotic arousal. Thus, where Vatsyayana's remarks could easily be read on a quite general level of aesthetics (what Yashodhara calls general *kama*), Yashodhara narrows them down to focus quite specifically on sexual pleasure (particular *kama*) and, within that category, on genital contact (primary *kama*), whether real or imagined.

Devadatta Shastri's Commentary, the Jaya

There are several published commentaries on the *Kamasutra* in modern Indian languages, including a Bengali translation and commentary published in Calcutta in 1909, a Tamil commentary published in Kumbhakonam in 1924, and a Telugu transcription of Yashodhara's *Jayamangala* commentary, together with a Telugu commentary and translation, published in Madras in 1924. Devadatta Shastri's Hindi commentary was published along with his translation of the text in 1964. His explanation (*vyakhya*), as he preferred to call his composition, reflects a traditionalist understanding of sexuality in contemporary Hindu India. He was a modern traditionalist in the sense that, although he had an old-fashioned Sanskrit education, he was also aware of the currents of Western sociological and psychological thought of his time. His commentary, he tells us, was written from the viewpoints of spiritual philosophy and modern social science.

Born in 1912 in a small village in the North Indian state of Uttar Pradesh, Devadatta was orphaned at an early age. In protest against ill treatment by his elder brother, he left home at the age of 12 and entered the Sanskrit College at Rajapur, from which he graduated with the title of Shastri. For a short while he was the editor of the Hindi newspaper *Hindustan*, published from Delhi, before he settled down in Allahabad to the life of a traditional scholar and a Tantric practitioner. He wrote 76 books on the Vedas, Tantras, Puranas and ancient Indian texts of political science. He died in 1982, leaving unfinished a volume on the identity of the author, date, and place of the *Kamasutra*, which he had announced in his commentary.

We have provided excerpts from his commentary, particularly his expansive summaries of each chapter, as an Appendix.

III. TRANSLATIONS INTO EUROPEAN LANGUAGES

Burton et al.

It is startling to realize that the *Kamasutra*, the Indian text best known, at least by name, to European and American readers,[58] was hardly known at all by such readers just a hundred years ago and even now is not really known, since the very first English translation, which remains the one most widely used and reused, long out of copyright and in the public domain, does not say what the Sanskrit says. Moreover, it is not even the work of the man who is known as its author, Sir Richard Francis Burton. This translation, published

---

[58] Amartya Sen remarked, 'There is a similar neglect [in the West] of Indian writings on nonreligious subjects, from mathematics, epistemology, and natural science to economics and linguistics. (The exception, I suppose, is the *Kama Sutra*, in which Western readers have managed to cultivate an interest)', Sen, 'East and West', 36.

in 1883,[59] was far more the work of Forster Fitzgerald Arbuthnot, whose name appears on the title-page with Burton's only in some editions, though Burton later referred to the *Kamasutra* translation as 'Arbuthnot's Vatsyayana'.[60] But the translation owed even more to two Indian scholars whose names do not appear on the title-page at all: Bhagavanlal Indrajit and Shivaram Parashuram Bhide.[61] (There is a pre–post-colonial irony in the fact that Arbuthnot later tried to get the censors off his trail by stating, in 1885, a half-truth that he almost certainly regarded as a lie: that the translation was done entirely by Indian pandits.[62]) It really should, therefore, be known as the Indrajit–Bhide–Arbuthnot–Burton translation, or perhaps the IBAB translation, but since Burton was by far the most famous member of the team, it has always been called the Burton transla-tion, and we will continue to refer to it in the conventional way.

Richard Burton was born in 1821 at Torquay, England, educated at Oxford, sent to Bombay in 1842 as an ensign in the Indian army, and posted to Sind, in Northwest India (now Pakistan). There he served with the infamous Sir Charles Napier, under whose com-mand he undertook a study of brothels staffed by 'boys and eunuchs'.[63] His biographers insist that he learned Hindustani, Sindi, Marathi, Gujarati, Sanskrit, Arabic and Persian, all in two years,[64] and then, in 1844, began moving about Indian society in native

---

[59] The title-page read: 'The Kama Sutra of Vatsyayana, Translated from the San-scrit. In Seven Parts, with Preface, Introduction and Concluding Remarks. Cosmopoli: 1883: for the Kama Shastra Society of London and Benares, and for private circulation only.'

[60] Archer, 'Preface', 36.

[61] This form of gentlemanly appropriation repeated itself almost a century later, when Alex Comfort, a doctor with no formal Sanskrit training, made a brief trip to India in 1964 and immediately published a quite erudite translation of the *Koka Shashtra*, complete with a preface by William G. Archer (who had written the preface to the first legal edition of the Burton *Kama Sutra* just one year earlier). Were there Indian scholars who did for Comfort the work that the two pandits did for Arbuthnot and Burton? When Comfort died, his obituary in the 29 March 2000 *New York Times* began: 'Dr. Alex Comfort, whose graphically illustrated 1972 book *The Joy of Sex* became the coffee-table Kama Sutra of the baby-boom generation, died on Sunday . . .' But the *Times* also stated with confidence that Comfort had translated the *Koka Shashtra* from the Sanskrit.

[62] Brodie, *The Devil Drives*, 357.

[63] Archer, 'Preface', 17; see also Doniger, ' "I have Scinde".'

[64] Even the author of *The Cartoon Kama Sutra* had her doubts: 'Burton . . . was reputed to speak over 50 languages, but [and she quotes a mistranslation from Burton's *Arabian Nights*]. So who knows what was written in the original Kama Sutra?'

disguise, like Rudyard Kipling's Kim. He left India in 1856, returning only for a brief visit in 1876. F. F. Arbuthnot (whom Burton used
to call 'Bunnie') was a retired Indian civil servant who had been born
near Bombay in 1833 and, after going to Europe for his education,
returned to India. Burton and Arbuthnot met either in India in
1853–4 or on Arbuthnot's furlough to London in 1859–60. They
remained friends, first in India and then in England (from 1879,
when Arbuthnot retired to Guildford and married, until Burton's
death in 1890).

Burton and Arbuthnot first produced a translation of a fifteenth-
century text, the *Anangaranga*, which they tried to publish (under
the title of *Kama Shastra*) in 1873; they disguised their names on the
title-page ('A.F.F. and B.F.R.') but ran into trouble with the printers
and ended up publishing only four proof copies, because the printer
allegedly panicked upon reading the proofs and refused to go on.[65]
They published it more successfully, and under its proper title of
Anangaranga (or, in their edition, *Ananga Ranga*) only in 1885. In the
preface to their translation of the *Kamasutra*, they wrote:

It may be interesting to some persons to learn how it came about that
Vatsyayana was first brought to light and translated into the English language. It happened thus. While translating with the pandits the 'Anunga
Runga, or the stage of love', reference was frequently found to be made to
one Vatsya. The sage Vatsya was of this opinion, or of that opinion. The
sage Vatsya said this, and so on. Naturally questions were asked who this
sage was, and the pandits replied that Vatsya was the author of the standard work on love in Sanscrit literature, and that no Sanscrit library was
complete without his work, and that it was most difficult now to obtain in
its entire state.[66]

This little anecdote is rich in paradoxes. If the text was the 'standard
work' on love, and essential to every library, why was it 'most difficult now to obtain'? (The Sanskrit text was first published by Pandit Durgaprasad in Bombay only in 1891, eight years after the translation.[67]) Why had Burton and Arbuthnot never heard of it, when
they had heard of the lesser, and much later, work, the *Anangaranga*?

[65] Archer, 'Preface', 28.

[66] Ibid. 28–9.

[67] The first edition was printed with the commentary of Yashodhara, except on Book
Seven. The new edition, published in Bombay in 1905, was edited by Kedara-Natha
Sarma, with Yashodhara's commentary on Book Seven.

There are several likely reasons. The *Anangaranga* was already far better known in India than the *Kamasutra* because it was a kind of *Kamasutra* lite, much shorter[68] and written in much more accessible Sanskrit. As in the case of the *Rig Veda* (the most ancient text) in India, or the Constitution in America, people had heard of the *Kamasutra* and genuflected to it, but the later versions and commentaries were what they actually used.[69] More particularly, the *Anangaranga* cuts to the chase, reducing the *Kamasutra* to very little that is not in Books Two and Seven, about sex and drugs; the ten chapters of the *Anangaranga* cover descriptions of women, erogenous zones, the size of sexual organs, types of women, regional peculiarities, ways of gratifying women (the longest chapter), magic recipes, eligible marriage partners, embracing and kissing, and sexual positions. This emphasis on Book Two of the *Kamasutra*, and particularly on the sexual positions, has persisted, so that most Americans and Europeans today think that the sexual positions are all there is to the *Kamasutra*. (The *New York Times* entitled Edward Hower's review of Sudhir Kakar's novel about Vatsyayana, 'Assume the Position', and Sanjeev Bhaskar's 2001 sex odyssey, via television documentary, about the *Kamasutra* is entitled *Position Impossible*.) The real *Kamasutra*, by contrast, is not the sort of book to read in bed while drinking heavily, let alone holding the book with one hand in order to keep the other free.

In fact, it is likely that other, better-read Sanskritists were well aware of the existence of the *Kamasutra* and might not have been quite so surprised as Burton was to hear 'Vatsya's' name dropped. Some British scholars may actually have known the text or, at the very least, have come across references to it in the erotic poetry that had been translated from the very start of the British colonial awareness of India (beginning with Kalidasa's *Shakuntala*, translated by Sir William Jones in 1789, five years before he translated Manu). Burton and Arbuthnot were not great Sanskrit scholars. Burton had buckled his swash through a great deal of 'Oriental' erotica but was not likely to have browsed through a lot of Sanskrit court poetry;

---

[68] The *Anangaranga* has only ten chapters, with a total of some 453 verses, in comparison with the *Kamasutra*'s 1,492 or 1,683 passages.

[69] Similarly, the *Laws of Manu* was not nearly so widely used as were its commentaries, which were more detailed and easier to read, unpacking all the tantalizing obscurities.

Arbuthnot wrote three short travel books but never published anything else about Sanskrit literature. It was therefore arrogant of Burton and Arbuthnot to assume that that *Kamasutra* 'was first brought to light' when they first saw it. They 'discovered' the *Kamasutra* only in the sense that Columbus discovered America; Indian scholars certainly, and European scholars probably, had landed on those shores long before. But scholars in the late nineteenth century, the end of the Victorian age, may have regarded such texts as pornographic and hesitated to write about them.[70]

In any case, once Burton found out about the existence of the *Kamasutra* he must have felt that he had at last found the erotic literary equivalent of the source of the Nile (for which he had searched, in vain, years before[71]). He set to work with Arbuthnot. The German Orientalist Georg Bühler, who was to publish a new translation of the *Laws of Manu* in 1886 and who had worked for years with Indian Sanskrit scholars, put Burton and Arbuthnot in touch with a pandit that Bühler himself had worked with, Bhagavanlal Indrajit, and his associate Shivaram Parashuram Bhide. Indrajit gathered the manuscripts, one each from Bombay, Calcutta, Benares, and Jaipur, some lacking parts of the complete text or the complete commentary.[72] The two Indian scholars prepared a version of the translation, which Arbuthnot then doctored and prepared in time for Burton's brief visit to India, with his wife Isabel, in 1876.[73] According to one of Burton's many biographers, Fawn Brodie, 'Burton apparently worked through the translation during his holidays in Arbuthnot's country house outside Bombay.'[74] Burton polished the text, possibly in consultation with the manuscripts; Arbuthnot wrote the introduction and preface.[75] Burton's main contribution, however, was the courage and determination to publish the work.[76] To get around the censorship laws, Burton and Arbuthnot set up an imaginary publishing house, the Kama Shastra Society of London

---

[70] A study of diaries and academic journals from this period might settle these questions one way or the other, but we know of no one who has done such a study.

[71] Brodie, *The Devil Drives*, 265–70.

[72] None of these texts, apparently, was cited in the later printed editions.

[73] Brodie, *The Devil Drives*, 357.

[74] Ibid. 358.

[75] Archer, 'Preface', 36, citing a note from Arbuthnot to H. S. Ashbee (apparently published in 1885 in *Catena Librorum Tacendorum*).

[76] In our day, the parallels that come to mind are Grove Press or even, perhaps, Larry Flynt.

and Benares, actually consisting of just the two of them, with printers said to be in Benares or Cosmopoli. Arbuthnot put up the money for the printing. The Kama Shastra Society later published other erotica that Burton translated from the Arabic, such as *The Perfumed Garden*, as well as Burton's great masterpiece, *The Arabian Nights*. But that is another story.

Burton did for the *Kamasutra* what Max Müller did for the *Rig Veda* during this same period.[77] Widespread public knowledge of the *Kamasutra*, in both India and Europe, begins with the Burton translation, which had a profound effect upon literature across Europe and America.[78] Even though it was not formally published in England and the United States until 1962, the Burton *Kamasutra* soon became 'one of the most pirated books in the English language',[79] constantly reprinted, often with a new preface to justify the new edition, sometimes without any attribution to Burton or Arbuthnot. It remains precious, like Edward Fitzgerald's *Rubaiyat*, as a monument of English literature, though not much closer to Vatsyayana than Fitzgerald was to Omar Khayyam.

For the Burton translation is seriously flawed. A detailed criticism of it, line by line, would be neither worth while nor possible, since without a precise knowledge of the text they used, one cannot say with any certainty where they deviated from that text. Nor can we know at what point along the line of transmission such slips occurred: with one of the original manuscripts, the choice of a particular reading among manuscripts, either of the two Indian pandits, Arbuthnot, or Burton. But there is every reason to believe that they used a text very like the one that was published just a few years later and that agrees in general with all the texts published since, and in broad terms it is easy enough to see what they left out, put in, and mistranslated. For instance, at 4.1.19–21 we have translated the text like this:

---

[77] Müller published the first volume of a selected English translation in 1869, and the second volume in 1891, having published the first complete edition of the Sanskrit text, with Sayana's commentary, in 1849 and the second edition in 1890. In perhaps sardonic appreciation for this 'discovery', Hindus often pun on Max Müller's name, calling him Moksha Mula, or 'the root of Release'.

[78] Unfortunately, it took longer for academics to make full use of the text. Sir Monier Monier-Williams, who composed, in 1899, the great Sanskrit–English dictionary still used by most scholars, lists Vatsyayana but not the *Kamasutra* as potential sources and seldom, if ever, cites a word from that text in his lexicon.

[79] Brodie, *The Devil Drives*, 358.

Mildly offended by the man's infidelities, she does not accuse him too much, but she scolds him with abusive language when he is alone or among friends. She does not, however, use love-sorcery worked with roots, for, Gonardiya says, 'Nothing destroys trust like that.'

The Burton translation here reads:

In the event of any misconduct on the part of her husband, she should not blame him excessively, though she be a little displeased. She should not use abusive language towards him, but rebuke him with conciliatory words, whether he be in the company of friends or alone. Moreover, she should not be a scold, for, says Gonardiya, 'there is no cause of dislike on the part of a husband so great as this characteristic in a wife.'

What is wrong with this picture? In the first place, the passage is watered down, padded, almost twice as long as the more direct translation. Secondly, the translators either had a very different reading or mistranslated the word for 'love-sorcery worked with roots' (*mulakarika*), which they render as 'she should not be a scold'.[80] Third, 'misconduct' is not so much a mistranslation as an error of judgement, for the word in question (*apacara*) does have the general meaning of 'misconduct', but in an erotic context it usually takes on the more specific meaning of 'infidelity', a choice that is supported both by the remedy that the text suggests (and rejects)—love-magic—and by Yashodhara's gloss (*aparadha*). But the most serious problem is the word 'not' that negates the wife's right to use abusive language against her straying husband, a denial only somewhat qualified by the added phrase, 'rebuke him with conciliatory words.' Was this an innocent error (and if so, whose?), or does it reflect a sexist bias (again, whose?)? We cannot know.

There are also pervasive patterns of mistranslation. The Burton translation has no commentary and only a few notes, but there is little need for them, for they are incorporated in the text. The pandits admitted relying heavily on Yashodhara's commentary,[81] which the Burton translation often simply inserted into Vatsyayana's text, a move that accounts for a good deal of the padding.[82] The Burton

---

[80] At 4.1.9, they translate the agentive form of the same word ('a magician who uses love-sorcery worked with roots') as 'witch', showing a basic understanding of the term.

[81] Archer, 'Preface', 30.

[82] This habit has unfortunately corrupted almost every translator except Richard Schmidt, the first to translate the commentary separately, thus freeing it from the text; Mylius, too, keeps the commentary out of the text.

translation also deprives the reader of two essential aspects of the formal construction of the text. First, the translators made almost all of the direct quotes into indirect quotes, thus losing the force of the dialogue that animates the work. And secondly, they failed to recognize most of the verses and printed them as prose, thus failing to alert the reader to the different voice presented by the verses. There are also countless miscellaneous errors, including anachronisms such as translating *aluka* (at 4.1.29) as potatoes, which did not exist in India in Vatsyayana's time.[83]

Most unfortunately, Burton and Arbuthnot, in Brodie's words, 'adroitly managed to escape the smell of obscenity' by using 'the Hindu terms for the sexual organs, *yoni* and *lingam*, throughout.'[84] To the extent that nineteenth-century writers regarded the words themselves, not the actual things that they designated, as obscene, the foreign words, devoid of any English connotations at all, were able to make an end-run around the obscene thought. But this decision of Burton's was problematic in several ways. First of all, these terms do not represent Vatsyayana's text, which only rarely uses *lingam* to refer to the male sexual organ and never refers to the female sexual organ as *yoni*.[85] Instead, Vatsyayana uses several different words, primarily the gender-neutral *jaghana* (which can be translated as 'pelvis', or 'genitals', or 'between the legs'[86]) or other terms (such as *yantra* or *sadhana*, 'the instrument') that are neither coy nor obscene. In some places, he circumvents, by indirection or implication, the need to employ any specific word at all. Where Vatsyayana does use *lingam* [2.1.1], the context suggests, and Yashodhara affirms, that it is (like *jaghana*) gender-neutral, meant to apply to both the male and female sexual organs.

Secondly, by Burton's time, the terms *lingam* and *yoni* had taken on strong religious overtones, as both Indian English and Indian vernacular languages used them primarily to designate the sexual organs of the god Shiva and his consort Parvati. The human and

---

[83] Monier-Williams tells us that it is a root, *Arum campanulatum* (probably arrow-root), 'in modern dialects applied to the yam, potato, etc.'

[84] Brodie, *The Devil Drives*, 359.

[85] Vatsyayana does use *lingam* for the male sexual organ in Book Seven, but that has an entirely different tone from the rest of the text. Yashodhara uses *lingam* and *yoni* more often, but he too uses several other words.

[86] *Jaghana* could most literally be rendered as 'bottom', but only in the British sense of the word (genital) rather than the American (anal).

divine facets of the term were sometimes explicitly compared, as in a text that argued that all creatures in the universe are marked with the signs of the god Shiva and his consort, since, just as Shiva's *lingam* is always placed in the *pindi* (a word for the base in which the *lingam* is supported), so, too, all females, who have *pindi*s, join with males, who have *lingam*s.[87] The exclusive application of these two terms to human genitals, therefore, may have had, at the very least, inappropriate overtones and, at the most, blasphemous implications for some Hindus.

More significantly, these terms had Orientalist implications for most English readers. The use of any Sanskrit term at all in place of an English equivalent anthropologized sex, distanced it, made it safe for English readers by assuring them, or pretending to assure them, that the text was not about real sexual organs, *their* sexual organs, but merely about the appendages of weird, dark people far away. This move dodged 'the smell of obscenity' through the same logic that allowed *National Geographic* to depict the bare breasts of black African women long before it became respectable to show white women's breasts in *Playboy*.[88] It enabled the authors to pretend that the book was not obscene because it was about India, when they really thought it was about sex, and knew that English readers would think so too.

In fact, the Burton translation is most accurate in the sections of Book Two that deal with the sexual positions, the topic for which the book became famous. Can this relative accuracy be explained by the fact that this is the part of the book most closely glossed by the *Anangaranga*? Or was it because this was what Burton cared about most, or worked on most carefully? Or was it because sex is easier to understand, being universal, than the cultural information that is specific to India? For the book is, really, about India after all, and this area, the realm of South Asian cultural assumptions built into the text, is where the Burton translation goes wrong most often.

---

[87] *Skanda Purana* 1.8.18–19; Doniger, *The Bedtrick*, 397. There are interesting parallels here with Plato's *Symposium*, which tells of a primeval androgyne that split into the ancestors of men and women, who therefore always try to get back together again.

[88] Indeed, in some instances *National Geographic* actually darkened the skin colour of a partially naked Polynesian woman 'in order to render her nudity more acceptable to American audiences' (Lutz and Collins, *Reading National Geographic*, 82).

Other Translations

Several other English translations have been published in India, some of them based on the Burton translation, some apparently original works, but these are not generally available outside India, nor is any of them a significant improvement on the Burton translation. In particular, most of the Indian translations lack the frankness about sexual matters that is the strong point of the Burton translation.[89] Two French translations (by Isidore Liseux in 1883 and by Pierre Eugène Lemairesse in 1891) were basically translations of the Burton translation. (Lemairesse also folded in other bits of erotic literature and used, as a preface, a text by the Marquis de Sade.) An original, far more accurate, and complete German translation, of both the text and Yashodhara's commentary, was published by Richard Schmidt in 1897.[90] Reprinted several times, it remains the best European translation, though its usefulness in our day is somewhat impaired by Schmidt's decision to haul out a Latin fig leaf to cover up what Monty Python used to call the naughty bits, mostly in Book Two. It was general practice in the nineteenth century to castrate the 'obscene' parts of Sanskrit texts (as Griffith did) or to translate them into Latin, and Schmidt's fastidiousness makes all the more remarkable the Burton translation's courage in rendering everything into English (everything but *lingam* and *yoni*). In fact, Burton and Arbuthnot remarked, 'It was at first our intention, after rendering the [*Anangaranga*] into English, to dress it up in Latin, that it might not fall into the hands of the vulgar',[91] but they decided to render it all into English, and damn the torpedoes.[92] Schmidt's translation lacks notes, for which he more than compensated by writing two massive and still authoritative books about sex in ancient India.[93] Klaus Mylius, in 1987, rendered the entire text (though not the commentary) into German, with excellent notes, producing a translation sometimes more accurate than Schmidt's, though never as readable.

[89] See the Bibliography.

[90] Schmidt, like the first printed edition of the Sanskrit text, lacked Yashodhara's commentary on Book Seven.

[91] Cited by Archer, 'Preface', 28.

[92] Lee Siegel's fictional Sanskritist, Roth, made a 'perverse endeavor to translate the section on fellatial procedures in a way that reverses the conventional nineteenth-century practice of rendering the transgressive texts of a foreign-language discourse into Latin, to put the clean parts in Latin and the dirty parts in English'.

[93] See Bibliography.

The most recent full translation into English (1994) is an English rendering of Alain Daniélou's 1992 French edition, complete with excerpts from both Yashodhara and Devadatta Shastri. This translation is sometimes ingenious (as we saw in Daniélou's reading of the genders in the passage about women playing the roles of men) but often departs too far from what the Sanskrit will allow.[94] Whatever its flaws, almost every translation has some ideas that open up a piece of this intriguing text, and in working on it a translator is privileged to stand on the shoulders of giants and pygmies alike, to be able to consult a number of friendly spirits: Vatsyayana/Yashodhara (with the help of various Sanskrit dictionaries); Devadatta Shastri (and a Hindi dictionary or Hindi-speaking friend); Indrajit–Bhide–Arbuthnot–Burton; the many Indian translators, especially Upadhyaya; Schmidt (and the Latin dictionary); Mylius (and the German dictionary); Syrkin (and the Russian dictionary), and even Daniélou.

The Present Translation

The translators of this edition bring complementary skills and backgrounds to the project: a woman and a man, an American and an Indian, a historian of religions and a psychoanalyst, a Sanskritist and a Hindi-speaker. The basic division of labour was that Wendy Doniger prepared a draft of the Sanskrit text, relevant parts of the Sanskrit commentary, and parts of the explanatory notes; Sudhir Kakar prepared a draft of the relevant parts of the Hindi commentary, shed Hindi insight on Sanskrit dilemmas, and supplied other parts of the explanatory notes. Each of the authors then made suggestions for revisions in the other's work. Similarly, Kakar drafted 'Psychology and Culture in the *Kamasutra*' in the Introduc-

---

[94] In translating the very first Yashodhara passage, for instance, Daniélou stumbles on the most basic step: separating the Sanskrit words (which are printed with the end of each word combined with the beginning of the next, changing both words in accordance with complex rules). Where the text reads *tam upayam achikhyasur acaryamallanaga*, which we render, 'wishing to explain that method, the scholar Vatsyayana Mallanaga . . .' Daniélou makes the break differently: *tam upayam achikhya asuracaryamallanaga*. This deprives the verb ('explain') of its desiderative ending and extracts the word *asura*, designating a kind of demon or anti-god, from a combination of that desiderative ending (*asur*, 'wishing to') and the beginning of *acarya* ('scholar'), with this result: 'the prophet of the Asuras, Vatsyayana Mallanaga . . . created this science, after studying its means of accomplishment.' A startling mythological assertion indeed, but, alas, not in the text.

tion, Doniger the rest of the introduction, and again each responded to the work of the other.[95]

The first task was to decide on a text to translate, for there is no critical edition of the *Kamasutra*. Burton and Arbuthnot put together manuscripts to establish their text (which we do not have), Schmidt reconstituted his, and we, too, have combined several printed versions, principally those of Shastri and of Goswami, for our own text.[96] We have generally used Shastri's readings of Vatsyayana, and his system of numbering the passages,[97] but occasionally Goswami's readings make better sense, and then we have used them (but continued to follow Shastri's numbering).[98] We have chosen Goswami's readings of Yashodhara more often, though not invariably.[99]

Our aim was to produce a clear, readable English translation that did not commit the besetting sin of our predecessors, moving the commentary up into the text. In general, we have left the text plain and given the reader the commentator's reading as one among possible options. Occasionally, however, we did have to expand a pronoun in the text with a noun, sometimes a noun taken from the commentary. Vatsyayana's non-sexist language,[100] for example, here

[95] Laura Desmond did the fundamental research for the bibliography and for the discussion of the history of the text and the translations, in the introduction. Ajay Rao tracked down the Latin and English names of the Sanskrit plants for Book Seven. Shubha Pathak hunted down all the books and articles we used in Chicago. Vibhuti Mishra of the Hindi Sahitya Sammelan provided the information on Devadatta Shastri. David Shulman, Patrick Olivelle, Sheldon Pollock, Dominik Wujastyk, and Richard Gombrich gave precious advice on some of the more recalcitrant parts of the Sanskrit text. We are indebted to Sarah Engel for producing, as her project in the Radcliffe Institute's summer publishing programme, a virtual publication of a mythical translation of the *Kamasutra* translation by Wendy Doniger, the blurbs for which were so persuasive that they inspired the production of this actual volume—life, as usual, mirroring art.

[96] Goswami's version of Vatsyayana's text differs from Shastri's only from time to time, and not always with a better reading, but it has a far more complete and less corrupt version of Yashodhara's commentary than Shastri has, particularly for Books Six and Seven.

[97] Shastri and Goswami number the passages differently, though they number the sections in the same way. Schmidt and Burton do not number the passages at all; Syrkin uses Goswami's system, while Mylius and most of the Indian translators use Shastri's.

[98] We have used Goswami's readings of Vatsyayana at 3.4.1, 4.2.45, 5.1.51, 5.3.28, 5.4.54–7, 5.6.19, 6.4.41, 6.5.7, 6.5.14, and 6.5.35.

[99] Since we have not aspired to a complete translation of Yashodhara, we did not think it necessary to specify which edition of the commentary we were using for each particular passage. Indeed, from time to time we have used the readings of Yashodhara in the edition by Ramanand Sharma.

[100] I owe this observation to Judith Butler, personal communication, January 2001.

poses a challenge for the English translation. Where Vatsyayana's pronouns lacked clear referents, we have supplied them; and where the passage assumes that a word or phrase is to be carried over from an earlier line, we have repeated it. For instance, throughout Book Two, especially in Chapters six and seven, it is clear that the woman's body is the one being manipulated, but it is not always so clear that she, rather than the man, is the one doing the manipulation, since Sanskrit verbs often lack subjects.[101] Yet the commentary suggests the gender of the subject in many verses, the author specifies it in others, and the context often strongly suggests a male agent or a female agent in passages adjacent to those that are ambiguous.[102] Vatsyayana assures us, for instance, that the basic pattern is for the man to slap and the woman to moan [2.7.23], and where there are pronouns or gendered noun-endings, they confirm this pattern, as does the commentary.[103] We have therefore supplied pronouns or possessive pronominal adjectives, in keeping with this pattern, to make sense of certain passages.[104] With these exceptions, however, we strove to keep the bare bones of the text separate from the commentary that fleshes it out.

Though the text often uses subjunctive or optative forms, we have generally translated the verbs in the indicative, which conveys the flavour of a novel or a play better than the subjunctive appropriate to a manual of instruction. (Burton usually uses an optative 'should', making the text sound moralistic where it is descriptive.) For Vatsyayana's 'should' is often lodged on an assumption of 'is', as if to say, 'If you decide to do this, you should do it like this . . . but you may not want to do it at all.'

We translated every Sanskrit word into English (if you count Brahmin as an English word), and this decision invariably involved

---

[101] Either the man or the woman may be the agent in 2.6.8, for instance.

[102] 2.6.3, 8, 10, 11, 13, 19, 20, 26, 27, 29, 30, 31, 32.

[103] 2.7.9–11, 14, 19; 2.7.15, 20Y.

[104] 2.7.8, 12–13, 15, 20–1. In Book Four, chapter two, the female protagonist is seldom named but is simply the assumed, unexpressed subject of the verb, while a demonstrative pronoun usually designates her rival. In our translation, we have generally used 'she' to designate the subject under discussion (first the senior wife, then the junior wife) and 'her' or 'the other woman' for her rival (first the junior wife, then the senior wife); sometimes we have supplied the full noun. And when the wife and the messenger are conversing [5.4.3–31], and only the context and the use of different Sanskrit pronouns (designating a person nearer or more distant) indicates who is speaking, we occasionally carried forward the referent noun from the previous line to replace the ambiguous pronoun.

some compromises. The English names of the more obscure plants, flowers, and drugs are very approximate indeed; as in a game of telephone, we moved first from the Sanskrit to Monier-Williams's Latin approximation, and then, since the rough Latin equivalents would hardly have any more meaning for most readers than the Sanskrit originals, we consulted botanical dictionaries to find English names by which the plants were known. The slippage at both points of transition effectively doubled the margin of error, giving the reader only an impressionistic, rough idea of the substances involved. But we thought that even that blur was preferable to the only alternative, which was to leave the words in incomprehensible Sanskrit or Latin. (Readers who want to know the original Sanskrit terms can find them in the Glossary.) We therefore warn the reader that ointments made following the recipes in this book will probably not have the same effects that were achieved by people who used the Sanskrit recipes in ancient India.

Sexually Explicit Vocabulary

A basic and pervasive problem was the translation of the words for sex, because, just as Eskimos are (apocryphally, apparently) said to have many more words for snow than we Anglos do, Sanskrit certainly has far more words for sex. The challenge is compounded by English's lack of a register corresponding to the matter-of-fact terminology of the Sanskrit text, a register midway between the obscene and the medical. The obscene will jar the English-speaking reader in an inappropriate way, and in any case, in this post-rap-and-David-Mamet age, the people who do use the word 'fuck' seldom use it to designate the sexual act. The medical is equally inappropriate for this imaginative and elegant text; though the use of 'glans' and 'foreskin' was unavoidable in the highly explicit description of fellatio, we have relegated the terms 'penis' and 'vagina' to the commentaries (and to Book Seven, which has a very different tone from the rest of the book); in the text proper, we have used terms like 'pelvis', 'sexual organ', or 'between the legs'. The *Kamasutra* itself notes [2.1.32] that there are numerous synonyms for both the sexual act and sexual pleasure. This is also true, if less true, of English, and in both languages, a single term may have different connotations. We hope that the text's own awareness of this problem justifies our practice of, on the one hand, translating several different Sanskrit nouns and verbs by one English word (such as 'sex' or 'pleasure') and, on the other hand, using several different English words to translate a single Sanskrit word (such as *priti*). For Sanskrit intermingles concepts of passion, love, and pleasure, which English tends to hold separate. Moreover, just as *dharma* is context-sensitive in Manu, requiring many different translations, so the words for sex/love/passion are context-sensitive in the *Kamasutra*, requiring many different English words.

Kama sometimes signifies 'pleasure', sometimes 'desire', sometimes 'a sexual affair', sometimes 'sexual pleasure', and sometimes just 'sex', thus overlapping with other terms such as *priti* (also pleasure, but also, sometimes, love, satisfaction, erotic joy, affection, or orgasm), *anuraga* (love for someone) and *rata* (the sexual act, sexual pleasure, or climax). We have generally used the English terms 'sex' or 'making love' or, sometimes, 'in bed', to translate several different Sanskrit terms for the sexual act (primarily *surata* and *samprayoga*). *Abhiyoga* means 'making advances' or, occasionally, 'wooing'; the person who does it is a 'suitor'. Sanskrit employs the same basic verb [*yunj*, 'to join', cognate with the English 'yoke' and 'yoga'] for both this word and the word for sex (*samprayoga*), but with the preposition 'to' [*abhi*] for preliminary wooing, and with the prepositions 'with' and 'for' [*sam* and *pra*] for the actual physical act. (A related form, *pra-yoga*, means 'practices' or 'techniques' and as a gerundive—*prayogya*—denotes the woman or man whom someone intends to enjoy sexually, which we have translated as 'the man [or woman] she [or he] wants'.) *Bhava* sometimes means 'emotion', sometimes 'orgasm', sometimes 'true feelings' or 'inclination'; occasionally (as in the title of 2.1 and in 2.1.33) it replaces *vega*, 'sexual energy'. *Sukha* can mean 'happiness', or 'sensual pleasure', or 'bliss', depending on the context. The verb *ranj* and its derivatives (*raga*, *anuraga*, etc.) sometimes means 'to experience pleasure' and sometimes 'to fall in love' or, in the causative, 'to give pleasure' or 'to make someone fall in love' or 'to charm'; sometimes [as in 7.2.1], it is best approximated by the old-fashioned euphemism, 'to pleasure'.

Contemporary Pleasures of the Text

In India as in Europe, once the *Kamasutra* became available in English, it was first regarded as pornography masquerading as Orientalism masquerading as literature and then became the object of prurient mockery and satire. Even the 1966 (Berkeley) edition of the Burton translation proclaims, on its cover, 'Still shocking after 15 centuries! Now complete and unexpurgated!' Once available only 'for private circulation' or 'for medical use', the Burton translation is now available online. One website offers *The Kamasutra of Pooh*, posing stuffed animals in compromising positions (Piglet on Pooh, Pooh mounting Eeyore, and so forth); a later website posed Kermit the Frog in action on an unidentified stuffed animal.[105] Lee Siegel offers us a board game, 'Kamasutra: The Game of Love', for 2 players, with 6 pawns (the 6 basic sexual sizes, elephant-cow, mare, etc.) and 64 cards. Since there is no patented 'Kamasutra™', the title is used for a wide array of products. In India it is the name of a condom. In America it is the name of a wristwatch that displays a different position every hour. The Red Envelope company advertises a 'Kama Sutra Pleasure Box' and 'Kama Sutra Weekender Kit', collections of oils and creams packaged in containers decorated with quasi-Hindu paintings of embracing couples. An anonymous fourteenth-century Catalan book about sex was published (in 1995) as *Le Kamasutra Catalan*.[106] A cartoon depicts 'The Kamasutra Relaxasizer Lounger, 165 positions'.[107] *Cosmopolitan* magazine published two editions of its 'Cosmo *Kamasutra*', offering '12 brand-new mattress-quaking sex styles', each with its numerical 'degree of difficulty', including positions called 'the backstairs boogie', 'the octopus', 'the mermaid', 'the spider web', and 'the rock'n' roll'.[108] There are numerous books of erotic paintings and/or sculptures called Illustrated *Kamasutras*,[109] including one, by Georges Pichard, in

[105] www.planetx.com/pooh/ or /pooh/images.phtml. Perversely, they insist that you must swear you are 18 years old or over to use this site—which is, after all, about a children's book.

[106] Anonyme du XIVe Siècle, *Le Kamasutra Catalan. Le Miroir du foutre*. Anatolia/ Le Rocher, 1995.

[107] Mr Boffo cartoon by Joe Martin, Inc., distributed by Universal Press Syndicate; published in the *Chicago Tribune* 29 September 2000. A salesman is saying to a customer, 'Most people just buy it to get the catalogue.'

[108] *Cosmopolitan*, September 1998, 'The Cosmo Kamasutra'; September, 1999, pp. 256–9, 'The Cosmo Kamasutra, 2'.

[109] One combines all of Burton's erotica: *The Illustrated KamaSutra, Ananga-Ranga, Perfumed Garden*. In America, where information comes in at the eye, like love according to the poet Yeats, a translator foolish enough to tell a friend that he or she is working on the *Kamasutra* is invariably and immediately asked, Will it have illustrations? This is, in part, because the descriptions of the positions are so stark that they are sometimes hard to visualize without the help of a detailed image.

which the woman is attacked with an actual needle, pincer, and scissors.[110] (In the film *Urban Legend* (1998), some giggling girls gleefully discover 'an early edition of the *Kamasutra*, WITH ILLUS-TRATIONS!!!') There are cartoon *Kamasutras*, in which the god Shiva plays a central role.[111] The Palm Pilot™ company has made available a pocket Sutra, 'The Kama Sutra in the palm of your hand', consist-ing of a very loose translation of parts of Book Two. A book called *The Popup Kamasutra* failed to take full advantage of the possibilities of this genre; the whole couple pops up.

The Onion ran a satire about a couple whose 'inability to execute The Totally Auspicious Position along with countless other ancient Indian erotic positions, took them to new heights of sexual dissatis-faction . . . Sue was unable to clench her Yoni (vagina) tightly enough around Harold's Lingam and fell off . . .'[112] Another satire proposes 'a *Kama Sutra* that is in line with a postpatriarchal, post-colonial, postgender, and perhaps even postcoital world'.[113] Here are some high points:

If the man feels that the Bull Elephant embrace is inappropriate—if it, for example, represents a macho stereotype that he is trying to transcend—he should express this perspective and explain why the Howler Monkey embrace would make him feel more comfortable . . . . When the lovers decide to join in any of the Animal Embraces mentioned above, and in others such as The Vulture Has Second Thoughts, The Mule Escapes Exploitation, and The Antelopes Form a Support Group, they first enter into deep meditation, facing one another, breathing deeply, and . . . then call into question the very idea of using animal names to describe human sexual activities. Rejecting this subtle mode of domination of the natural world, they separate, enter once again into profound meditation, and fall asleep. . . . As the moment of union approaches, however, their awareness grows that . . . vows that suggest that Shiva and Shakti are 'primordial' or 'universal' may be deeply offensive to members of other faith com-munities. In a spirit of profound respect for religious pluralism, they draw apart, and the man's lingam withers.[114]

Feminism, ecology, and religious pluralism, all noble causes, can be

---

[110] Pichard, *The Illustrated Kama Sutra*, i, 72, presumably illustrating 2.7.24.

[111] Tolputt, *The Cartoon Kama Sutra*, and *Manara's Kama Sutra*.

[112] *The Onion*, 30 March–5 April 2000, 8, 'Tantric Sex Class Opens up Whole New World of Unfulfillment for Local Couple'.

[113] Jon Spayde, 'The Politically Correct Kama Sutra', 56.

[114] Ibid. 57.

tacked onto the sexist, ecologically innocent, and narrowly Hindu text; but the lingam withers.

What use is the *Kamasutra*? In our time, when sexually explicit novels, films, and instruction manuals are available everywhere, the parts of the *Kamasutra* that have previously been most useful are now the least useful: the positions described in Book Two. Today they can inspire only a few reactions: 'I already do that' or 'I've thought of doing that' or 'I never thought of that, and wouldn't want to try it now' or 'I never thought of doing that, and I think I'll try it now.' Book Seven, too, is hardly practical. Yashodhara's comment on 7.1.25 ('Do this in such a way that the woman you want does not realize, "A man with something spread on his penis is making love to me"') has inspired at least one reader to remark, 'Any woman who would let you make love to her with all that stuff smeared on you would have to be madly in love with you already.' Some of it, like the magic formulas, remains truly foreign to us, or accessible only through rather distant analogies. Betel, for instance, such a basic part of the erotic scene in ancient India, can best be understood by analogy with the overtones that champagne has in Europe, or the post-coital cigarette. It evokes the cigarette foreplay of Bogart and Bacall in *To Have and Have Not* and *The Big Sleep* or the cigarette sublimation shared by Bette Davis and Paul Heinreid in *Now Voyager*. Betel, the life in the harem, the world of courtesans—these parts of the text make you think, 'How very different these people are from us.'

But then you come across the passage in which the boy teases the girl when they are swimming together, diving down and coming up near her, touching her, and then diving down again [3.4.6], and you are in familiar personal territory. You must surely also recognize the man who tells the woman on whom he's set his sights 'about an erotic dream, pretending that it was about another woman' [3.4.9], and the woman who does the same thing [5.4.54]. Sometimes the unfamiliar and the familiar are cheek by jowl; the culture-specific list of women the wife must not associate with (including a Buddhist nun and a magician who uses love-sorcery worked with roots [4.1.9]) is followed in the very next passage by the woman who is cooking for her man and finds out, 'This is what he likes, this is what he hates, this is good for him, this is bad for him', a consideration that surely resonates with many contemporary anglophone readers.

One part of the text that speaks to the modern reader is Book Five, on the seduction of other men's wives. In the earlier meditations on reasons to do this [1.5], there are a few details, such as the commission to kill the king's enemy, that do not survive the cross-cultural journey. But for the most part, this passage brilliantly represents the self-justifying arguments of the adulterer, and of the adulterous wife, in ways that rival the psychologizing of John Updike and Gustave Flaubert. Book Six has an even more basic relevance for modern women and men, since this is the one section of the text that imagines both men and women as more or less free agents, constrained by the man's lust and the woman's need for money, it is true, but not by an assumption of the natural passivity of the woman (an assumption that colours the rest of the text and is made explicit at 2.1.26). In Book Six the woman's thoughts on such subjects as how to get a lover, how to get rid of him, or how to tell when he is cooling toward her, ring remarkably true in the twenty-first century. Vatsyayana himself often calls the courtesan here 'the woman', and her lover 'the man', and when he does so Yashodhara remarks (at 6.1.12–13, for instance) that these passages often have a more general application. This may mean that they apply to any relationship in which the woman may have the upper hand, not merely the particular case of the courtesan. This part of the text is not just about sex for money, but about sex for love, particularly for people who are free to choose their partners; which means it is for us. The *Kamasutra* has attained its classic status because it is at bottom about essential, unchangeable human attributes—lust, love, shyness, rejection, seduction, manipulation—and it is fascinating for us to see ourselves mirrored in it even as we learn deeply intimate things about a culture that could well be described as long ago and in a galaxy far away.

A NOTE ON PRESENTATION

An asterisk in the main text and in Yashodhara's commentary indicates a note at the back of the book. Notes solely to Yashodhara's commentary are prefixed by [Y] in these Explanatory Notes. In Yashodhara's commentary V stands for Vatsyayana (the author of the *Kamasutra*).

References are in the form: 1.3.5 (meaning Book One, Chapter Three, passage 5). In the main text superior figures mark the beginning of each passage, and the numbering in Yashodhara's commentary relates to the passage numbers. The running headlines to every page show the passages that appear on that page.

The sixty-four sections are not part of this numbering reference system; their numbers are, however, shown in square brackets to the left of their headings, which also appear as running headlines.

KAMASUTRA

BOOK ONE · GENERAL OBSERVATIONS

[1]   *Summary of the Text*

RELIGION
POWER
PLEASURE

¹ WE bow to religion, power, and pleasure, ²because they are the subject of this text,* ³and to the scholars who made known the mutual agreement among the three, ⁴because those subjects are

———

YASHODHARA'S COMMENTARY

¹ Those who talk about pleasure say that pleasure is the most important of the three aims of human life,* because it is both the cause and the result of the other two, religion and power. And realizing that nothing happens without a method to make it happen, and wishing to explain that method, the scholar Vatsyayana Mallanaga created this text, always taking into consideration the opinions of scholars. You can, of course, learn about pleasure from other teachings, just as you can read meaning into a hole shaped like a letter of the alphabet that a bookworm has eaten out of a page, but you do not understand what you should do and what you should not do. And so people say:

A man should not be congratulated
if he happens to succeed at something without knowing its science,
for it is pure chance, like a bookworm eating a hole
in the shape of a letter of the alphabet.

² The three aims of human life are the three divinities in charge of this work; if they were not divinities it would not be right to bow to them. And there is textual evidence that they are in fact divinities. For the historian tells us: 'When King Pururavas went from earth to heaven to see Indra, the king of the gods, he saw Religion (Dharma) and the others embodied. As he approached them, he ignored the other two but paid homage to Religion, walking around him in a circle to the right. The other two, unable to put up with this slight, cursed him. Because Pleasure (Kama) had cursed him, he was separated from his wife, Urvashi, and longed for her in her absence. When he had managed to put that right, then, because Power (Artha) had cursed him, he became so excessively greedy that he stole from all four social classes. The Brahmins, who were upset because they could no longer perform the

integral to the text. ⁵For when the Creator emitted his creatures, he first composed, in a hundred thousand chapters, the means of achieving the three aims of human life, which is the vital link with what sustains those creatures. ⁶Manu* the son of the Self-born One made one part of this into a separate work about religion, ⁷Brihaspati* made one about power, ⁸and Nandin, the servant of the Great God Shiva, made a separate work of a thousand chapters, the *Kamasutra*, ⁹which Shvetaketu Auddalaki cut down to five hundred chapters. ¹⁰And then Babhravya* of Panchala cut this down further to a hundred and fifty chapters in the following seven parts: General Observations, Sex, Virgins, Wives, Other Men's Wives, Courtesans, and Erotic Esoterica.

¹¹Dattaka made a separate book out of the sixth part of this work,

---

> sacrifice or other rituals without the money he had stolen from them, took blades of sharp sacrificial grass in their hands and killed him.'

⁵ Desire brings happiness and children, but hatred brings neither, and what sustains someone who has neither happiness nor offspring is like a blade of grass.

⁷ Brihaspati composed the text called the *Arthashastra*.

⁸ This is not some other person named Nandin, for the scripture says: 'While the Great God Shiva was experiencing the pleasures of sex with his wife Uma for a thousand years as the gods count them, Nandin went to guard the door of their bedroom and composed the *Kamasutra*.'*

⁹ Shvetaketu Auddalaki was the son of Uddalaka. Once upon a time, there was so much seduction of other men's wives in the world that it was said:
>   Women are all alike,
>   just like cooked rice, your majesty.
>   Therefore a man should not get angry with them
>   nor fall in love with them, but just make love with them.
> But Auddalaki forbade this state of affairs, and so people said:
>   The son of the guru
>   forbade Brahmins to drink wine,
>   but the seer, Uddalaka's son, even forbade common people
>   to take other people's wives.
>   Then, with his father's permission,
>   Shvetaketu, who had amassed great ascetic power,
>   happily composed this text, which distinguishes
>   those who are eligible or ineligible for sex.*

¹¹ A certain Brahmin from Mathura was living in Pataliputra. In his old age he had a son, whose mother died giving birth to him. The father

about courtesans, which the courtesans de luxe of Pataliputra* commissioned. [12] In response to this, Charayana made a separate book about general observations, Suvarnanabha about sex, Ghotakamukha about virgins, Gonardiya about wives, Gonikaputra about other men's wives, and Kuchumara about erotic esoterica. [13] When many scholars had divided it into fragments in this way, the text was almost destroyed. [14] Because the amputated limbs of the text that Dattaka and the others divided are just parts of the whole, and because Babhravya's text is so long that it is hard to study, Vatsyayana condensed the entire subject matter into a small volume to make this *Kamasutra*.

[15] Here is an overview of its sections and chapters:*

[16] The first book, on General Observations, has five sections in five chapters: summary of the text, the means of achieving the three aims of human life, exposition of the arts, the lifestyle of the man-about-town,* and the work of the man's male helpers and messengers.

[17] The second book, on Sex, has seventeen sections in ten chapters: sexual typology according to size, endurance, and temperament, types of love, ways of embracing, procedures of kissing, types of

---

gave him to another Brahmin woman to be her own son and, in time, went to the other world. She named him Dattaka ('little gift'), because he had been given to her, and she raised him; he learned all the arts and sciences in a short time. One day he had the idea of learning the finest ways of the world, best known by courtesans. And so he went to the courtesans every day, and learned so well that they asked *him* to instruct *them*. A woman named Virasena, speaking on behalf of the courtesans de luxe, said to him, 'Teach us how to give pleasure to men.' And because of that commission he made a separate book; so the story goes. But another quite plausible story is also widely believed: Dattaka once touched Shiva with his foot in the course of a festival to bless a pregnant woman, and Shiva cursed him to become a woman; after a while he persuaded Shiva to rescind the curse and became a man again, and because of that double knowledge he made the separate book. If he had simply made a separate work out of what Babhravya had said, how would his own book have demonstrated such originality that people would say that he knew both flavours? But if the author of the *Kamasutra* had known that he had such double knowledge, then he would have said, 'Dattaka, who knew both flavours, made a separate book.'

[13] The text referred to here is Babhravya's text.

scratching with the nails, ways of biting, customs of women from different regions, varieties of sexual positions, unusual sexual acts, modes of slapping and the accompanying moaning, the woman playing the man's part, a man's sexual strokes, oral sex, the start and finish of sex, different kinds of sex, and lovers' quarrels.

¹⁸ The third book, on Virgins, has nine sections in five chapters: courting the girl, making alliances, winning a virgin's trust, making advances to a young girl, interpreting her gestures and signals, the advances that a man makes on his own, the advances that a virgin makes to the man she wants, the advances that win a virgin, and devious devices for weddings.

¹⁹ The fourth book, on Wives, has eight sections in two chapters: the life of an only wife, her behaviour during his absence, the senior wife, the junior wife, the second-hand woman, the wife unlucky in love, women of the harem, and a man's management of many women.

²⁰ The fifth book, on Other Men's Wives, has ten sections in six chapters: on the characteristic natures of women and men,* causes of resistance, men who are successful with women, women who can be won without effort, ways of becoming intimate, making advances, testing her feelings, the duties of a female messenger, the sex life of a man in power, the life of the women of the harem, and the guarding of wives.

²¹ The sixth book, on Courtesans, has twelve sections in six chapters: deciding on an eligible lover, reasons for taking a lover, getting a lover, giving the beloved what he wants, ways to get money from him, signs that his passion is cooling, getting him back when his passion has cooled, ways to get rid of him, getting back together with a discarded lover, weighing different kinds of profits, calculating gains and losses, consequences and doubts, and types of courtesans.

²² The seventh book, on Erotic Esoterica, has six sections in two chapters: making luck in love, putting someone in your power, stimulants for virility, rekindling exhausted passion, methods of increasing the size of the male organ, and unusual techniques.

²³ Thus the text has sixty-four sections, in thirty-six chapters, in seven books, consisting of 1,250 passages.* That is the summary of the text.

> ²⁴ Now that it has been summarized briefly,
>   it will be described in detail,
>   since wise men of the world like to have things told
>   in both a contracted and an expanded form.

CHAPTER TWO

[2]   *The Means of Achieving the Three Aims of*
Human Life

¹ A man's lifespan is said to be a full hundred years.* By dividing his time, he cultivates the three aims in such a way that they enhance rather than interfere with each other. ² Childhood is the time to acquire knowledge and other kinds of power,* ³ the prime of youth is for pleasure, ⁴ and old age is for religion and release.* ⁵ Or, because the

---

¹ A man is the main subject here; women's lack of freedom makes their pursuit of the three human goals dependent upon men. The three aims of human life are combined in the following ways: When a man who wants children unites with his legal but unattractive wife in her fertile season, religion is combined with power. When a man who wants children unites with his legal and attractive wife in her fertile season, religion is combined with pleasure. When an unmarried man takes an unattractive virgin of his own class, power is combined with religion. When a married man takes an attractive virgin of a lower class, power is combined with pleasure. When a man unites with his legal and attractive wife, not in her fertile season but because she is tormented by desire, pleasure is combined with religion. When a married man who has nothing unites with an attractive woman of any class, pleasure is combined with power. These are the single combinations.

When an unmarried man joins, in the proper manner, with an attractive woman of his own class who has had no other man before him, religion is combined with pleasure and power. When an unmarried man gets an attractive virgin of his own class, power is combined with religion and pleasure. When an unmarried man gets a woman who has money and beauty, and they desire one another, pleasure is combined with religion and power. These are the double combinations.

² There is a saying:

> Until the age of sixteen a man is a child,
> as long as he eats rice cooked in milk;
> he is middle-aged until he is seventy;
> and after that he is said to be old.

⁴ There are four classes in this world,* the Brahmins and the three others, and there are four stages of life: the chaste student, the householder, the forest dweller, and the renouncer. But since release (*moksha*)

lifespan is uncertain, a man pursues these aims as the opportunity arises, ⁶but he should remain celibate until he has acquired knowledge.*

⁷Religion consists in engaging, as the texts decree, in sacrifice and other such actions that are disengaged from material life, because they are not of this world and their results are invisible; and in refraining, as the texts decree, from eating meat and other such actions that are engaged in material life, because they are of this world and their results are visible.* ⁸A man learns about it from sacred scripture* and from associating with people who know about religion. ⁹Power, in the form of wealth, consists in acquiring know-ledge, land, gold, cattle, grain, household goods and furniture, friends, and so forth, and increasing what has been acquired. ¹⁰A man learns about it from 'The Tasks of the Superintendent',* and from merchants who know about trades and markets. ¹¹Pleasure, in general, consists in engaging the ear, skin, eye, tongue, and nose each in its own appropriate sensation, all under the control of the mind and heart driven by the conscious self. ¹²Pleasure in its primary form, however, is a direct experience of an object of the senses, which bears fruit and is permeated by the sensual pleasure of erotic arousal that results from the particular sensation of touch.* ¹³A man learns about pleasure from the *Kamasutra* and from associating with the circle of men-about-town.

¹⁴When these three aims—religion, power, and pleasure—compete, each is more important than the one that follows.

––––––

is out of the question for householders, whether they are Brahmins or of other classes, for them the human goals remain a trinity.

⁶ He must not pursue pleasure until he has completed his mastery of knowledge. Otherwise, he will violate religion, thereby producing an obstacle to gaining pleasure, and he will fail to get knowledge and power. But there is no rule against acquiring something such as land during this period.

⁹ 'And so forth' includes jewellery and clothing.

¹² This experience bears fruit because, when it goes on uninterrupted, it results in an emission of semen and, simultaneously, pleasure and bliss.

¹⁴ Power is more important than pleasure, since pleasure can only be achieved with power; and religion is more important than power, since power can only be achieved with religion.

¹⁵ But power, in the form of wealth, is the most important goal for a king—because it is the basis of social life—and for a courtesan.* Those are the means of achieving the three aims.

[handwritten margin note: Sex is natural. why a book?]

¹⁶ Scholars say:* 'It is appropriate to have a text about religion, because it concerns matters not of this world, and to have one about power, because that is achieved only when the groundwork is laid by special methods, which one learns from a text. ¹⁷ But since even animals manage sex by themselves, and since it goes on all the time, it should not have to be handled with the help of a text.' ¹⁸ Vatsyayana says: Because a man and a woman depend upon one another in sex, it requires a method, ¹⁹ and this method is learned from the *Kamasutra*. ²⁰ The mating of animals, by contrast, is not based upon any method:

---

¹⁵ The basis of social life is the behaviour of the four classes and the four stages of life. It is the religious duty of the king to protect this, knowing that it must not change. And he can do that only if he has political power, and his political power lies in his treasury, his law enforcers, and his army, all of which come from power and money. As for a courtesan, she will give up religion (in the form of a lovesick Brahmin) or pleasure (in the form of an attractive man-about-town), thinking, 'Both of them will come later', and take up instead with a man even if she does not desire him, thinking, 'This one will give me money.'

¹⁷ Even animals like cows, whose intellects are shrouded in torpor, visibly manage sex without instruction from a textbook; how much more must this happen among humans, whose intellects consist primarily of passion?* As it is said:

> For desire is satisfied without instruction,
> and does not have to be taught.
> Who is the guru for deer and birds, for the methodology
> to give and take pleasure with those they desire?

And desire goes on all the time, because the qualities of wanting and hating are always there in the soul. These scholars are people who talk about religion, power, and release.

²⁰ There is no guarding or any other form of concealment, because the females of the species are loose. Animals mate only during their fertile season. Humans who want children, however, do it during a woman's fertile season but also outside her fertile season,* in order to enjoy and please the woman. So animals and humans are not the same. And so the law book says:

> You may have sex with a woman in her fertile season
> —or any time when it is not expressly forbidden.

because they are not fenced in, they mate only when the females are in their fertile season and until they achieve their goal, and they act without thinking about it first.

[21] Materialists say:* 'People should not perform religious acts, for their results are in the world to come and that is doubtful. [22] Who but a fool would take what is in his own hand and put it in someone else's hand? [23] Better a pigeon today than a peacock tomorrow, and

> [24] "Better a copper coin that is certain
> than a gold coin that is doubtful."'

[25] Vatsyayana says: People should perform religious acts, because the text cannot be doubted; because, sometimes, black magic and curses are seen to bear fruit; because the constellations, moon, sun, stars, and the circle of the planets are seen to act for the sake of the world as if they thought about it first; because social life is marked by the stability of the system of the four classes and four stages of life; and because people are seen to cast away a seed in their hand for the sake of a crop in the future.

[26] Fatalists say:* 'People should not act to gain power and wealth, for even when these are energetically pursued they are not always achieved, while even when they are not sought at all, they may come by chance. [27] "It all happens as fate decrees", people say, [28] for fate is what leads men to gain and loss, victory and defeat, happiness and unhappiness.

Cārkī

And animals engage in sex just until they achieve a climax; they do not wonder, 'Has he reached his climax or not?' and therefore wish to mate a second time. And so, since the goal of animals and humans is not the same, animals need no method for sex. Animals, moreover, do not first think, before engaging in sex, 'What will happen to religion, power, sons, relatives, and the prosperity of our faction?' Sex just happens to animals in their own way.

[21] Materialists (*Lokayatikas*) are people whose thinking is limited (*ayata*) to this world (*loka*).

[22] Someone will take money in his own hand and put it in someone else's hand, thinking, 'In time of need I myself might go there and get back what I lost and use it to get something to eat', but in fact he is throwing it far away. In precisely the same way, someone who engages in an act such as sacrifice, thinking, 'I will enjoy this in another life', actually throws it far away.

> [29] Fate made Bali into
> an Indra, king of the gods,
> and fate hurled Bali back down,
> and fate is what will make him an Indra again.'*

[30] Vatsyayana says: All undertakings are based upon a method, because they presuppose a man's exertions. [31] Even wealth and power that must inevitably arise in the future presuppose a method. Nothing good happens to a man who does nothing.

[32] Pragmatists say:* 'People should not indulge in pleasures, for they are an obstacle to both religion and power, which are more important, and to other good people. They make a man associate with worthless people and undertake bad projects; they make him impure, a man with no future, [33] as well as careless, lightweight, untrustworthy and unacceptable. [34] And it is said that many men in the thrall of desire were destroyed, even when accompanied by their troops. [35] For instance, when the Bhoja king named Dandakya* was

---

[29] Even though Bali was unworthy, because he was a demon, and should have been spurned, he ascended to the throne of Indra, king of the gods, and established himself there until the wheel of fortune turned around, and he was thrown out of that seat and hurled back down into hell. But when the wheel of fortune turns back around again, it will once again send him out of hell and back onto the throne of Indra. And so people say:

> Time ripens and cooks all beings,
> time absorbs all creatures,
> time is awake when all are asleep,
> for no one can fight against time.

[32] Good people, experienced in knowledge or in asceticism, abandon a man who is attached to desire. Bad projects would involve going out to meet a woman at night, jumping over walls, and so forth. A man without a future has lost his strength with venereal diseases like 'Desire's donkey'.

[35] Dandakya was out hunting when he saw the daughter of the Brahmin Bhargava in his hermitage. Overwhelmed by passion, he took her up in his chariot and carried her off. When Bhargava returned with the fuel and sacred grass that he had gone off to fetch, and did not see her, he meditated to learn what had happened and then he cursed the king. As a result, Dandakya and his entire family and kingdom were covered by a dust-storm and died. Even today they sing about that place, the Dandaka Wilderness.

aroused by a Brahmin's daughter, desire destroyed him, along with his relatives and his kingdom. [36] And Indra the king of the gods with Ahalya, the super-powerful Kichaka with Draupadi, Ravana with Sita, and many others afterwards were seen to fall into the thrall of desire and were destroyed.' [37] Vatsyayana says: Pleasures are a means of sustaining the body, just like food, and they are rewards for religion and power. [38] But people must be aware of the flaws in pleasures, flaws that are like diseases.* For people do not stop preparing the cooking pots because they think, 'There are beggars', nor do they stop planting barley because they think, 'There are deer.'* [39] And there are verses about this:

———

[36] The king of the gods, Indra, was aroused by Ahalya; for when he saw her in the hermitage of her husband Gautama, he desired her.* When Gautama returned with the fuel and sacred grass, his wife Ahalya hid Indra in the womb of the house, but just at that moment Gautama took his wife into the inside of the house, with an invitation to make love. Then he realized, with the magic gaze that he had achieved through yoga, that Indra had come there, and seeing that a third seat had been drawn up for him he said, 'What is this for, since only the two of us, my wife and I, are here?' Then he became suspicious, and by meditation he saw what had happened; in fury he cursed Indra: 'You yourself will have a thousand vaginas!' And so, even though Indra was the king of the gods, desire brought him to this sorry state, which was regarded as his destruction. Even to this day that mark that makes people call him 'Ahalya's Lover' has not vanished. As for Kichaka, he is said to have been superpowerful because he had the strength of a thousand elephants; but even he was destroyed by desire, for Bhima killed him when he lusted after Draupadi.

[38] People must be aware in order to take preventive measures, just as they take measures against the diseases of the body such as indigestion. And there is a saying:

> 'The existence of men who hate pleasure
> is meaningless as the existence of blades of grass.
> But one must avoid its fatal flaws.'
> Scholars made this a fixed rule.

[39] But atheists, those who lack all ambition, and those who hate pleasure win a happiness that does have thorns, because each of these three groups lacks one of the three aims of human life.

> A man who serves power, and pleasure,
> and religion in this way
> wins endless happiness that has no thorns,
> in this world and the next.
> 40 Knowledgeable people undertake a project
> that does not make them worry,
> 'What will happen in the next world?'
> Or 'Is this a pleasure that will not erode my power?'
> 41 Undertake any project that might achieve
> the three aims of life, or two, or even just one,
> but not one that achieves one
> at the cost of the other two.

CHAPTER THREE

[3]   *Exposition of the Arts*

¹ A man should study the *Kamasutra* and its subsidiary sciences as long as this does not interfere with the time devoted to religion and power and their subsidiary sciences. ² A woman should do this before she reaches the prime of her youth, and she should continue when she has been given away, if her husband wishes it.

³ Scholars say: 'Since females cannot grasp texts, it is useless to teach women this text.' ⁴ Vatsyayana says: But women understand the practice, and the practice is based on the text.* ⁵ This applies beyond this specific subject of the *Kamasutra*, for throughout the world, in all subjects, there are only a few people who know the text, but the practice is within the range of everyone. ⁶ And a text, however far

---

⁴¹ For example, through too much generosity, religion impedes power and pleasure; power, when it overrides all else, impedes religion and pleasure (as it did for Pururavas); and pleasure destroys the other two when it involves women of a higher class (as in the case of Dandakya) or other excesses.

² The prime of her youth is the period while she is still in her father's house.

⁶ If just one person who knows the text practises it, another learns it from him, and another from him, and so on, no matter how far removed.

Practice
vs.
literature

removed, is the ultimate source of the practice. ⁷'Grammar is a science', people say. Yet the sacrificial priests, who are no grammarians, know how to gloss the words in the sacrificial prayers.* ⁸'Astronomy is a science', they say. But ordinary people perform the rituals on the days when the skies are auspicious. ⁹And people know how to ride horses and elephants without studying the texts about horses and elephants. ¹⁰In the same way, even citizens far away from the king do not step across the moral line that he sets. The case of women learning the *Kamasutra* is like those examples.

¹¹And there are also women whose understanding has been sharpened by the text: courtesans de luxe and the daughters of kings and ministers of state. ¹²A woman should therefore learn the techniques and the text, or at least one part of it, from a trusted person, in private. ¹³And alone, in private, a virgin should practise the sixty-four techniques that take practice. ¹⁴But the people qualified to teach a virgin are: a foster-sister who grew up with her and has already made love with a man; or a girlfriend* who has had the same experience and with whom she can converse without risk; one of her mother's sisters who is her age; an old servant woman who is trusted and can take that aunt's place; a female renunciant with whom she has previously been intimate; and her own sister, if that sister takes her into her confidence about her own love-making.

¹⁵The sixty-four fine arts that should be studied along with the

---

⁸ Even people who are not astronomers pick up the information from somewhere or other. But in this case, too, the text is the ultimate source.

¹⁴ The word 'but' is used to distinguish women from men, who, because of their independence, easily find instructors. The foster-sister is the daughter of her wet-nurse. Her own sister, that is, her older sister, can teach her if she trusts her enough to make love with another man right under her eyes. Otherwise a sister would not want to teach even her own sister, because of their rivalry.

¹⁵ They cut shapes out of the leaves of trees such as birches, to decorate their foreheads; they make lines in the form of designs on the jewelled floors of temples of Sarasvati or the god Kama, with rice-powder of various colours. Unusual techniques are various spells to make someone stop loving someone else, or to reduce someone to a single sense organ, or turn his hair grey, and so forth, as will be described in the discussion of 'Erotic Esoterica' [Book Seven]. They complete words by putting on the final syllable; difficult words can be tongue-twisters or anagrams;

Kamasutra are: singing; playing musical instruments; dancing; painting; cutting leaves into shapes; making lines on the floor with rice-powder and flowers; arranging flowers; colouring the teeth, clothes, and limbs; making jewelled floors; preparing beds; making music on the rims of glasses of water; playing water sports; unusual techniques; making garlands and stringing necklaces; making diadems and headbands; making costumes; making various earrings; mixing perfumes; putting on jewellery; doing conjuring tricks; practising sorcery; sleight of hand; preparing various forms of vegetables, soups, and other things to eat; preparing wines, fruit juices, and other things to drink; needlework; weaving; playing the lute and the drum;* telling jokes and riddles; completing words; reciting difficult words; reading aloud; staging plays and dialogues; completing verses; making things out of cloth, wood, and cane; woodworking; carpentry; architecture; the ability to test gold and silver; metallurgy; knowledge of the colour and form of jewels; skill at nurturing trees; knowledge of ram-fights, cock-fights, and quail-fights; teaching parrots and mynah birds to talk; skill at rubbing, massaging, and hairdressing; the ability to speak in sign language; understanding languages made to seem foreign; knowledge of local dialects; skill at making flower carts; knowledge of omens; alphabets for use in making magical diagrams; alphabets for memorizing; group recitation; improvising poetry; dictionaries and thesauruses; knowledge of metre; literary work; the art of impersonation; the art of using clothes for disguise; special forms of gambling; the game of dice; children's games; etiquette; the science of strategy; and the cultivation of athletic skills.

———

they complete verses by adding the last quarter to a verse of four parts. Woodworking is useful for making things like sex tools, carpentry for making things like chairs and beds. Massage done with the feet is called rubbing, massaging the head with the hands is called hairdressing, and massaging the rest of the body with the hands is called massage. Languages made to seem foreign are strings of real words, which, by the transposition of syllables, become devoid of real meaning and can be used as a secret code. Alphabets for memorizing are textbooks that teach the technique for remembering what has been heard or written; literary work consists in making poetry and poetical ornaments. Clothes are used to disguise something small to make it look big, and something big to make it look small. Athletic skills include things like hunting.

(¹⁶The sixty-four arts* of love that come from Babhravya of Panchala are different. We will return to them and speak of their techniques in the discussion of sex, for they are an essential element of pleasure.)

¹⁷A courtesan* who distinguishes herself in these arts
and who has a good nature, beauty, and good qualities,
wins the title of Courtesan de Luxe
and a place in the public assembly.

¹⁸The king always honours her,
and virtuous people praise her.
Men seek her, approach her for sex,
and she is a standard for other courtesans to strive for.

¹⁹The daughter of a king or of a minister of state,
if she knows the techniques,
can keep her husband in her power
even if he has a thousand women in his harem.

²⁰And if she is separated from her husband
and in dire straits, even in a foreign land,
by means of these sciences
she can live quite happily.

²¹A man who is accomplished in these arts,
eloquent, and skilled at flattery,
even if he is not well known,
finds the way to women's hearts right away.

²²Luck in love* comes
from learning the arts;
but a man should consider the right time and place
before he uses, or does not use, a technique.

---

¹⁷ While a prostitute is generally called by the common title of courtesan (*veshya*), this woman wins the special title of courtesan de luxe (*ganika*), because she has these special marks of a courtesan de luxe.

²⁰ She can make a living by teaching these sciences.

CHAPTER FOUR

[4]   *The Lifestyle of the Man-about-town*

[1] When a man has become educated, he enters the householder stage of life and begins the lifestyle of a man-about-town,* using the money that he has inherited, on the one hand, or obtained from gifts, conquest, trade, or wages, on the other, or from both. [2] He settles down in a city, a capital city, a market town, or some large gathering where there are good people, or wherever he has to stay to make a living. [3] And there he makes his home in a house near water, with an orchard, separate servant quarters, and two bedrooms. [4] This is how the house is furnished: In the outer bedroom there is a bed, low in the middle and very soft, with pillows on both sides and a white top sheet. (There is also a couch.) At the head of the bed there is a grass mat and an altar, on which are placed the oils and garlands left over from the night, a pot of beeswax, a vial of perfume, some bark from a lemon tree, and betel.* On the floor, a spittoon. A lute, hanging from an ivory tusk; a board to draw or paint on, and a box of pencils. Some book or other, and garlands of amaranth flowers. On the floor, not too far away, a round bed with a pillow for the head. A board for dice

---

[1] If he is a Brahmin, he gets his money from gifts; a king or warrior, from conquest; a commoner, from trade; and a servant, from wages earned by working as an artisan, a travelling bard, or something of that sort.

[4] The inner bedroom is where the wives sleep. The outer bedroom is for sex. The couch is for the man to sleep on after sex. That is what decent people do; but the lovers of courtesans sleep together with them in the bedroom, and have no need for a couch. And so there is a saying:

> The lover makes love with his beloved
> wherever he happens to be,
> but a wise man, a pure man,
> does not sleep there on that polluted bed.

The lemon bark is chewed to dispel the bad taste in the mouth and prevent bad breath; about this there is a saying:

> The lover who, in the evening, sucks
> a stick of lemon bark, smeared with honey,
> is not plagued by foul breath
> when he is caught in the net of his woman's arms.

The book is understood to be a book of recent poetry, to read aloud.

and a board for gambling. Outside, cages of pet birds. And, set aside, a place for carpentry or woodworking and for other games. In the orchard, a well-padded swing in the shade, and a bench made of baked clay and covered with flowers.

⁵ He gets up in the morning, relieves himself, cleans his teeth, applies fragrant oils in small quantities, as well as incense, garlands, beeswax and red lac, looks at his face in a mirror, takes some mouth-wash and betel, and attends to the things that need to be done. ⁶ He bathes every day, has his limbs rubbed with oil every second day, a foam bath every third day, his face shaved every fourth day, and his body hair removed every fifth or tenth day. All of this is done without fail. And he continually cleans the sweat from his armpits. ⁷ In the morning and afternoon he eats; 'In the evening, too', says Chara-yana. ⁸ After eating, he passes the time teaching his parrots and mynah birds to speak; goes to quail-fights, cock-fights, and ram-fights; engages in various arts and games; and passes the time with his libertine, pander, and clown.* And he takes a nap. ⁹ In the late afternoon, he gets dressed up and goes to salons to amuse himself.

¹⁰ And in the evening, there is music and singing. After that, on the bed in a bedroom carefully decorated and perfumed by sweet-smelling incense, he and his friends await the women who are slipping out for a rendezvous with them. ¹¹ He sends female messengers* for them or goes to get them himself. ¹² And when the women arrive, he and his friends greet them with gentle conversation and courtesies that charm the mind and heart. ¹³ If rain has soaked the clothing of women who have slipped out for a rendez-vous in bad weather, he changes their clothes himself, or gets some of his friends to serve them. That is what he does by day and night.

---

⁵ He uses oil in small quantities, because he is no man-about-town if he uses large amounts. He colours his lips with a ball of moist red lac and fixes it with a small ball of beeswax. He puts a ball of sweet-smelling mouth-wash in his cheek and takes some betel in his hand to use later. He does what needs to be done to accomplish the three goals of human life.

⁶ He has the hair shaved from his hidden place with a razor every fifth day, and then, every tenth day, has his body hair pulled out by the roots, because it grows so fast. The sweat that breaks out after any activity must be constantly removed with a rag, to prevent a bad smell and a consequent lack of sophistication.

¹⁴ He amuses himself by going to festivals, salons, drinking parties, picnics, and group games.

¹⁵ On a specified day at half moon or full moon, there is always an assembly of invited guests at the temple of the goddess Sarasvati.* ¹⁶ Visiting players also come and give an audition for them, and on the second day they are rewarded with a fixed fee. Then they may give a performance or be dismissed, according to their reception. In case of a disaster or an occasion for celebration, they substitute for one another. ¹⁷ They honour and protect visitors who join them. Those are the customs of theatrical companies. ¹⁸ The festivals dedicated to this or that particular deity can be described in this same way, taking into consideration the different circumstances.

¹⁹ A salon takes place when people of similar knowledge, intelligence, character, wealth, and age sit together in the house of a courtesan, or in a place of assembly, or in the dwelling-place of some man, and engage in appropriate conversation with courtesans. ²⁰ There they exchange thoughts about poems or works of art, ²¹ and in the course of that they praise brilliant women whom everyone likes, and they bring in women who love all men equally.* ²² They have drinking parties at one another's houses. ²³ There the courtesans get the men to drink, and drink after them, wine made from honey, grapes, other fruits, or sugar, with various sorts of salt, fruit, greens, vegetables, and bitter, spicy, and sour foods.

²⁴ Picnics can be described in this same way. ²⁵ Early in the morning, men dress with care and go out on horseback, attended by servants and accompanied by courtesans. They enjoy the daytime events there and spend the time at cock-fights, gambling, theatrical

---

¹⁶ Visiting players are actors and dancers who arrive from somewhere else. If one of the visiting players falls ill or is in mourning, or attends a celebration such as a wedding, one of the invited players takes his place, in order not to cancel the performance, or if one of the invited players has a misfortune or a celebration, one of the visiting players takes his place.

¹⁷ Visitors are men who have the standing of men-about-town and come from somewhere else to see the festival. They honour them with such things as garlands and perfumed oils, and protect them by giving them assistance in case of disaster. The companies are made up of the players and men-about-town, invited and visiting.

spectacles, and appropriate activities, and then in the afternoon they go back again in the same way, taking with them souvenirs of the pleasures of the picnic. ²⁶ And in the same way, in the summer, people enjoy water sports, in pools built to keep out crocodiles.

²⁷ Then there are Goblin Night, Full Moon Vigil, and the Spring Festival. ²⁸ The group games are breaking open mangoes, eating roasted grains, eating lotus stems, playing with new leaves, water-fights, doing imitations with puppets, playing the 'one silk-cotton tree' game, and mock-fighting with the red-orange flowers of the 'morningstar' tree.* They play at these various widespread and local games, different from those of the common people. ²⁹ A single man, if he can afford it, ³⁰ a courtesan de luxe, and the woman with her girlfriends and men-about-town can also do what has been described here.

³¹ But the man called a libertine* has no wealth, indeed has nothing but his body; his only possessions are his collapsible chair, his soap, and his astringent. He comes from an honourable part of the country and is skilled in the arts, and by teaching them he introduces himself into society and into the sort of gatherings frequented by courtesans.

---

²⁷ Here he mentions the general games: Goblin Night is a night of pleasure, on which, because the goblins are near, most people light lamps. Full Moon Vigil takes place on the night of the full moon when the moon is in the Pleiades (October–November), when the moon is especially bright, and people play with swings and lamps. The Spring Festival is the festival of the god Kama, which people celebrate by playing, dancing, singing, and making music. Those are the widespread games.

²⁸ Here he describes the regional games. The game of lotus stems is played near ponds; people play games with new leaves in the forests, after the first rain; 'one silk-cotton tree' is a game, played in Vidarbha, in which they find one single, great silk-cotton (*shalmali*) tree laden with blossoms and play with its blossoms. The festivals and so forth are just for the men-about-town, while the public games are for both the common people and the men-about-town.

³¹ He is said to have nothing but his body because he has no son or wife. His collapsible chair is a small seat on sticks that swings down from his back to support his body. The libertine is called a *pithamarda* ('stool-crusher') because he gives his instructions while 'crushing' a collapsible chair called a 'stool'. With this, he lives the life of a scholar.

³² The man called a pander,* by contrast, has used up his wealth but has good qualities and is married. Well respected among courtesans and society people, he lives off them. ³³ But the man called a clown,* or a comedian, has just a fragmentary knowledge of the arts. He is a prankster and a trusted friend. ³⁴ These are the 'advisers' whom courtesans and men-about-town employ in their battles and truces.* ³⁵ Included among these are beggar women,* women with shaved heads, low-caste women, and old courtesans de luxe, sophisticated in the arts.

³⁶ A man who lives in a village stirs up his clever and curious relatives, describing to them the lifestyle of the set of men-about-town and inspiring their longing for that life. He emulates it himself, organizes gatherings, and charms the people by his contact with them. He ingratiates himself with them by helping them in their projects and does favours for them.

That is the lifestyle of the man-about-town.

³⁷ The man who tells stories in society,
  neither too much in Sanskrit
  nor too much in the local dialect,*
  becomes highly regarded in the social world.

³⁸ A wise man will not descend
  to a society that people hate,
  or one that slips out of control
  or is malicious to others.

³⁹ An educated man succeeds in society
  when he moves with a set of people
  who incline to the ways of the world
  and regard playing as their one and only concern.

---

³² He is called a *vita* ('pander') because he 'makes a noise' (*vitati*), that is to say, he tells stories, between one person and another.

³³ He has no wealth or has used up his wealth, has nothing but his body or has a wife, is a local or a visitor, and cannot live as he used to do.

³⁵ A beggar woman (*bhikshuki*) is the wife of a male beggar (*bhikshuka*). All of these types of women are sophisticated in the arts, for they, too, are always procuring things for battles and truces, and so they are called Procuresses.

CHAPTER FIVE

Reasons for Taking Another Man's Wife

¹Pleasure enjoyed according to the texts, with a woman who is of the man's own class, and who has not been with another man before, is a means of getting sons, a good reputation, and social acceptance. ²But with women of higher classes or with women married to other men, pleasure will achieve none of these things, and it is forbidden. And it is neither encouraged nor forbidden with courtesans, second-hand women, and women of lower classes who have not been expelled from society, because the only purpose of such liaisons is pleasure.*
³In this respect, women who may be lovers* are of three sorts: virgins, second-hand women, and courtesans.

⁴Gonikaputra says: 'There is a fourth sort of woman who may be a lover: under the pressure of some other reason, a woman who aids his cause may become his lover, even if she is married to another man.' ⁵The man may think, 'This is a loose woman. ⁶She has already ruined her virtue with many other men. Even though she is of a class

---

¹ These are legitimate sons.
² Sex with women of classes lower than his own caste is not forbidden, nor is it encouraged with such women even if they have not been expelled, that is, excluded from sharing dishes; for there are some women who, when they eat from a dish, pollute it so that it cannot be purified simply by being cleaned. And so it is said:
   Traditionally, only a servant woman can be the wife of a
   servant;
   she and one of his own class can be the wife of a commoner;
   these two and one of his own class for a king;
   and these three and one of his own class for a Brahmin.
   A second-hand woman is one who had another man before, lost her virginity, then became a widow, and, because the flesh is weak, took another man, again.
⁴ 'Some other reason' would be a reason other than a son or pleasure. But otherwise, without such a reason, he should not desire married women; this is what V implies, following the opinion of the followers of Babhravya. V has already said that Gonikaputra wrote the book about other men's wives. There Gonikaputra gives the example cited in this passage.
⁶ He thinks: 'Just as she would shatter her virtue if she made love with me, so she has already done with others, with many lovers.'

higher than mine, I can go to her as I would
without offending against religion. She is a se
[7] Since another man has kept her before me, th
hesitate about this.' [8] Or, 'This woman has h
under her control, and he is a great and powerf
ate with my enemy. If she becomes intimate with me,
affection for me she will make him reverse his allegiance.' [9] Or, 'That
powerful man has turned against me and wishes to harm me; she will
bring him back to his former nature.' [10] Or, 'If I make him my friend
through her, I will be able to do favours for my friends, or ward off
my enemies, or accomplish some other difficult undertaking.' [11] Or,
'If I become intimate with this woman, and kill her husband, I will
get for myself the power of his great wealth, which ought to be
mine.' [12] Or, 'There is no danger involved in my having this woman,
and there is a chance of wealth. And since I am useless, I have
exhausted all means of making a living. Such as I am, I will get a lot
of money from her in this way, with very little trouble.' [13] Or, 'This

---

[8] He thinks: 'Since her affection will grow as a result of making love, she
will make him turn away from the enemy who wants to harm me, and
he will have special feelings for me. Otherwise, my enemy will get
support from that great and powerful man and kill me before I have
experienced all four of the aims of human life.'

[9] He thinks: 'That powerful man is her husband.'

[10] He thinks: 'For a man would give up his life's breaths for a friend, or
even enter hell. And I must ward off my enemies to save my own body.'

[11] He thinks: 'Her husband is my enemy; I will kill him silently, with a
stick. Otherwise, I will find that he will kill my family, or take them
from me by violence and enjoy them himself, by force. And since he has
raised a weapon to kill me, killing him does not violate religion.'*

[12] He thinks: 'There is no guard, and she will give me the money out
of affection. Since I am unable to support my family, I will use her
enormous wealth to do deeds for the sake of religion, and so forth.

> For Manu says a man should support
> An old mother, a father, a good wife, and a little son,
> even by doing a hundred things
> that should not be done.'*

[13] He thinks: 'She desires me, when we are face to face. But [behind my
back] she will say, "He lusts after the kingship", and so people will
think, "He is working schemes against the king."'

. is madly in love with me and knows all my weaknesses. If I
. her, she will ruin me by publicly exposing my faults; [14] or she
.ll accuse me of some fault which I do not in fact have, but which
will be easy to believe of me and hard to clear myself of, and this will
be the ruin of me; [15] or she will cause a break between me and her
husband, who is a man with a future and under her control, and she
will get him to join my enemies; [16] or she herself will become intimate
with them.' Or, 'This woman's husband is the seducer of the women
of my harem; I will pay him back for that by seducing *his* wives, too.'
[17] Or, 'By the king's command, I will kill his enemy, who is hiding
inside.' [18] 'Another woman, whose desire I desire, is in the power of
this woman. I will get to that one by using this one as a bridge.' [19] Or,
'This woman will get me an unattainable virgin, rich and beautiful,
who depends on her.' [20] Or, 'My enemy is united with this woman's
husband. Through her, I will get him to drink a potion.' For these
and similar reasons one may seduce* even the wife of another man.
[21] But nothing rash should be done merely because of passion. Those
are the reasons for taking another man's wife.

[22] Charayana says: 'For these very reasons, there is also a fifth

---

[14] He thinks: 'People will say, "He is an adulterer", and that will be the
ruin of me.'

[15] He thinks: 'He does what she tells him to do. And when my enemies
have gained power through him, they will kill me.'

[16] He thinks: 'She will get my enemies to kill me.' Or, 'He corrupts the
women I have married, by seducing them. And it is said, "An enemy's
cruelty should be paid back in kind."'

[17] He thinks: 'The king has hired me to spy inside the house; since there is
no other means, I will become intimate with his wife, who does not trust
him, and get him to come outside.'

[19] He thinks: 'She will bring me a girl that I cannot attain because I have
no money, a girl who is both beautiful and rich and therefore a source of
the three aims of human life. Or, when I am making love to this one, she
will think, "He will get us both together", and I will seduce, at the same
time, some woman or other and the woman who is the real thing.'

[20] He thinks: 'My enemy, who would steal my life's breaths, sits, lives,
drinks, and eats with her husband. (Above [1.5.8], it was just a matter of
being intimate in a general way.) Through her, when I have become
intimate with her, I will get him to drink a poison that will steal his life's
breaths in a short time.'

woman who can be a lover, a widow who is kept by a minister of state or by the king and comes to him only part of the time, or some other widow who can accomplish a man's purposes.' [23] Suvarnanabha says: 'There is a sixth: a woman just like that, who is a wandering ascetic.'* [24] Ghotakamukha says: 'There is a seventh: a servant woman, or the daughter of a courtesan de luxe, who has not had a man before.' [25] Gonardiya says: 'A young woman of good family who is no longer a child is an eighth, because she is treated differently.' [26] Vatsyayana says: These women* should be counted with the others, because there is no difference in the purposes for which they are used. And so there are just four sorts of women who can be lovers. [27] Some people say: 'The third nature is a fifth sort of woman who can be a lover, because she is different.'*

[28] Now, there is one kind of male lover, and everyone knows him

———

[25] A young woman of good family, married, and now in the prime of youth, can no longer be treated like a virgin. For a man uses a virgin subtly and with techniques applied one at a time, while he uses a girl who has reached the prime of youth blatantly and with everything at once.

[26] There is no difference between her and the other four: virgins, second-hand women, courtesans, and the wives of other men. The widow [1.5.22] and the wandering woman ascetic [1.5.23] can be regarded like the wives of other men, because there are other reasons for taking them; the servant girl and the daughter of the courtesan de luxe [1.5.24] are like courtesans, because they are taken for pleasure; the young woman of good family [1.5.25] is like a virgin, taken for the sake of a son and family.

[27] A member of the third nature is a non-male, who is different from both men and women because she is neither a man nor a woman. Or else one could regard her as a kind of courtesan, because the reason for sex with her is pleasure, obtained through oral sex.

[28] Because there are no distinctions among male lovers as there are for female lovers, the one kind of lover is involved with virgins, second-hand women, and courtesans, and everyone knows him well. But when that same lover seeks an excessive pleasure with the wives of other men, in order to get something special, he becomes the second kind of lover, concealed. The best kind has all the good qualities, the middling kind has half, and the worst kind has just a quarter; a man who lacks all of the good qualities is no lover at all. 'Both' refers to both male and female lovers.*

well. But a second kind conceals himself in order to get something special, and he is known, according to his good qualities or lack of good qualities, as best, worst, or middling. We will explain the good qualities and lack of good qualities in both of them in the discussion of courtesans. [29] But the following women are not eligible to be lovers: a leper, a lunatic, a fallen woman, a woman who tells secrets, who asks for it in public, whose prime of youth is almost entirely gone, who is too light or too dark, bad-smelling, a relative, a woman friend, a wandering female ascetic, or the wife of a relative, of a friend, of a Brahmin who knows the Veda, or of a king. [30] The followers of Babhravya say: 'Any woman who is known to have had five men is eligible.' [31] But Gonikaputra says, '—except for the wife of a relative, of a friend, of a Brahmin who knows the Veda, or of a king.'

---

[29] The 'but' means that these women are not eligible even for the reasons discussed above. A leper is marked by a disgusting disease. A lunatic can do anything but finds no pleasure in it. A woman fallen from her own caste because of some major crime makes any man who associates with her fallen, too. A woman who tells secrets embarrasses her lover. A woman who expresses, in public, her desire for her lover shames him and causes trouble for him. A woman whose prime of youth is almost entirely gone destroys the lifespan and vigour of the man who serves her. A woman who is bad-smelling in her hidden places and in her mouth turns a man away from sex. A woman friend is a contemporary of his wife. A wandering woman ascetic, who has taken a vow under some order or other, is forbidden because having her would obstruct both religion and power. And so it is said:

> A man who sheds his seed in the womb that was his own,
> or in maidens, low-caste women,
> or the wives of his son or friend,
> is equal to a man who defiles his teacher's marriage-bed.*

[30] If, besides her own husband, she has five men as husbands, she is a loose woman and eligible for everyone who has a good reason. Draupadi,* however, who had Yudhishthira and the others as her own husbands, was not eligible for other men. How could one woman have several husbands? Ask the authors of the Epic!

[5] *The Work of the Man's Male Helpers ar*

[32] Someone who played in the sand with you, who is a favour, who has the same character and vices, wh with you, who knows your vulnerable spots and vulnerable spots and secrets you know, your foster-b̶ ̶ ̶ ̶ ̶ ̶ ̶ ̶ ̶ ̶,̶ ̶o̶r̶ ̶s̶o̶m̶e- one who grew up with you, is someone you can regard as a friend. [33] The conditions that make a friend are that his father and grand- fathers were friends with yours, that he does not break his word, is steadfast, is under your control, firm, not greedy by nature, cannot be won over by someone else, and does not leak confidences. [34] Vatsyayana says: A friend may be a washer-man, barber, florist, perfumer, wine-merchant, beggar, cowherd, betel-seller, goldsmith, libertine, pander, or clown, and so forth; and men-about-town can be friends with the wives of these men, too.* [35] The work of the messen- ger is done by someone who has the friendship and respect of both partners, but is especially well trusted by the woman. [36] The qualities to look for in a messenger are glibness, audacity, a knowledge of signals and gestures that reveal emotions, a knowledge of the right moment for deception, an understanding of what is possible, and a light approach to method. [37] And there is a verse about this:

> A man who knows himself and has friends,
> who is well trained, knows about emotions,
> and recognizes the right time and place,
> can win over, effortlessly, even an unattainable woman.*

---

[32] A foster-brother is a child who drank milk at the wet-nurse's breast along with the man. He is like the friend who played in the sand with him but is mentioned separately because of the intensity of his affection.

END OF BOOK ONE

BOOK TWO · SEX

CHAPTER ONE

[6]   *Sexual Typology According to Size, Endurance,*
and Temperament

[1] The man is called a 'hare', 'bull', or 'stallion', according to the size of his sexual organ; a woman, however, is called a 'doe', 'mare', or 'elephant cow'. [2] And so there are three equal couplings, between sexual partners of similar size, [3] and six unequal ones, between sexual

---

[1]   The sexual organ is called the 'sign' (*lingam*), because it is the sign of femaleness and so forth. From texts and from experience it is known that the male organ is convex and the female organ concave. If the man's penis is small, like a hare's, he is called a 'hare'; if medium, a 'bull'; if large, a 'stallion'. The word 'however' indicates that women are distinct; they have a different nomenclature because they have a different sexual organ. Knowing this, scholars called them 'doe' and so forth instead of 'female hare' and so forth. And they spoke of the distinguishing marks in this way:

> The size of the penis is divided
> into the three categories of 'hare' and so forth,
> according to the length, in graduated order:
> six, nine, and twelve [fingers].*
> Its circumference should measure
> equal to its length.
> But some say, 'There is no fixed rule
> about the circumference.'
> Women are divided in the same way
> in common parlance:
> 'does' and so forth, just like 'hares' and so forth,
> with regard to both length and circumference.

[2]   The three equal couplings, characterized by the equal size of the opening and the inserted organ, are between a 'hare' and 'doe', 'bull' and 'mare', and 'stallion' and 'elephant cow'.

[3]   These are the six unequal couplings: The harder way (when the penis, because of its greater size, can enter the opening only with difficulty) is

partners of dissimilar size. Among the unequal ones, when the man is larger there are two couplings with the two sexual partners immediately smaller than him and one, when he is largest, with the smallest woman. But in the opposite case, in a coupling when the man is smaller, there are two sorts of couplings with the two women immediately larger than him and one, when he is smallest, with the largest woman. Among these, the equal couplings are best, the largest and the smallest are worst, and the rest are intermediate.* ⁴Even in the medium ones, it is better for the man to be larger than the woman.* Thus there are nine sorts of couplings according to size.

⁵A man has dull sexual energy if, at the time of making love, his enthusiasm is indifferent, his virility small, and he cannot bear to be wounded, ⁶and a man has average or fierce sexual energy in the

----

with the two women immediately beneath the man (1. 'bull' with 'doe'; 2. 'stallion' with 'mare'), and with the woman farthest beneath him (3. 'stallion' with 'doe'). The easier way (when the penis, because of its smaller size, works inside the opening, but cannot fill it fully) is with the two women immediately above him (4. 'hare' with 'mare'; 5 'bull' with 'elephant cow') and with the woman farthest above him (6. 'hare' with 'elephant cow').

⁴ In the largest coupling, a woman's itch is most satisfactorily relieved; she accommodates the large penis inside her by assuming a position such as the 'wide open' [2.6.7 ff.], stretching her vagina. But in the smallest coupling, even when she contracts her vagina by assuming a position such as the 'cup' [2.6.13 ff.], there is no relief for her. V will speak later about ways of changing the size of the sexual organ, in which the woman stretches hers by the use of her arms and shoulders [2.6.7], and the man uses devices to increase his [7.1–2]. But it is said:

> But if a lover has a small penis,
> no matter how long the man works,
> women, they say, do not grow very fond of him,
> because he does not relieve their itch.

And the saying is right.

⁵ He might be wounded when she bites or scratches or slaps him.

⁶ The two opposite circumstances are, first, when he has average sexual energy (his enthusiasm is average, his virility average, and he can bear to be somewhat wounded) and, secondly, when he has fierce sexual energy (his enthusiasm is very great and he can bear, to the extreme, serious wounds).

opposite circumstances. The same goes for the woman. ⁷And so, just as with size, so with temperament, too, there are nine sorts of couplings.

⁸And similarly, with respect to endurance, men are quick, average, and long-lasting. ⁹But there is an argument about women in this matter.

¹⁰Auddalaki says:* 'A woman does not reach a climax as a man does. ¹¹But she has an itch, which the man, during sex, scratches continually. ¹²And when this scratching is combined, in addition, with the sensual pleasure of erotic arousal, it produces a different feeling,* and this is what she thinks of as sensual pleasure. ¹³Someone might

---

¹⁰ A man experiences sensual pleasure when he ejaculates, but a woman does not have that kind of sensual pleasure, because she does not have semen. Why, then, does she make love with the man? To answer this, he says the next passage.

¹¹ There is a verse about this:
> Tiny worms, born of menstrual blood,
> some with mild powers, some average, some terrible,
> cause an itch in the abodes of erotic love,
> according to their strength.

The itch is scratched continually when the penis goes on moving without interruption.*

¹² Scratching the itch is just like scratching an ear with a twig. The different feeling is a different sensual pleasure, caused by the scratching of the itch combined with kissing and so forth. She thinks, 'What sensual pleasure I feel!' But the scratching of the itch is not a true perception of sensual pleasure, and the difference is that this experience bears no fruit, because she has no seed. And so the two sexes are not alike in the matter of their form or their timing, and therefore there are not nine couplings with respect to endurance and climax.

¹³ Since the workings of someone's mind are not accessible to someone else's sense perceptions and cannot be recognized by an eyewitness, what man can know a woman's different feeling? The word 'and' indicates, 'a woman's ecstasy, too'. When a woman acts the part of a man and produces her own ecstasy by her own movements, how can he know what her ecstasy is in its very essence, since he cannot perceive this sensually? And no one can ask, 'Does your sensual pleasure come from an ejaculation, like ours, or from something else?' Since the woman cannot sensually perceive the sensual pleasure of ejaculation, and the

ask, "But since no one can know a man's ecstasy, and since no one can be asked, 'What sort of sensual pleasure do you feel?' [14] how can this be known?" The answer would be: Because when a man reaches a climax, he stops of his own accord and pays no attention to the woman; a woman, however, is not like that.'

[15] This objection might be raised about that argument: Women love the man whose sexual energy lasts for a long time, but they resent a man whose sexual energy ends quickly, because he stops before they

---

man cannot sensually perceive a different form of sensual pleasure, it is not possible for one to ask the other about this. Even if someone could speak of it, the other would have no experience through which to understand the perception. To answer this doubt, Auddalaki describes, in the next passage, a means by which one person can know another's sensual pleasure.

[14] When a man has ejaculated he has accomplished what he set out to do and stops moving, even if she is still working quite hard at it. And if a woman experienced the sensual pleasure of ejaculation like a man, she would then loosen his penis from her and stop. But this does not happen. When the man stops, she wants another man. For sometimes when a woman has made love with one man she may make love with other men who happen to be there. And so it is said:

> A fire is never sated by logs,
> nor the ocean by the rivers that flow into it;
> death cannot be sated by all the creatures in the world,
> nor a fair-eyed woman by men.

Therefore, since a woman does not stop of her own accord, she does not reach a sensual pleasure of ejaculation like a man's sensual pleasure just before ejaculation.

[15] The man whose sexual energy lasts for a long time thrusts inside the woman for a long time before he reaches the sensual pleasure of ejaculation and stops. With him, women become affectionate, just as they become wet.* So the love of the women shows that they have achieved their sensual pleasure, and their hatred shows that they are unhappy because they have not achieved their sensual pleasure. For even men whose sexual energy lasts for a long time achieve sensual pleasure and experience love if the woman plays the man's part and works for a long time before she stops. But if she stops suddenly, the men lose their passion for her, since they are unhappy because they have not achieved their sensual pleasure. The fact that women experience love for long-lasting men shows that, like men, they know the sensual pleasure of ejaculation.

reach a climax at the conclusion. And all of that is a sign that they either do reach a climax, with the long-lasting man, or do not, with the quick man.

¹⁶ 'Not so. For the scratching of an itch also feels good for a long time. That is evident. And because of this ambiguity, the preference that women have for long-lasting men is no sign of a climax.

> ¹⁷ A man scratches a woman's itch
> when they make love;
> and when that is enhanced by erotic arousal
> it is called sensual pleasure.'

¹⁸ The followers of Babhravya say: 'A young woman reaches a climax

---

¹⁶ Because of this ambiguity—'Has she just had her itch scratched or achieved her climax?'—the resentment that women have for quick men is no sign that women do or do not achieve the sensual pleasure of ejaculation.

¹⁷ He expresses this opinion by quoting a verse from the 'Song of Auddalaki'.

¹⁸ Both he and she experience the sensual pleasure of ejaculation, but hers takes place from the very beginning, from the moment when he penetrates her with his penis, and goes on continually, without any interruption. For as the man moves inside her, she gradually gets wet; water flows from her as it flows from a broken pot. This is evident from eyewitnesses. And so she ejaculates from the very start, like a man. But he has his climax only at the end, when he emits his semen. And so, since the timing of the two of them is different, there are not nine couplings with regard to endurance, but there are nine according to climax, because of the similarity in the sensual pleasure of ejaculation.

For the physician Charaka says that 'satisfaction and keeping the semen in her womb are among the signs that a woman has just become pregnant', and by satisfaction he means climax. That is, conception is not possible without the ejaculation of semen. Now, some people say, 'She emits a menstrual discharge, not semen. For it is said:

> When a man and women mingle their bodies together mutually
> and their hearts are heated by the flame of desire,
> the embryo is churned out of the mixture of semen and menstrual blood,
> like fire by the twirling of the two fire sticks.'

But if the woman had no semen, how could she conceive? For a woman can be impregnated by making love with another woman just as she can by making love with a man. As Sushruta says:

continually, from the very beginning of lovemaking; a man, by contrast, only at the end. That is even more clearly evident. For surely no embryo would be conceived if she did not achieve a climax.'

[19] There could be a further doubt and confutation about that argument, too. [20] This objection may be raised about it: If a woman achieved this feeling continually, it would not be evident, as it is, that at the beginning her mind is indifferent and she cannot bear much, but gradually her passion grows greater and she has no regard for her body, and at the end there is a wish to stop.

[21] 'Not so. For when a potter's wheel or a spinning top whirls about

---

> 'When a woman and a woman
> make love together,
> and emit semen into one another,
> a child is born without bones.'*

For blood is formed out of the basic liquid of the body and becomes, under certain circumstances, menstrual blood, while semen is formed out of the marrow of the bones.

[19] Women love producing the climax even if it takes a long time, because the climax is the most important thing. Women hate a quick man because he cannot take a long time to produce the climax. Indeed, women want a climax that takes a long time to produce, because their desire is eight times that of a man. Given these conditions, it is perfectly right to say that 'a fair-eyed woman cannot be sated by men', but this is true because men's desire is just one-eighth of women's, not because women do not experience the sensual pleasure of ejaculation.

[20] These entirely different conditions of a woman would *not* be evident if she achieved this feeling constantly.

[21] A top is a wooden toy that little boys spin with a long string. In the same way, although a woman's sensual pleasure in ejaculation, caused by the man's thrusts, remains the same at the beginning, middle, and end of love-making, at the beginning she experiences only a dull sexual energy and gentle sexual pleasure but gradually she achieves full sexual energy and the greatest sexual pleasure.

But if her climax continues without interruption, why is there a wish to stop? Because the fluids are used up. When the erotic climax begins, the fluid, that is, the semen, falls from its own place and moves through its own channel. Because it flows constantly from the very start, eventually it is used up, and then all passion is stilled and there is a desire to stop.

in the same way, at the start it whirls with dull energy and then gradually increases to its full energy. That is evident. And the "wish to stop" occurs because the fluids are used up.* So this is not a convincing objection.

> [22] Men's sensual pleasure comes at the end of sex,
>   but women's is continual.
>   And the wish to stop occurs
>   only when fluids are used up.'

[23] Vatsyayana says: It is clearly apparent from this very argument that the sensual experience of a woman is manifested just like that of a man. [24] How could two people of the same species who are striving toward a single goal achieve different climaxes? [25] One might argue: because they differ in their methods and in their erotic arousal. [26] But what causes the difference in their methods? Their different physical natures. By his physical nature, the man is the active agent and the young woman is the passive locus; the agent contributes to the action in one way and the locus in another. And the difference in their erotic arousal comes from this difference in their methods that comes from their physical natures. The man is aroused by the thought, 'I am taking her', the young woman by the thought, 'I am being taken by him.'

[27] This objection may be raised about that argument: 'Why do they not differ in their climaxes just as in their methods?'

Not so. The difference in their methods has a cause, namely, the different characteristics of the active and passive roles. But, logically, there can be no difference in their climaxes since that has no cause. For they are not of different species.*

[28] This objection may be raised about that argument: 'The

---

[22] He makes this point by quoting a verse from the 'Song of Babhravya'.

[24] Two people of different species, such as a man and a mare,* would have different kinds of sensual pleasure; and so he specifies the same species, the human species. But even two people of the same species might have different goals, such as bathing or eating, and so he specifies a single goal, namely sex.

[26] Men and women are created differently: the organ of one goes in, and of the other, out; one swallows and the other is swallowed.

[28] The two cases, of a sexual couple (man and woman) and a grammatical sentence (with an active subject and passive locus) are not analogous at

different parts of a sentence (subject and locus) cohere in producing a single meaning, but these two people, by contrast, are each intent upon achieving separate personal goals. So this analogy is inappropriate.'

[29] Not so. Several agents may achieve their goals at the same time, as we see when two rams batter one another, or two wood apples* strike one another in a game, or two wrestlers are locked together in a fight.

Someone might object: 'But there is no distinction between the two actors in these cases.'

Nor is there any distinction between the essence of the subjects in this case, the man and woman. The difference in their methods just comes from their physical natures, as has already been established in this argument. And so the two of them also experience a similar sensual pleasure.

> [30] Since there is no difference in the species
> of a couple, they seek a similar sensual pleasure.
> Therefore the woman should be treated in such a way
> that she achieves her sexual climax first.*

---

all. For, in the sentence, 'Devadatta is using logs to cook rice in a pot', the rice is produced through the combined action of the various case relations such as nominative (Devadatta), instrumental (logs), locative (a pot), and so forth.* But the man and the woman are acting upon one another, since the woman, who is the passive locus, depends on the action of the man in achieving her object, namely pleasure in her own offspring, and the man, who is the active agent, is dependent upon the woman. And their sensual pleasures are separate and dissimilar because their timing and their natural forms are different, even though they are of the same species.

[30] As it is said:

> A woman's sensual pleasure is twofold:
> the scratching of an itch and the pleasure of melting.
> The melting, too, is twofold:
> the flowing and the ejaculation of the seed.
> She gets wet just from the flowing,
> and her sensual pleasure of ejaculation comes from being churned.
> But when a woman is carried away by her sexual energy,
> she ejaculates at the end, it is said, just like a man.

The best case is when the man and woman achieve their sexual pleasure at the same time, because that is an equal coupling. But if it does not

³¹ Since the similarity in climaxes has been proved in this way, there are nine forms of sex keyed to endurance, too, in terms of the time to climax, just as there are nine in terms of size and temperament.

³² The synonyms for sexual pleasure (*rati*) are sexual feeling (*rasa*), sexual pleasure or ecstasy (*rati*), love or ecstasy (*priti*), emotion, temperament, or climax (*bhava*), passion (*raga*), sexual energy (*vega*), and satisfaction (*samapti*). The synonyms for the sexual act (*surata*) are sex or making love (*samprayoga*), mating or coupling (*rata*), the secret act (*rahas*), going to bed together (*shayana*), and seduction (*mohana*).*

³³ Since there are nine kinds of sex according to each of the criteria of size, endurance, and temperament, when they are combined it is not possible to enumerate all the forms of sex. There are just too many. ³⁴ Vatsyayana says: After deliberating about these forms, a man should choose the appropriate sexual practices.

———

happen at the same time, and the man reaches his climax first, his banner is no longer at full mast, and the woman does not reach her climax. Therefore, if the coupling is unequal rather than equal, the woman should be treated with kisses, embraces, and so forth, in such a way that she achieves her sexual pleasure first. When the woman reaches her climax first, the man, remaining inside her, puts on speed and reaches his own climax.

³¹ Otherwise, because of the dissimilarity between the sensual pleasure of scratching an itch and the sensual pleasure of ejaculation, how could there be nine forms of sex with regard to climax?

³³ There are nine forms of each of the three categories, making twenty-seven possibilities for each man and the same number for each woman. If these mate in all possible combinations, the total comes to 729 (27 × 27).

³⁴ There are some verses of Babhravya about this:

> Endurance is the most important factor of all,
> because, in time, even a 'hare'
> can touch deeply, everywhere,
> inside the vagina of an 'elephant cow'.
> But a 'stallion' is said
> to make up for the endurance that a 'doe' needs,
> and therefore some say that
> size is what is absolutely more important.
> And others say that sexual energy is more important,

³⁵ In the first coupling, the man's sexual energy is fierce but he lasts just a short time; in later ones, it is just the opposite. On the other hand, it is just the other way around for a woman, until the fluids are used up.* ³⁶ And it is commonly said: 'The man runs out of fluid before the woman runs out of fluid.'

³⁷ 'Women achieve their sensual pleasure quickly
   if they are naturally delicate
   and can be strongly stimulated.'
   That is what scholars agree upon.

[7]   *Types of Love*

³⁸ Up to this point, sex has been explained
   for experts; from now on,
   a detailed description will be elaborated
   to enlighten the slow-witted.*
³⁹ People who know the science say
   that love takes four forms,
   arising out of habit, erotic arousal,
   transference, and the objects of the senses.

———————

since even a 'stallion', if he lacks sexual energy,
cannot accomplish the goal;
sexual energy makes up for length of endurance.
But even a woman whose sexual energy is dull
should not worry about this,
for a man must find out the strengths and weaknesses
of the sensuality of each woman.
A man who lacks sexual energy and size,
or who has sexual energy but lacks endurance,
or who lacks endurance and size,
can succeed by using the one that is left.

³⁶ He runs out of fluids first because the woman has eight times as much fluid as a man.* And so it is commonly said [see 14, Y]: 'A fair-eyed woman cannot be sated by men.'

³⁷ She may be strongly stimulated externally, by kissing and so forth, and internally, by the work of the fingers. The implication is that these women have quick sexual energy, and that, in the opposite case, the women have average or long-lasting sexual energy. This applies to men, too.

³⁹ The people who know the science are those who know the *Kamasutra*.

⁴⁰ The love that comes from habit
   is marked by the constant repetition of certain actions;
   it can be recognized in the course of activities like hunting,
   and is expressed in words and other manifestations.
⁴¹ The love that comes from erotic arousal
   arises from the imagination,
   not in response to any object of the senses,
   nor in activities that have previously become a habit.*
⁴² It can be recognized in the course of
   oral sex with a woman
   or with a person of the third nature,
   or in various activities such as kissing.
⁴³ Those who know the science call it
   the love that comes from a transference
   when someone says, referring to another object of desire,
   'This one here, not the other one from the past, is the one I love.'*
⁴⁴ The love that comes from the objects of the senses,
   right before one's eyes, is well known in the world;

———

⁴⁰ Hunting is an athletic art like dancing, singing, playing a musical instrument, and cutting shapes out of leaves.

⁴² Oral sex means using the mouth as a vagina; the person on whom the act is performed experiences a physical love in response to the object of the senses, over and over again. Erotic arousal also comes from kissing, embracing, scratching, biting, slapping, and so forth; at the moment of sexual pleasure, the person performing these acts experiences a mental love, and the woman for whom they are done also experiences a mental, rather than merely physical, love, because of the imaginative power of passion directed to each spot that is being stimulated.

⁴³ When someone says, 'This one is that one', referring to some other man or woman who was always an object of desire in the past, the past love is transferred to some other man or woman. The idea is, 'The qualities, the causes of love, in the person I loved in the past are also here in this one.' And so they call this past love a transferred love. Thus V will say [at 6.1.17], 'resemblance to someone loved is a reason for taking a lover.'

⁴⁴ Since this type of love is well known, there is no need to give signs by which it can be recognized. It is, moreover, the type of love intended in the discussion of the various occasions in the lifestyle of the man-about-town. The most important fruit is the enjoyment of the pleasures of visible sense-objects.

and because it yields the most important fruit,
it is the goal of the three others, too.
⁴⁵ When a man learns about the types of love from the text,
and recognizes each type from the signs that the text describes,
he will make use of each emotion in the way
appropriate to the manner in which it arises.

CHAPTER TWO

[8]   *Ways of Embracing*

¹ Some people call the part* of this text about sex 'the sixty-four'.
Because it has sixty-four sections, ² scholars have called the whole
text 'the sixty-four'.* ³ Or, because the arts number sixty-four and
are a part of sex, 'the sixty-four' may refer to the aggregate of the

---

⁴⁵ When she inclines toward one of the four forms, arising from habit and
so forth, he will work with that form, to achieve the love that comes
from that form. If he uses that love in the wrong way, he will find a form
of love he does not want, or no love at all.

¹ 'Some people' refers to scholars. The word 'sixty-four' applies to the
whole text or to a part of the text, but in both cases it refers to the part
about the sexual act.

³ These are the sixty-four fine arts, singing and so forth, which are a part
of sex as a whole. Or they may be the sixty-four arts of love described in
one particular part of the text, about sex, for they are called 'the sixty-
four arts that come from Babhravya of Panchala' [1.3.16]. A great sage
from Panchala composed sixty-four hymns of the *Rig Veda*. And
Babhravya of Panchala [1.1.10] spoke about embracing and so forth in
the book about sex that he himself made. The *Rig Veda*, which is
divided into ten 'circles', is called 'the sixty-four'. In the case of the
Kamasutra, too, in the part about sex, the number 'sixty-four' is connected with the ten circles of the *Rig Veda*, because the *Kamasutra* book
about sex has ten sections, as the saying goes:

> They say there are ten parts:
> embracing, kissing, biting, scratching,
> moaning, slapping, sexual positions,
> a man's sexual strokes,
> oral sex, and the woman playing the man's part.

arts. Some people say: 'Because the verses of the *Rig Veda* (which are divided into ten sections) are called "the sixty-four", that number connects this text with that one. And because both of these texts are connected with Panchala, those who know the many verses of the *Rig Veda* use the name of "the sixty-four" to honour the *Kama-sutra*.'* ⁴The followers of Babhravya say: 'Sixty-four is eight eights, the eight theoretical varieties of each of the eight parts: embracing, kissing, scratching, biting, sexual positions, moaning, the woman playing the man's part, and oral sex.' ⁵But Vatsyayana says: Since the division into eight theoretical varieties is too few for some categories and too many for others, and since sex involves other categories, too, such as slapping, screaming, a man's sexual strokes, and unusual sexual acts, this is merely a manner of speaking, just as we speak of the 'seven-leaf' devil tree or the 'five-colour' offering of rice.

⁶When a man and woman have not yet made love together, they use four sorts of embraces to reveal the signs of their love: 'touching', 'stabbing', 'grinding', and 'pressing'. ⁷Generally, the exact meaning of the name precisely describes the action. ⁸On some pretext, he moves close to the woman he wants, when she is facing him, and touches limb to limb. This is 'touching'. ⁹She makes as if to take something from the man she wants, when he is standing or sitting in a deserted place, and stabs him with her breast, and the man also grasps her and presses in response. This is called 'stabbing'. ¹⁰These two embraces are for a couple who have not yet spoken much together. ¹¹In a dark or crowded or deserted place, the two of them move slowly and grind their bodies against one another for not too brief a time. This is 'grinding'. ¹²The very same action with a wall or a pillar used as the other leg of a pair of tongs, pressing extensively, is called 'pressing'. ¹³These two embraces are for a couple who have already understood one another's signals.

¹⁴Four embraces are used while making love: the 'twining vine', 'climbing the tree', 'rice-and-sesame', and 'milk-and-water'. ¹⁵As a vine twines around a great dammar tree, so she twines around him and bends his face down to her to kiss him. Or, raising it up again,

---

⁷ This applies more generally, to things like kissing, as well.

¹⁴ These four embraces are for a couple who have already become moist while making love.

she pants gently, rests on him, and gazes at him with love for a while. This is the 'twining vine'. [16] She steps on his foot with her foot, places her other foot on his thigh or wraps her leg around him, with one arm gripping his back and the other bending down his shoulder, and panting gently, moaning a little, she tries to climb him to kiss him. This is called 'climbing the tree'. [17] These two embraces are done standing up. [18] Lying on a bed, their thighs entangled and arms entangled, they embrace so tightly that they seem to be wrestling against one another. This is 'rice-and-sesame'.* [19] Blind with passion, oblivious to pain or injury, they embrace as if they would enter one another; she may be on his lap, seated facing him, or on a bed. This is called 'milk-and-water'. [20] These two embraces are used in moments of passion. [21] Those are the ways of embracing closely, according to the followers of Babhravya.

[22] But Suvarnanabha describes an additional four close embraces of a single part of the body: [23] The thighs are used as a pair of tongs to press the partner's thigh, or both thighs, between them, squeezing as hard as possible. This is called the 'close embrace of the thighs'. [24] The woman, her coiffed hair flying loose, leaps on top of the man and presses his pelvis with her pelvis, to scratch, bite, slap, and kiss him. This is the 'close embrace of the pelvises'. [25] She presses her two breasts into his chest and transfers their full weight to him. This is called the 'embrace of breasts'. [26] One partner touches the other, mouth to mouth, eyes to eyes, forehead to forehead. This is the 'embrace of foreheads'.

[27] Some people think that massaging is also a kind of close embrace, because it involves touching. [28] But Vatsyayana says: No. For a massage takes place at a particular time set aside, has a different use, and is not enjoyed by both partners in the same way.

---

[18] When the woman is lying on her left side, the man on his right side, he places his left thigh between her two thighs, and his left arm under her right armpit; and she does the same to the man. And the opposite, if they lie on the opposite sides.

[22] These are in addition to the eight forms of embracing according to Babhravya.

[28] Both partners engage in an embrace at the same time, without stopping; but a massage, whether done by a man or by a woman, is not shared in the same way.

²⁹ When men ask about all the ways of embracing,
    or hear about them,
    or tell stories about them,
    they want to make love.
³⁰ Some sexual embraces, not in this text,
    also intensify passion;
    those, too, may be used for love-making,
    but only with care.
³¹ The territory of the texts extends
    only so far as men have dull appetites;
    but when the wheel of sexual ecstasy is in full motion,
    there is no textbook at all, and no order.

CHAPTER THREE

[9]   *Procedures of Kissing*

¹ There is no order of precedence for kissing, scratching, or biting, because they involve passion. They are generally used before sex, and slapping and moaning during sex. ² Vatsyayana says: Everything at any time, because passion does not look before it leaps.

³ These techniques should be used one at a time and not blatantly, in the first coupling with a trusting woman, given the nature of her passion. After that, they may be used quite quickly, in particular combinations, to enflame passion. ⁴ People kiss on the forehead, hair, cheeks, eyes, chest, breasts, lips, and the inside of the mouth; ⁵ the people of Lata also kiss where the two thighs join the torso, on the armpits, and on the Mound of Venus. ⁶ Vatsyayana says: There are all sorts of places to kiss, in the sway of passion and according to local customs, but not all of them are for all people.

⁷ There are three sorts of kisses for a virgin, called the 'casual', the 'throbbing', and the 'brushing'. ⁸ When he grasps her by force and

---

³ For, at the beginning, her passion is dull and her mind is indifferent, and she cannot bear much [20], and the technique should be suited to that condition. After the beginning, her passion grows greater and she has no regard for her body, and a different technique is suited to that condition.

she places her mouth on his mouth but does not move, that is called the 'casual' kiss. [9] When she is still a bit shy but wants to grasp his lower lip after he has pressed it into her mouth, and she makes her lower lip throb but cannot bear to do this with her upper lip—that is called the 'throbbing' kiss. [10] When she grasps him gently, closes her eyes, covers his eyes with her hand, and brushes him with the tip of her tongue, that is the 'brushing' kiss.

[11] And there are four more kisses: the 'equal', the 'sideways', the 'turned-around', and the 'pressing'. [12] There is also a fifth, called the 'pressing hard': cupping the fingers to squeeze the partner's lips into a ball, one partner presses hard with the cup of the lips, but without using the teeth.

[13] Then a lover can play a game: [14] the winner is the one who first grasps the other's lips. [15] If she loses, she pretends to cry, waves her hand about, pushes him away, bites him, and turns away from him; if he drags her to him by force, she disputes the loss and says, 'Let us wager again.' If she loses that time too, she comes at him twice as much as before. [16] If he becomes overconfident or careless, she grasps his lower lip and holds it with her teeth so that he cannot get it out; then she laughs, shouts, makes fun of him, leaps, exults, dances, and says whatever she pleases, mocking him, raising her eyebrows and rolling her eyes. This is the kissing-game quarrel. [17] In this same

---

[10] She brushes him with her mouth, touching him everywhere as she moves about.

[11] There are five ways of grasping the partner's lower lip with the cup formed by the two lips. When the partners are face to face, that is the 'equal grasping'. When one of them grasps the other by bending the cup of the lips sideways to make a circle, that is the 'sideways grasping'. When one grasps the other by the chin and the head and turns the face around, so that they can grasp one another's lower lips, that is the 'turned-around grasping'. And in the fourth, unlike the first three, the lips are pressed hard together, which is why it is called the 'pressing'. The 'pressing' kiss takes two forms: When both partners press hard, it is called 'basic pressing'. When the tip of the tongue is also used, it is called 'licking-and-pressing'. (This latter form has two other names: 'sucking' and 'lip-drinking'.)

[12] So there are eight forms of lower-lip-kisses: three kisses for virgins and five grasping-kisses.

[17] Whoever is first to scratch, and so forth, is the winner.

manner, there are mock-quarrels for scratching, biting, and slapping.
¹⁸ But these fierce methods are suitable only for two people whose sexual energy is fierce, because they suit their natures.

¹⁹ He grasps her upper lip while she is kissing him; this is called 'kissing the upper lip'. ²⁰ One partner grasps the other's two lips with the tongs made of the two lips; this is called the 'bowl', and can be done to a woman or to a man who does not yet show the signs of sexual maturity. ²¹ In this kiss, one partner may rub the tongue over the other's teeth, palate, or tongue; and this is called the 'battle of tongues'. ²² It may also involve giving and receiving hard blows on the mouth and teeth. ²³ Kisses may be applied moderately, with pressure, with curved lips, or gently, on other parts of the body, each according to the particular place. Those are the varieties of kisses.

²⁴ When a woman gazes at the mouth of her sleeping lover and kisses him because she desires him, this is the 'kiss that kindles passion'. ²⁵ The 'stirring kiss' is used to wake up a man who is inattentive, quarrelsome, looking in another direction, or inclined to sleep. ²⁶ A man who comes home late at night and finds his woman asleep in bed may give her an 'awakening kiss', because he desires her. ²⁷ But if she wishes to know her man's mood, she may pretend to be asleep when she knows he has come back.

²⁸ He may kiss the reflection or shadow of the woman he wants, in a

---

²⁰ Now he tells how to kiss both lips at the same time. This can be done by a man to a woman, because her lips have no hair on them, and by a woman to a man who has not yet sprouted a beard. Otherwise, a mouthful of hair would destroy the pleasure.

²¹ Now he describes how to kiss the inside of the mouth, within the category of the 'bowl'.

²³ These kisses are for parts of the body other than the lips and the inside of the mouth. Kisses may be applied moderately, neither with pressure nor too gently, where the thighs join the torso, on the armpits, and on the chest; with pressure on the cheeks, the base of the armpits and the base of the navel; with curved lips on the forehead, chin, and around the armpits; and with just a gentle touch on the forehead and the eyes.

²⁴ Those same kisses take on other names according to the circumstances in which they are used.

be used on any place. ¹⁸ If it is curved and applied right up to the nipple of the breast, it becomes a 'tiger's claw'. ¹⁹ A 'line' facing toward the nipple, made by all five fingers facing one another, is the 'peacock's foot'. ²⁰ With a woman praised for her love-making, he uses the 'hare's leap', making five 'peacock's foot' scratches close together right on the nipple of her breast. ²¹ A mark in the form of a lotus leaf, on the upper part of the breast or around the hips, is called a 'lotus leaf'. ²² When a man is about to depart on a journey, he marks three or four lines on her thighs or on the upper part of her breasts, to make her remember him. Those are the ways of using the nails.

²³ And he may also make other scratches, in various forms. ²⁴ Scholars say: 'Because the things people can imagine are infinite, and there are infinite kinds of dexterity, and one can learn anything by practice and repetition, and passion is at the very heart of cutting with the nails, who could survey all the forms?' ²⁵ Vatsyayana says: For even passion demands variety. And it is through variety that partners inspire passion in one another. It is their infinite variety that makes courtesans de luxe and their lovers remain desirable to one another. Even in archery and in other martial arts, the textbooks insist on variety. How much more is this true of sex! ²⁶ But a man should not scratch marks of such variety on the wives of other men—except for special marks on concealed places, to increase their passion and make them remember.

> ²⁷ When a woman sees the scars
>   that nails have made on her hidden places,
>   her love even for someone given up long ago
>   becomes as tender as if it were brand new.
> ²⁸ When passions have been given up long ago,
>   love may disappear
>   unless there are wounds made by nails
>   to prompt memories of the abodes of passion.
> ²⁹ Passion and respect arise
>   even in another man who sees,
>   from a distance, a young girl
>   with the marks of nails cut into her breasts.

---

²³ He may make scratches in the various forms of a bird, flower, water-pot, leaf, creeper, and so forth.

²⁸ The seats of passion are beauty, youth, and good qualities.

³⁰ And a man who is marked
with the signs of nails in various places
generally disturbs a woman's mind
no matter how firm it may be.
³¹ There are no keener means
of increasing passion
than acts inflicted
with tooth and nail.

CHAPTER FIVE

Quality of Teeth

[11]   *Ways of Biting*

¹ The places for kissing are also for biting, except for the upper lip, the inside of the mouth, and the eyes. ² Teeth of good quality are even and of the right size, with a shiny, reflective surface, sharp edges, no chips, and the ability to retain colours. ³ Teeth of bad quality are blunt, marked with lines, rough, uneven, soft, broad, and separated by spaces. ⁴ The different kinds of biting are: the 'hidden', the 'swollen', the 'dot', the 'garland of dots', the 'coral and jewel', the 'garland of jewels', the 'scattered clouds', and the 'gnawing of the wild boar'.* ⁵ The 'hidden' bite is perceptible through a not-too-bloody, barely red mark, ⁶ and this becomes 'swollen' when it is done with force and pressure. ⁷ These two form a 'dot' when they are applied to the middle of the lower lip. ⁸ The 'swollen' bite and the 'coral and jewel' bite can be made on the cheek. ⁹ The 'earring kiss' and wounds made by both scratching and biting are adornments for the left cheek. ¹⁰ The 'coral and jewel' is so-called because it is made by

---

³¹ There is no keener means in the world, not even making love.

² The teeth retain colours from chewing betel leaf and so forth.

⁵ It is not too bloody because there is no wound; it is made with the tip of just one front tooth.

⁹ This mark beautifies the left cheek just like an earring.

¹⁰ The upper teeth (like a white jewel) and the lower lip (like red coral) press on the spot again and again without making a wound, but leaving a mark.

bringing the teeth and lip together repeatedly. [11] This same mark, repeated to form an ensemble, makes the 'garland of jewels'. [12] The 'dot' is so called because it is made on a very small patch of skin with a pincer formed by a pair of teeth. [13] And repeated to form an ensemble, it makes the 'garland of dots'. [14] Both of these 'garlands' can be made on the neck, armpit, or flanks, [15] but the 'garland of dots' can also be made on the forehead and thighs. [16] The 'scattered clouds', on the top of the breasts, form a kind of circle with uneven peaks. [17] The 'gnawing of the wild boar', only on the top of the breasts, is a series of many rows of long tooth-marks close together, with crimson between them. [18] The last two are only for two people whose sexual energy is fierce. Those are the ways of biting.

[19] When a man applies scratches, bites, and so forth to a forehead decoration, an earring, a bouquet of flowers, betel, or a sweet-smelling cinnamon bay-leaf used by the woman he wants, he is making advances.

[12]   *Customs from Different Regions*

[20] A man should treat a woman according to the nature of the region she comes from. [21] The women from central India are mostly noble-women with pure habits; they hate kissing, scratching, and biting, [22] and so do the women of Bahlika and Avantika, [23] though they are fond of unusual sexual acts. [24] Women from Malava and Abhira like embracing, kissing, scratching, biting, and sucking, and although they do not like to be wounded they can be won over by slaps. [25] The women who live in the land watered by the Indus and the other five rivers like oral sex. [26] The women of the West and of Lata are capable of fierce sexual energy, and they moan softly. [27] In the land where women rule,* and in Kosala, the women like to be slapped hard and generally use sex tools, for their sexual energy is very rough indeed. [28] The women of Andhra are delicate by nature but have coarse habits and are very fond of sexual ecstasy and impure delights. [29] The

---

[11] One mark is made, and then another right next to it, until it becomes a garland.

[25] The other five rivers are the Vipash, Shatadru, Iravati, Chandrabhaga, and Vitasta.

women of Maharashtra are aroused by all of the sixty-four tech-niques, enjoy dirty, coarse talk, and take the initiative impetuously in bed. [30] The women of the city are just like that, but they reveal it only in private. [31] And when Dravidian women are stimulated with fore-play they only very slowly become wet. [32] The women of Vanavasa have average sexual energy and will endure everything, but they hide their bodies, laugh at other people's bodies, and cannot abide any-thing objectionable, dirty, or rough. [33] The women of Gauda speak delicately, have delicate bodies, and tend to fall in love.

[34] Suvarnanabha says, 'The nature of the individual is more important than the nature of the region.' Local customs are not relevant to this matter. [35] And in the course of time, practices, styles of clothing, and games move from one region to another; and a person should know that, too. [36] In the list that begins with close embraces, each kindles more passion than the one that follows but is more commonly used.

[37] Whatever wound a man inflicts on a woman,
      even when she tries to restrain him and cannot bear it,
      she should do that very thing to him
      twice as hard.
[38] The response to a 'dot' is a 'garland',
      and to a 'garland', a 'scattered cloud'.
      Pretending to be angry, this is how
      a woman picks a quarrel.
[39] She grabs him by the hair
      and bends down his face and drinks from his mouth;
      she pounces on him and bites him
      here and there, crazed with passion.

---

[30] The women of the city are the daughters of Pataliputra.

[31] Before a man enters a woman of Karnataka, he stimulates her with embraces and so forth, both externally and internally. Then her limbs relax and she very slowly emits a very little bit of fluid, but she does not faint with sensual pleasure, for she never becomes intoxicated. But then, at the end, she is carried away by her sexual energy and ejaculates. And she spends her passion through just that one sexual act.

[36] The list of the six external actions is: embracing, kissing, scratching, biting, slapping and moaning. Unusual acts are twisted acts.

⁴⁰Resting on the chest of the man she loves,
   she raises his head and bites him on the neck
   with the 'garland of jewels'
   or any other bite she knows.
⁴¹When she sees the man, even in the daytime,
   in the midst of a group of people, displaying the mark
   that she herself made on him, she laughs,
   unnoticed by the others.
⁴²Then, pretending to wrinkle her face,
   and pretending to rebuke the man,
   as if in jealousy, she displays
   the marks made on her own body.
⁴³When two people behave in this way
   with modesty and concern for one another's feelings,
   their love will never wane,
   not even in a hundred years.

[handwritten marginal note: How is that modest?]

CHAPTER SIX

[13]   *Varieties of Sexual Positions*

¹At the moment of passion, in a coupling where the man is larger
than the woman, a 'doe' positions herself in such a way as to stretch
herself open inside. ²And in a coupling where the man is smaller, an
'elephant cow' contracts herself inside. ³Where the union is in

---

⁴¹ She laughs, thinking, 'This is a fitting punishment for that wicked
   man.' She is unnoticed both by the others and by him.
⁴² Pretending to wrinkle her face, she puckers up her mouth as if to give a
   kiss, but does not give it; pretending to rebuke the man, she gives a
   signal by raising her brows and rolling her eyes.
¹ At the moment of passion, when the penis is erect, she positions herself
   so that his penis and her sexual organ can join together.
² She contracts by squeezing her thighs together, to pucker up the mouth
   of her vagina.
³ With no need either to contract or to extend, the back of her vagina
   remains flat.

harmony, she just lies flat on her back. [4] What has been said of these two women also applies to the 'mare'. [5] As she is doing this, the woman receives the man inside her. [6] Sex tools may also be used, especially in a coupling where the man is smaller than the woman.

[7] A 'doe' generally has three positions to choose from: the 'wide open', the 'yawning', or the 'Junoesque'. [8] Her head thrown down, her pelvis raised up, she is 'wide open'. [9] This position must allow a way for the man to slide back. [10] Without lowering her thighs, suspending them while spreading them wide apart, she receives him in the 'yawning' position. [11] Parting her thighs around his sides, at the same time she pulls her knees back around her own sides, in the

---

[4] The 'mare', too, stretches when she makes love with a 'stallion' in the coupling with a larger man, contracts when she makes love with a 'hare', and remains the same in an equal coupling, with a 'bull'.

[5] In all three sexual positions—contracting, extending, or flat on her back—she receives him when his penis is not yet inside her.

[6] In an equal coupling, the woman neither contracts nor expands to receive an artificial penis that resembles the penis itself, and even if it is larger than the penis, she can expand to receive it. If he is larger than she is, there is no need for sex tools.

[7] In an equal coupling, the general practice is learned from talk, not from texts. For people generally say that there is a difference between the way they do it in the country and in the city, two ways for the woman to position herself when she is flat on her back. And so it is said:

> The country way: the woman places her thighs
> on the thighs of her seated lover;
> the city way: the two lotus feet of the woman
> stand on the thighs of the man.

[9] When she is making love with the man's penis inside her, she should slide back with her hips; or when the man is making love with her he should slide back little by little, so that they do not press together too tightly. For if he moves inside her too roughly, she can be injured, and the man's foreskin can be torn off, which physicians call 'ruptured foreskin.'

[11] She puts her thighs around his sides, so that her shins closely embrace his thighs, and places her knees around her own sides, on the area below her armpits. And in this way, grasping her thighs with her upper arms and keeping them in place, she opens more widely than before. This, too, must allow a way for him to slide back.

'Junoesque'* position, which can only be done with practice. [12] This position can also be used in the coupling in which the man is largest.

[13] She receives him with the 'cup' in a coupling when the man is smaller, [14] and even in the coupling when he is smallest. An 'elephant cow' [15] may use the 'cup', the 'squeeze', the 'circle', and the 'mare's trap'. [16] In the 'cup', both partners stretch out both of their two legs straight. [17] There are two variants: the 'cup lying on the side' or 'the cup supine', according to the way the act is done. [18] But if he is lying on his side, he should have the woman lie on her right side; this applies to everyone.* [19] If, as soon as he has penetrated her in the 'cup', he squeezes her two thighs together tightly, it becomes the 'squeeze'. [20] If she then crosses her thighs, it becomes the 'circle'. [21] In the 'mare's trap', which can only be done with practice, she grasps him, like a mare, so tightly that he cannot move.* [22] This is generally

---

[12] A 'doe' can use the 'Junoesque' position not only with a 'bull', but also with a 'stallion'. Moreover, in the 'wide open' and 'yawning' positions, too, a 'doe' can receive a 'bull', and with those same two positions a 'mare', too, can receive a 'stallion'.

[13] With the 'cup', an 'elephant cow' can receive a 'bull'.

[14] An 'elephant cow' can even receive a 'hare' and, as can be inferred from the previous passage, a 'mare' can also receive a 'hare'.

[16] They stretch out in such a way that he can penetrate her.

[17] How does he penetrate her in this position? It is so easy that there is nothing to worry about!* But Katyayana describes the 'cup' somewhat differently:

> The man's hips press on the thighs of the woman,
> whose breasts crush against him
> as he faces her, making a human triangle.
> This is what is traditionally called the 'cup'.

And so he says: Because the thighs are held tightly, the vagina does not contract. And so it should not be used on an 'elephant cow', in a coupling where the man is smaller, but in equal couplings, as in the common practice in which the thighs are positioned naturally.

[18] In order to sleep, all women, 'does' and so forth, lie on their right side, and the man lies on his left side. But at the time of sexual pleasure, it is just the opposite: he lies down on his right side so that he can use his left hand to touch her hidden places.

[19] He does this with either the 'cup lying on the side' or the 'cup supine'.

[21] She grasps his penis with the 'cup' formed by the lips of her vagina.

employed among the women of Andhra. Those are the forms of the sexual positions according to the followers of Babhravya.

²³ Now for those of Suvarnanabha: ²⁴ When both thighs of the woman are raised, it is called the 'curve'. ²⁵ When the man holds her legs up, it is the 'yawn'. ²⁶ When he does that but also flexes her legs at the knees, it is the 'high-squeeze'. ²⁷ When he does that but stretches out one of her feet, it is the 'half-squeeze'. ²⁸ When one of her feet is placed on the man's shoulder and the other is stretched out, and they alternate again and again, this is called 'splitting the bamboo'. ²⁹ When one of her legs is raised above her head and the other leg is stretched out, it is called 'impaling on a stake', and can only be done with practice. ³⁰ When both of her legs are flexed at the knees and placed on her own abdomen, it is the 'crab'. ³¹ When her thighs are raised and crossed, it is the 'squeeze'. ³² When she opens her knees and crosses her calves, it is the 'lotus seat'. ³³ When he turns around with his back to her, and she embraces his back, that is called 'rotating', and can only be done with practice.*

³⁴ Suvarnanabha says: 'One can practise the more unusual techniques in water—standing, sitting, or lying down—because it is easier that way.' ³⁵ Vatsyayana says: But this is forbidden, because learned men do not include it in the tradition.*

---

²³ These are the positions described by Suvarnanabha for an 'elephant cow'.

²⁴ The woman, on her back, raises both thighs, pressed closely together. And the man, on his left knee, embraces her with his two thighs and moves inside her; her thighs are raised so that he does not slip out.

²⁵ He places the woman's knees on his shoulders.

²⁶ The man places her two feet on his chest, and, encircling her neck with the noose made of his arms, he moves inside her. Her two feet, with the legs bent above them, remain on his chest and do not slip down.

²⁹ Placing her left leg on the man's shoulder, after just a moment she lowers her right leg and stretches it out; this is the first position. Then, in alternation, she places her right leg on his shoulder and stretches out the left.

³⁰ The crab moves with its front feet bent like that.

³¹ It is called the 'squeeze' because it squeezes her vagina.

³³ The man enters her and, without pulling out, turns around his upper body, turning his back to her while making love.

[14] *Unusual Sexual Acts*

[36] The following are unusual sexual acts. [37] Two young people lean against a wall or a pillar or one another and embrace standing up. This is called, 'sex standing up'. [38] He leans against a wall, and she throws the noose of her arms tightly around his neck and sits on the cage made by his two hands clasped together; she wraps the noose of her thighs around his pelvis in a circle and swings from one side to the other by shifting from one foot to the other on the wall. This is called 'sex suspended'. [39] When she gets on the ground on all fours and he mounts her like a bull, that is 'sex like a cow'. [40] In this position, he does on her back the things that he usually does to her chest. [41] He may also consider various other special matings of this sort, not previously mentioned, imitating the behaviour of a dog, stag, or billygoat, the donkey's assault, the cat's pounce, the tiger's spring, the elephant's crush, the boar's friction, or the stallion's mounting.

[42] With two women who are fond of one another, it is 'sex in a cluster'. [43] Done with many women, it is 'sex with a herd of cows'. [44] Water sports, and sex in the manner of a goat or in the manner of a stag, imitate the acts of animals. [45] In regions where there are villages

---

[37] The woman leans against a wall or a pillar, and her partner leans on her.

[42] This is sex with two women who trust one another and one man. On one bed, the man can make love simultaneously with a pair of women. For all the while he is quenching the passion of one woman by moving inside her, he awakens the passion of the other woman at the very same time, by kissing her and so forth. And then he slakes the passion of that woman and re-awakens the passion of the one whose passion he has just extinguished.

[43] One man making love with many women who are fond of one another is like a bull in a herd of cows.

[44] A man can take his pleasure with women in the water like an elephant with elephant cows. And just as one man can have sex with two women or many women, so a woman can have sex with two men or many men. For 'sex in a cluster' also intends to indicate sex between one woman and a cluster of men, such as two men embraced by one woman playing the man's part. And in 'sex with a herd of bulls', one woman acts like a cow with a herd of men as bulls.

of women, or where women rule, and in the region of Bahlika, many young men serve each woman sexually, as if they were her harem. [46] They pleasure her one by one or all together, according to what suits her temperament and is feasible. [47] One of the men holds her, while another uses her sexually: one between her legs, another in her mouth, yet another on the middle of her body, and they do these things by turns, alternating, one after the other. [48] Like such a woman, a courtesan has sexual relationships with an entire company of men, and men are said to provide sexual services for the women who belong to the king.*

[49] The people in the South indulge in 'sex below', even in the anus. Those are the unusual sexual acts.

[50] We will describe a man's sexual strokes in the discussion of the woman playing the man's part.

[51] And there are two verses about this:
> A man who understands the heart should
> enlarge his repertory of techniques for sexual ecstasy
> by this means and that, imitating the amorous movements
> of tame animals, wild animals, and birds.

[52] When these various erotic moods are evoked
> according to the particular nature of the woman
> and of her region, they inspire
> women's affection, passion, and respect.

CHAPTER SEVEN

[15]   *Modes of Slapping* and
[16]   *The Accompanying Moaning*

[1] They say that sex is a form of quarrelling, because the very essence of desire is argument, and its character is perverse. [2] Therefore a part of sex is slapping—on the shoulders, on the head, between the breasts, on the back, between the legs, and on the sides—[3] in four ways: with the back of the hand, the outstretched hand, the fist, or the flat palm of the hand.

[4] Moaning arises out of this, since it expresses pain, and moaning takes several forms. [5] There are eight kinds of screaming:

that is dangerous. [28] The King of the Cholas killed Chitrasena, a courtesan de luxe, by using the 'wedge' during sex. [29] And the Kuntala king Shatakarni Shatavahana killed his queen, Malayavati, by using the 'scissor'. [30] Naradeva, whose hand was deformed, blinded a dancing-girl in one eye by using the 'drill' clumsily.* [31] And there are verses about this:

> This is no matter for numerical lists
> or textbook tables of contents.
> For people joined in sexual ecstasy,
> passion is what makes things happen.
> [32] The emotions and fantasies
> conjured up in a moment
> in the midst of sexual chaos
> cannot be imagined even in dreams.
> [33] For, just as a horse in full gallop,
> blinded by the energy of his own speed,
> pays no attention to any post
> or hole or ditch on the path,
> so two lovers blinded by passion
> in the friction of sexual battle,
> are caught up in their fierce energy

---

[28] He embraced Chitrasena so tightly, at the start of their love-making, that she suffered greatly, because she was so delicate. And even when he realized her condition, and knew that she had to be handled delicately, he was so blind with passion that he did not take account of his own strength and destroyed her by using a 'wedge' on her chest.

[29] Shatakarna's son Shatavahana, born in the territory of Kuntala, saw his queen, Malayavati, one day when she had not long recovered from an illness and did not have her full strength, but was dressing for the festival of Kama. Passion arose in him and he made love to her, but his mind was carried away by passion and by using an excessively powerful 'scissor' on her chest, he killed her.

[30] Naradeva was the general of the Pandya king. His hand had been deformed by a blow from a sword. When he saw Chitralekha, a dancing girl, dancing at the king's residence, his passion was aroused, and when he made love with her, blind with passion, he used the 'drill' clumsily because of his lame hand; he missed her cheek and instead hit her eye, blinding her in that eye. The 'tongs' is not mentioned here, because by its very nature it is not too dangerous.

and pay no attention to danger.

³⁴ And so a man who understands the text
will apply it only after he has come to know
the delicacy, ferocity, and strength of his young woman,
and his own strength.

³⁵ The sexual techniques cannot be used
at all times and on all women.
The method must be chosen according to
the part of the body, the region, and the time.

[handwritten annotation: ROLE OF REGION]

CHAPTER EIGHT

[17]   *The Woman Playing the Man's Part*

¹ When she sees that the man has become exhausted by continuous repetition, but that his passion is still not quenched, she may, with his permission, roll him under her and give him some help by playing the man's part herself. ² Or she can do it out of her own desire to do something she has only imagined doing, ³ or to satisfy the man's erotic curiosity. ⁴ To play the man's part, when he is inside her, she gets on top and puts him underneath her. In this way they can make love continually without interrupting the flow of love-making. This is one way of doing it. ⁵ The second way is to begin again and let her do this from the very start. ⁶ With the flowers from her hair strewn

---

³⁵ As for the part of the body: the place between the breasts can be slapped with the back of the hand, the head slapped with the outstretched hand, and so forth. As for the region: slapping is for a woman from Malava, oral sex for a woman from Abhira, and so forth. And as for the time: when he is inside her, he can slap her with the back of his hand; when she is seated on his lap, he can slap her with his fist, and so forth.

⁵ There is no third way. In the interval, he withdraws his penis, and then she begins from the very start in the man's part.

⁶ Her breathing is hard because of the unaccustomed activity and her exhaustion. She joins her face to his, and bends her head down, in shame, not in order to kiss or bite him. She uses the 'embrace of breasts' [2.2.25]. All of this activity is said to be done with a woman's natural talent [2.7.22]. The acts he demonstrated before are acts that he executed with roughness and ferocity, the man's natural talent; she now

about, her laughter interrupted by her hard breathing, pressing his chest hard with her breasts to join her face to his, bending her head down again and again, she does to him in return now whatever acts he demonstrated before. She says, 'You threw me down, and now I am throwing you down in return', laughing at him and threatening him and hitting him. And, at the same time, she indicates that she is embarrassed and exhausted and wishes to stop. She moves on him with precisely the sexual strokes* of a man. ⁷We will explain these:*

[18]   *A Man's Sexual Strokes*

⁸When the woman is lying on the bed, the man distracts her attention, as it were, with conversation and loosens her waistband. If she argues against this, he overwhelms her by kissing her cheeks. ⁹When he becomes hard, he touches her here and there. ¹⁰If it is the first time that they have been together, he caresses her between her tightly closed thighs. ¹¹And if she is a virgin, ¹²he caresses her

---

does these acts against the current of her own natural talent. She hits him hard, with the back of her hand and so forth, demonstrating her ferocity. And so, in order to express the woman's natural talent, even though she is not embarrassed, nor exhausted, and does not wish to stop, she indicates that she is embarrassed and exhausted and wishes to stop.

'Playing the man's part' (*purushayitva*) takes two forms, external and internal. This passage explains the first kind, the behaviour of a woman acting like a man (*purusha*). But 'playing the man's part' also refers to a man's sexual strokes (*purusha-upasarpanam*), and a woman can do these, too. When the man is the active one it is called 'a man's sexual strokes' and when a woman is the active one it is called 'playing the man's part'.

⁷ There are two kinds of sexual strokes of a man, external and internal. To describe the external strokes, he says the next passage.

⁹ He becomes hard because his passion is aroused. If her passion, too, is aroused, the action can succeed. But if not, then to arouse her passion, he touches the woman with his hand, on her armpits, thighs, breasts, and so forth.

¹⁰ Her thighs are tightly pressed together out of embarrassment; he caresses them to make her open them.

¹¹ Her breasts are tightly pressed together by the corset made of her arms.

breasts, which she has tightly pressed together, and her hands, armpits, shoulders, and neck. [13]If she is a loose woman, he does what is suitable and feasible. He catches hold of her by her hair, mercilessly, to kiss her, and cups his fingers to grasp her chin. [14]This embarrasses his partner and makes her close her eyes if it is the first time they have been together, or if she is a virgin. [15]And thinking, 'How can I arouse her passion for me?' he observes what she does when they are united in love-making. [16]When he is moving inside her, and her eyes roll when she feels him in certain spots, he presses her in just those spots.* Suvarnanabha says, 'This is the secret of young women.' [17]The signs that a woman is reaching her climax are that her limbs become limp, her eyes close, she loses all sense of shame, and she takes him deeper and deeper inside her. [18]She flails her hands about, sweats, bites, will not let him get up, kicks him, and continues to move over the man even after he has finished making love. [19]Before

---

[13] A loose woman is one whose boldness is full-blown and who does whatever she wants, indulging in sex without shame. The meaning here is that she is the one who makes the advances.

[15] Now he describes the internal sexual strokes of a man. When he is inside her making love, he observes how she moves in reaction to the external sexual strokes in order to determine how to stroke her with the internal ones.

[16] When she feels his penis moving in a certain spot inside her vagina, the pleasure of that touch makes her eyes whirl around in a circle; he strokes her with his penis very hard on that very spot, and from that pressure she quickly achieves her sexual ecstasy. This remains secret because women do not make it known. There is some argument about this. Some people say that, when the man is stroking inside her, whatever place the woman looks at, either specifically or vaguely, that is the place where he should press her. Others say that, if she looks at many places, he should press her in one place after another. Or, whatever place she looks at very hard is the place where he should press her very hard.

[17] She takes him very deeply inside her by attaching her sexual organ to his extremely closely, and that is a sign that she has reached her climax or is very close.

[18] The sign of a climax that has been ignited (but not quenched) is that, when the man has reached his climax, she is still active with her own vagina.

Animal analogues

he enters her, he puts his hand, like an elephant's trunk, inside her and agitates her until she becomes soft and wet, and then he enters her.

²⁰ A man's sexual strokes are 'moving around', 'churning', the 'dagger', 'grinding down', 'pressing', the 'blast of wind', the 'boar's thrust', the 'bull's thrust', 'frolicking like a sparrow', and the 'cup'. ²¹ Regular, straight sex is called 'moving around'. ²² When he takes his sexual organ in his hand and rotates it in all directions, it is called 'churning'. ²³ When he lowers her pelvis and thrusts into her from above, it is called 'the dagger'. ²⁴ When he raises her pelvis and thrusts into her from below, violently, it is called 'grinding down'. ²⁵ When he stabs her deeply and remains there, pressing her, for a long time, that is called 'pressing'. ²⁶ When he pulls out quite far and then plunges down into her fast and hard, it is called the 'blast of wind'. ²⁷ When he reams her many times just on one side, that is the 'boar's thrust'. ²⁸ When he does this to both sides, alternating, it is the 'bull's thrust'. ²⁹ When he enters her once and, without pulling out entirely, thrusts into her two, three, four times, and does this

---

¹⁹ He notices how she is moving before he enters her, and realizes that if he himself reaches his climax first, then the emotional flow of her climax will be interrupted. Women's vaginas are said to be of four kinds:

> The best part of a woman
> is like a lotus petal to touch inside,
> or like a small globe, or wrinkled,
> or rough as a cow's tongue.

All but the first kind need to be agitated because the itch is so extensive. For when her vagina has become soft and wet, she reaches her climax quickly once he moves around inside her. Thus it is said:

> The ring finger and the index finger,
> joined with the middle finger closely at the tip,
> form an artifice so like the tip of an elephant's trunk
> that people have given it that name.

²² He rotates his penis deep inside her vagina, as if he were churning.

²³ He lowers her hips and thrusts from above into the top part of the inside of her vagina, with his penis like a dagger.

²⁴ He thrusts from below into the lower part of her vagina, violently, because the itch is most extensive in the lower part of the vagina.

²⁵ He penetrates with his penis right to the very root, continuing for as long as the penis is able to rise up and sink down.

repeatedly, it is called 'frolicking like a sparrow'. [30] The 'cup', which has been described, is the method used when passion is ending.* [31] A man should choose from these sexual strokes and use the one particularly suited for each woman.

[32] But when the woman plays the man's part, there are, in addition, the 'tongs', the 'spinning top', and the 'swing'. [33] When she grasps him in the 'mare's trap' position and draws him more deeply into her or contracts around him and holds him there for a long time, that is the 'tongs'. [34] When she keeps him inside her and twists around him like a wheel around an axle, that is called the 'spinning top', and can only be done with practice.* [35] When she is doing this, her partner thrusts up his own pelvis under her. [36] When she twists around him while swinging her pelvis back and forth in all directions, that is the 'swing'.* [37] She may rest, with him still firmly within her, by laying her forehead on his forehead. [38] And when she has rested, the man turns over on top again. That is how the woman plays the man's part.

[39] And there are verses about this:

> Even when a sensual woman
> covers up her own feelings and hides her signals,
> she unveils her own feelings completely
> when her passion drives her to get on top.

[40] A man can learn everything
> —a woman's personality,
> what sort of sex excites her—
> from the ways she moves on top.

[41] But he should not make a woman act the man's part

---

[30] This is the time of the actual state of ejaculation.

[33] She uses the lips of the vagina as a tongs.

[34] With his penis inside her vagina, she bends her knees to put her feet on the man's chest and whirls around like a potter's wheel, supporting her body with her hands.

[35] To make it easier for her to do the 'spinning top', and to keep his penis from slipping out, the man raises his own pelvis upward.

[36] She swings forward and back, and from side to side. But if she twists around in a full circle, it is a variation of 'churning'.

[37] She does this so that his penis does not slip out of her, when passion is not yet extinguished.

[41] If she has her period, she may not conceive; or, on the other hand, if the

if she has her period, or has recently given birth,
or if she is a 'doe' woman, or pregnant,
or very fat.

꜀꜀꜀

CHAPTER NINE

[19]   *Oral Sex*

[1] There are two sorts of persons of the third nature, in the form of a woman and in the form of a man. [2] The one in the form of a woman imitates a woman's dress, chatter, grace, emotions, delicacy, timidity, innocence, frailty, and bashfulness. [3] The act that should be done in the sexual organ is done in her mouth, and they call that 'oral sex'.* [4] She gets her sexual pleasure and erotic arousal as well as her livelihood from this, [5] living like a courtesan. That is the person of the third nature in the form of a woman.

[6] The one in the form of a man, however, conceals her desire when she wants a man and makes her living as a masseur. [7] As she massages the man, she caresses his two thighs with her limbs, as if she were embracing him. [8] Then she becomes more boldly intimate and familiar and touches the places where his thighs join his torso, and his sexual organ. [9] If she notices that he has become hard as a result of this, she stimulates him by using her hand as a churn, pretending to tease him about how easily he becomes excited and laughing at him. [10] If the man does not urge her on, even when he has given this clear sign and even when it is obvious that he is aroused, she makes advances to him

------

man gets on top again and she does conceive, a little boy and little girl may be born with reversed natures.* If she has recently given birth, uterine blood may flow out. If she is a 'doe', a 'bull' or 'stallion' may split her apart. If she is pregnant, she may have a miscarriage. And if she is very fat, it is not possible for her to make active sexual strokes.

[9] She teases him, saying, 'You are so easy to excite, you get an erection just from being touched on your thighs!'

[10] If he does not say, 'Excite me with your mouth', despite the clear sign of an erection caused by being touched where the thighs join the torso and on the penis, and when it is known that he can be excited by oral sex, she makes advances without being urged on.

on her own. [11] If the man urges her to go on, she argues with him and only unwillingly continues.

[12] Oral sex involves eight acts, one after the other: [13] the 'casual', 'biting the sides', 'the outer tongs', 'the inner tongs', 'kissing', 'polishing', 'sucking the mango', and 'swallowing'. [14] As she finishes each one, she expresses her wish to stop, [15] and when each one is finished, the man asks her to do the next one, and when that one is finished, the one after that. [16] In the 'casual' act, she holds it with her hand, places it on her lips, pierces her mouth with it and moves it back and forth. [17] She bares the glans with her hand, nibbles at its sides with her two lips, keeping her teeth away, and she tantalizes him by saying, 'This is as far I as go.' That is 'biting the sides'. [18] When the man urges her to do more, she closes her lips, presses them down on the glans and kisses him as if drawing it out. That is called 'the outer tongs'. [19] Begging her to go on doing this, he pushes a little deeper into her mouth, and she squeezes the glans with her lips and then spits it out. That is called 'the inner tongs'. [20] Then she holds it in her hand and grasps it as if it were his lip. That is 'kissing'. [21] After she has done that, she licks it all over with the tip of her tongue and then pierces the glans. That is called 'polishing'. [22] When it is in precisely this state, driven halfway inside her mouth through the force of passion, she mercilessly presses down, and presses down again, and lets it go. That is called 'sucking the mango'. [23] Only when the man asks for it does she swallow it up and press until the climax. That is called 'swallowing'. [24] Groaning and slapping may also be

---

[16] She holds it with her hand to keep it from bending down, forms her lips into a ring, and pierces her mouth with the tip of it.

[17] She makes her hand into a fist.

[18] When he urges her to bite the sides, or to do something else, she closes her lips around the glans. Then she sucks it out and releases it again, using her lips like a tongs outside the foreskin.

[19] When she is performing the 'outer tongs', he presses further inside her mouth. This is the 'inner tongs' because her mouth acts like a tongs on the glans without its sheath.

[20] Once it is no longer covered by the foreskin, she grasps it as she would grasp his lower lip with her two lips.

[21] She pierces the glans, on the opening hole, with the tip of her tongue.

[22] In this state, the glans is no longer covered by the foreskin.

used, as they are called for. That is oral sex with a person of the third nature.

²⁵ Promiscuous women, loose women, servant girls, and masseuses also perform oral sex. ²⁶ Scholars say: 'But it should not be done, because it is opposed by the moral code and is not done in proper society, and because if a man has contact again with the mouth of these women, he himself may be troubled.' ²⁷ But Vatsyayana says: This is not a mistake for a man who loves courtesans, though it should also be avoided for other reasons. ²⁸ Therefore people in the East do not make love with women who practise oral sex. ²⁹ And the people of Ahichattra do not make love with courtesans, but when they do, they avoid the act of the mouth with these women. ³⁰ The men of Saketa do not worry about anything when they make love. ³¹ The

---

²⁶ It is forbidden by *dharma* texts: 'Do not ejaculate in a mouth.' For if he performs in the mouth of one of these women (the promiscuous woman and the others) the act that should be done in the vagina, then, at the time when the act is done in the vagina, if he again touches her mouth, in the throes of passion, he himself will be disturbed, saying, 'I have been debauched', but the woman will not be disturbed by this.

²⁷ Promiscuous women and so forth are varieties of courtesans. Oral sex is not a mistake on the grounds of being opposed by the moral code. It is, however, a mistake to have oral sex with one's wife. As Vasishtha says:

> 'But a man who copulates
> in the mouth of his wife
> causes his ancestors to starve
> for fifteen years.'*

But it should be avoided for other reasons: because it is not done in proper society, because of the dangers involved in contact with the mouth, because it is done secretly, and because one also eats food with the mouth. But it might not be a mistake for someone according to the customs of a particular region, and therefore might not have to be avoided.

²⁹ Even though they have never seen or heard of oral sex, they still imagine it among these women. When they do somehow make love with these women, in the throes of passion, they avoid the act of the mouth with them, that is, kissing them.

³⁰ In making love or doing the act of the mouth with courtesans, they do not think about what is pure and not pure.

³¹ The city is Pataliputra.

men of the city* do not indulge in oral sex themselves, [32] but the people of Surasena do everything, without the slightest hesitation. [33] For this is what they say: 'For who can have any faith in women's good character, purity, good behaviour, good practices, reliability, or words? For by their very nature they have a dirty gaze, but they need not be rejected. Therefore the religious tradition tells us to regard them as pure. And so they say:

> "A calf is unpolluted while the milk is flowing,
>   as is a dog when it catches a wild animal,
>   a bird when it knocks down a fruit,
>   and a woman's mouth in the ecstasy of sex." '*

[34] Vatsyayana says: Since learned men disagree and there are discrepancies in what the religious texts say, one should act according to the custom of the region and one's own disposition and confidence.

[35] And there are verses about this:

> Even young men, servants
>   who wear polished earrings,
>   indulge in oral sex
>   only with certain men.
> [36] And, in the same way, certain men-about-town
>   who care for one another's welfare
>   and have established trust
>   do this service for one another.
> [37] Sometimes men even perform
>   this act upon women,
>   transposing the procedure
>   for kissing a mouth.

---

[32] They do everything: love-making, oral sex, and the act of the mouth.

[36] Certain men-about-town, the ones who are practically women, take one another, in friendship, and give one another the sensual pleasure of ejaculation. They say, 'You do it for me now, and I will do it for you later.' Or both of them do it at the same time, by turning their bodies head to foot, losing all sense of time because of their passion. Thus there are two ways of doing it. Women, too, can do this. As it is said:

> 'Certain women in the harem,
>   unable to get any tools,
>   trusting in one another, excite one another
>   with their mouth on the vagina.'

³⁸ Sometimes a man and woman may turn their bodies
head to foot, so that they can make love
to one another at the same time;
and that is known as 'sex in the manner of crows.'*

³⁹ It is for this that courtesans
reject virtuous, clever, generous men,
and become attached to scoundrels,
servants, elephant-drivers, and so forth.

⁴⁰ But a wise Brahmin, or a minister of state
or a man on whom the king depends
or any man in whom people confide,
should not indulge in oral sex.

⁴¹ For the statement that 'There is a text for this'
does not justify a practice. People should realize
that the contents of the texts apply in general,
but each actual practice is for one particular region.

⁴² Medical science, for example,
recommends cooking even dog meat,
for juice and virility;
but what intelligent person would eat it?

⁴³ There are some men,
and there are certain sorts of regions,
and there are times when
these practices are not without their uses.

⁴⁴ Therefore, when a man has considered
the region, and the time, and the technique,
and the textbook teachings, and himself,
he may—or may not—make use of these practices.

⁴⁵ But because this matter is secret,
and because the mind and heart are fickle,
who could know who should do what,
and when and how?

---

³⁸ At the same moment, each has a mouth on the sexual organ of the other. The man and the woman are like crows because they are taking something unclean in the mouth.

⁴³ These practices, of oral sex, can be done just like kissing a mouth.

⁴⁵ Oral sex is secret, and people are especially fickle when passion is involved.

CHAPTER TEN

[20]   *The Start and Finish of Sex*

[1] In a room of his house dedicated to sex, a room decorated, full of flowers, and fragrant with perfume and incense, the man-about-town, surrounded by his friends and servants, receives the woman, when she has bathed and adorned herself and has drunk the proper amount; he puts her at ease and offers her another drink. [2] He sits down on her right side and touches her hair, the fringe of her sari, and the knot of her waistband. He embraces her gently with his left arm to prepare to make love.

> [3] They talk together about things
>   that they have done together before,
>   joking and titillating, touching upon
>   all sorts of things hidden and obscene.

[4] Then there may be singing and instrumental music, with or without dancing, and conversation about the fine arts, and then he entices her with another drink. [5] When her feelings for him have been aroused, he sends away the other people, giving them flowers, scented oils, and betel, and when they are alone together he makes advances to her with the embraces and so forth that have already been described, beginning with loosening the knot of her waistband. And that is the beginning of sex.

[6] As for the end of sex, when their passion has ebbed, the man and woman go out separately to the bathing place, embarrassed, not looking at one another, as if they were not even acquainted with one another. When they return, they sit down in their usual places without embarrassment, and chew some betel, and he himself rubs sandalwood paste or some other scented oil on her body. [7] He embraces her with his left arm and, holding a cup in his hand, persuades her to drink. Or both of them may drink some water or eat some bite-sized snacks or something else, according to their temperament and inclination: [8] fruit juice, grilled foods, sour rice-broth, soups with small pieces of roasted meats, mangoes, dried meat, citrus fruits with sugar, according to the tastes of the region. As he tastes each one he

---

[4] The remaining arts are sketching and so forth.

tells her, 'This one is sweet' or 'delicate' or 'soft', and offers it to her. ⁹Sometimes they sit on the rooftop porch to enjoy the moonlight, and tell stories that suit their mood. As she lies in his lap, looking at the moon, he points out the rows of the constellations to her; they look at the Pleiades, the Pole Star, and the garland of Seven Sages that form the Great Bear. That is the end of sex.

¹⁰And there are these verses about this:

> Even at the end, love
>   enhanced by thoughtful acts
>   and words and deeds exchanged in confidence
>   gives rise to the highest ecstasy.
> ¹¹Responding to their feelings about themselves,
>   inspiring mutual love,
>   at one moment turning away in anger,
>   at another moment looking with love,
> ¹²they play the 'plough-handle' game, sing,
>   and dance in the Lata way;
>   they look at the circle of the moon
>   with eyes moist and flickering with passion.
> ¹³They talk about it all, about the desires they felt
>   when they first saw one another long ago,
>   and the unhappiness they felt
>   when they were later separated.
>   And when they finish talking
>   they embrace and kiss with passion.
>   Through these and other feelings
>   the young couple's passion grows again.

[21]   *Different Kinds of Sex*

¹⁴The different kinds of sex are 'passionate sex', 'excitable passion', 'artificial passion', 'transferred passion', 'sex with a coarse servant', 'sex with a peasant', and 'unfettered sex'. ¹⁵When the passion of a

---

¹² It is said of the 'plough-handle' (*Hallishaka*):

> The 'plough-handle' is a dance
> with the women in a circle
> and one man the leader,
> like Krishna with the cow-herd women.*

man and a woman grows great from the moment that they see one another, and they get together only with great effort, or one of them returns after a long journey, or they reunite after a separation caused by a quarrel—that is 'passionate sex'; [16] this kind of sex goes on according to their inclination, until the climax. [17] When two people begin with average passion but then become more passionate toward one another, that is an 'excitable passion'; [18] in this kind of sex, the man stimulates the passion, kindling it and rekindling it with those of the sixty-four techniques that suit their inclinations. [19] When two people make love for the sake of a particular goal or are attached to others, that is an 'artificial passion'; [20] in this kind of sex, the man employs all together the techniques learned from the textbooks. [21] But when a man, placing in his mind another woman who is dear to his heart, superimposes or transfers her onto his actual partner from the moment he begins to make love until he reaches a climax, that is a 'transferred passion'. [22] 'Sex with a coarse servant'* takes place with a lower-class female water-carrier or house-servant, until the climax; [23] in this kind of sex, he does not bother with the acts of civility. [24] Similarly, 'sex with a peasant' takes place between a courtesan and a country bumpkin, until the climax, [25] or between a man-about-town and women from the countryside, cow-herding villages, or countries beyond the borders. [26] 'Unfettered sex' takes place between two people who trust one another, since each does whatever the other likes. Those are the different kinds of sex.

---

[18] The man stimulates both his own passion and the woman's.

[19] Their particular goal might be to gain something, or to reverse a loss, but they are not acting out of passion. The woman may be attached to another man, and the man to another woman.

[21] A woman can do this too.

[22] A coarse servant is a 'non-male' who has the characteristics of both sexes.

[24] This is similar to the kind of sex just described because it, too, involves sex with someone quite unlike the man.

[22]   *Lovers' Quarrels*

²⁷ Now, a woman who has grown fond of a man cannot bear it if he utters the name of a co-wife or casually refers to her or accidentally calls the woman by the other woman's name,* or if the man plays her false. ²⁸ Then there is a great quarrel, with weeping, anguish, tossing hair, slaps, falling from the bed or chair onto the ground, tearing off garlands and jewellery, and sleeping on the floor. ²⁹ When she does this, he remains calm in his own mind and heart and wins her over with appropriate words of conciliation or by falling at her feet, and he lifts her back onto the bed. ³⁰ She answers his words by getting even angrier, grabbing his hair and pulling his face up, kicking him once, twice, three times, on his arms, head, chest, or back. Then she goes to the door and sits down there and bursts into tears. ³¹ Dattaka says, 'But even if she is very angry indeed, she does not actually go beyond the door, because then she would be at fault.' For when she has been properly won over, still at that spot, she wishes for reconciliation; and even when she has been reconciled, she pummels him, as it were, with harsh words, but she wants to make love with her reconciled lover, and the man embraces her. ³² When, however, a woman who lives in her own house has quarrelled for some reason, she approaches the man with the same sorts of actions. ³³ Then the man engages libertines, panders, and clowns to assuage her anger, and they are the ones who win her over, and the ones with whom she goes to his house, and there she stays. Those are the lovers' quarrels.

   ³⁴ And there are verses about this:

>   The lover who employs in this way
>   the sixty-four arts of love that Babhravya taught
>   is successful with the best women.
>   ³⁵ Even if he can talk about other sciences,

---

²⁷ He plays her false by going to the house of a co-wife, or sending betel and so forth to that woman, or making love with her; the woman who is fond of him cannot bear it if the man is unfaithful.

²⁸ Sleeping on the floor means that she is not sleeping with him.

²⁹ He does not reveal any emotional disturbance.

³⁵ Their learning and conversations are about the three aims of human life.

if he lacks the sixty-four arts of love
he is not very well respected in conversations
in the assembly of learned men.

[36] But if he is adorned with the sixty-four arts of love,
even if he lacks other sorts of knowledge,
he penetrates to the very top place
in conversations in the society of men and women.

[37] Wise men delight in it,
even the dregs of society delight in it highly,
and the troupes of courtesans de luxe delight in it;
who does not delight in this Source of Delight?

[38] Scholars, in their texts,
say that this Source of Delight
is loved by women and brings
fortune, success, and luck in love.

[39] Virgins, other men's wives,
and courtesans de luxe
look with warm feelings and respect
on the man who is skilled in the sixty-four arts of love.

———

[36] These conversations are about the *Kamasutra*.

[37] Wise men, who know the three aims of human life, rejoice in this triad because it is a means of protecting women. The dregs of society delight in it because it explains the way things actually are for them; the courtesans de luxe, because that is how they make their living. People call the *Kamasutra* by this name because it gives them delight.*

[38] Women love it because it brings joy to them, especially. It brings fortune, because all householders use it; success, because, like magic, it gives power over people; and luck in love, because it makes both a woman and a man lucky in love.

[39] Second-hand women are subsumed under other men's wives.* He might have said 'courtesan' instead of 'courtesan de luxe', but he wanted to indicate that she is a woman skilled in the sixty-four arts of love.

END OF BOOK TWO

BOOK THREE · VIRGINS

CHAPTER ONE

[23]   *Courting the Girl*

[1] In a woman who is of the same class, who has not been with another man before, and who has been taken in accordance with the texts, a man finds religion, power, sons, connections, the growth of his faction, and straightforward sexual pleasure.* [2] Therefore he should cultivate a virgin of noble stock whose mother and father are living and who is at least three years younger than he. She should come of a family that is respectable, wealthy, well connected, and rich in relatives who get along well with one another. Her mother and father should come from powerful factions. She should have beauty, good character, and lucky marks on her body, and her teeth, nails, ears, hair, eyes, and breasts should be neither insufficient nor excessive, and undamaged. She should not be sickly by nature. He himself should have precisely these qualities, and Vedic learning, too. [3] Ghotaka-mukha says, 'A man should regard himself as fulfilled when he has taken such a woman, and his peers cannot fault him for courting her.'

[4] His father and mother and relatives help him court her, as do friends who are connected with both sides* and who confirm his words. [5] They allude to her other suitors' faults, both those apparent now and those to come, and reveal the man's good qualities, both of his family and of his personal manliness, qualities that will increase the parents' inclination to give him the girl, and especially those qualities, both present and future, that the girl's mother likes. [6] One of these friends dresses up as a fortune-teller and describes the man's future good luck and prosperity by interpreting the flights of birds, omens, the influence of the planets according to their positions in the zodiac, and the lucky marks on his body.* [7] Others drive the girl's

---

[4] The two sides are those of the mother and the father.

[7] The other friends, also dressed as fortune-tellers, say, 'They want to give him the rich, beautiful, and highly esteemed daughter of this

mother crazy with worry that he will get another girl elsewhere, by some special means. [8] He courts the girl, and receives her, at a time when fate, omens, bird signs, and overheard conversations are favourable.* [9] 'Not just by preference, which is merely human', says Ghotakamukha.

[10] Firmly reject a girl who, at the time of courtship, falls asleep, cries, or goes out, [11] and reject any girl who has been given a name that is not recommended, who is kept hidden, who has already been given away, who is tawny,* pimply, stooped, bow-legged, or like a bull, whose forehead bulges, who is promiscuous or pregnant, a friend, a girl who has started menstruating, whose purity has been defiled, who is too close in age, or who sweats profusely.

[12] Never court a girl
    with a disgusting name
    that is a constellation, a river, a tree,
    or ends in a syllable beginning with 'l' or 'r'.*

[13] Some people say, 'A man will do well with a woman who catches and binds his mind and heart and his eyes. He should not consider any other woman.'

[14] And so, when it is time to give the girl away, her people dress her in her finest and bring her out. Every afternoon, she gets dressed up and amuses herself with her girlfriends, and her people eagerly display her at crowded events such as sacrifices and weddings and at

------

general. And so we have been asked to consider the fit between the two horoscopes, tomorrow.'

[8] Fate consists in the good and bad karma amassed in previous lives, especially as revealed by the planets and constellations.

[11] A pimply girl is one marked with whiteheads, a condition which destroys wealth and kills her husband. A bull-like girl looks like a man and has a bad nature. When a girl starts menstruating, the blood breaks her maidenhead. She should not be less than three years younger. For it is said:

> A man should woo and marry
> a recommended virgin who is
> four to eight years younger,
> or else she is too old.

[12] He should avoid such names as Kamalu, Vimalu, Caru, and Taru.

[14] The people of the girl's faction also do all this at the time of courtship.

similar festivals, because she is just like any other piece of merchandise. ¹⁵ They receive with ceremony the men who come there to court her, if those men are nice-looking, well spoken, and accompanied by their relatives. ¹⁶ And they find some other pretext to show them the girl when she is all dressed up. ¹⁷ They set a limit to the period in which they will ascertain and test the workings of fate and the gods and then, at the end, they make the decision about giving her away. ¹⁸ When they are invited to bathe and so forth, those making the choice of bridegroom say, 'All of that will happen', but they do not agree to do it on the very day of the invitation.

¹⁹ According to the customs of the place and in keeping with the texts, a man should marry by a wedding in the manner of Brahma, of the Lord of Creatures, of the Sages, or of the Gods. Those are the rules of courtship.*

[24]   *Making Alliances*

²⁰ And there are verses about this:
> A man should engage in group games such as
> completing verses,* and in marriages and alliances,
> only with his equals,
>   not with people above or below him.
> ²¹ When the man marries a girl
> and lives with her like a servant,
> they call this an 'upward alliance'*
>   and wise men avoid it.

---

¹⁷ They say, 'It is in the lap of the Lord of Creatures.' And, 'Let us carry out the tests with the help of our friends and relations.'
¹⁹ As it is said:
> In a wedding in the manner of the god Brahma,
> a man summons his well-adorned daughter and gives her away.
> In a wedding in the manner of the Lord of Creatures,
> a man says, 'May the two of you together fulfil your *dharma*.'
> In the manner of the Sages,
> he gives wealth and a cow and bull.
> But in the manner of the Gods,
> he gives her to a priest performing the ritual at the altar.

²² Good people also despise
   the worthless 'downward alliance',
   in which his own in-laws defer to him
   and he behaves like a master.
²³ The best alliance plays the game
   so that both sides taste one another's happiness
   and treat one another
   as unique individuals.
²⁴ Even when a man has made an 'upward alliance',
   he must later bow low among his in-laws;
   but he simply must not make a 'downward alliance',
   which good people despise.

CHAPTER TWO

[25]   *Winning a Virgin's Trust*

¹ For the first three nights after they have been joined together, the couple sleep on the ground, remain sexually continent, and eat food that has no salt or spices. Then, for seven days they bathe ceremonially to the sound of musical instruments, dress well, dine together, attend performances, and pay their respects to their relatives. All of this applies to all the classes. ² During this ten-night period, he begins to entice her with gentle courtesies when they are alone together at night.

³ The followers of Babhravya say, 'If the girl sees that the man has not made conversation for three nights, like a pillar, she will be discouraged and will despise him, as if he were someone of the third nature.'* ⁴ Vatsyayana says: He begins to entice her and win her trust, but he still remains sexually continent. ⁵ When he entices her he does

---

²² His in-laws are his father-in-law, brother-in-law, and so forth.

² There are two kinds of maidens, those ready for sex and those not ready. The trust of the first sort is won by paying attention to the act of love-making, and of the second sort, by taking care to dispel her fear and embarrassment.

³ If he does not speak or move, she thinks, 'I have married a dumb peasant!'

not force her in any way, ⁶for women are like flowers, and need to be
enticed very tenderly. If they are taken by force by men who have not
yet won their trust they become women who hate sex. Therefore he
wins her over with gentle persuasion.* ⁷But to penetrate her
defences, he uses any means, even a trick, that enables him to make
an advance.

⁸He uses an embrace that she likes because it does not last for too
long. ⁹He begins by embracing her upper body, because this is easy to
endure. ¹⁰He does this by the light of a lamp, if she has reached the
prime of her youth and has already became familiar with him, or in
the dark, if she is still a child and has no previous experience. ¹¹When
the woman has accepted his embrace, he gives her betel with his
mouth. If she does not accept it, he gets her to take it through
conciliating words, oaths, repeated requests, and falling at her feet.
(Even a bashful or very angry woman cannot resist a man falling at
her feet; this is a universal rule.) ¹²While giving her the betel, he
kisses her softly, calmly, without a sound.

¹³When she has been won over in this way, he gets her to talk. ¹⁴In
order to hear her talk, he asks her, as if he did not know it, about
something or other that can be expressed in just a few syllables. ¹⁵If
she does not respond to that, he asks her again, many times, while
soothing her, never distressing her. ¹⁶If she still says nothing, he
should persevere in urging her. ¹⁷For, says Ghotakamukha, 'All girls
put up with a man's words, but they will not utter a word themselves,
even in small-talk.' ¹⁸When she is urged, however, she gives her
replies by nodding or shaking her head, except that, in a quarrel, she
does not even move her head.

¹⁹When he asks her, 'Do you want me or do you not want me? Do I
please you or do I not please you?' she remains still for a long time,
and when he urges her she nods or shakes her head to indicate her
inclination; but if he asks her yet again, she argues with him. ²⁰If she
is already familiar with him, he may carry on a conversation with her
through the mediation of a girlfriend whom both of them trust but
who inclines toward him. During this conversation, the girl smiles
with her head down, and if the friend says too much, she scolds her

---

⁸ Once he has embraced her in this way, he can stop immediately, before
it begins to upset her.

and argues with her. The friend, however, may say, just for a joke, 'This is what she said', even if she did not say it. The girl sends the friend away because of this, and remains silent even when he asks her to reply. But when he insists, she says, 'I am not saying anything of the sort', mumbling with indistinct syllables and unclear meaning. And smiling at the man, she glances at him sideways from time to time. That is how he gets her to talk.

²¹ And when she has become accustomed to him in this way, without speaking she places near him the betel, scented oil, and garland that he has asked for. Or she ties them up in his upper cloth. ²² While she is occupied in doing this, he touches her nipples with the 'goose-flesh' scratch.* ²³ And if she stops him, he says, 'Embrace me, and then I will not do this', and so he embraces her. And he moves his hand as far as her navel and back again. And gradually he gets her onto his lap and goes farther and farther. If she does not accept his advances, he threatens her, ²⁴ saying, 'I myself will put the marks of my teeth on your lower lip, and the scratches of my nails on the upper part of your breasts. And I will do the same to myself, and, in front of your girlfriends, I will tell the story that you did it. What will you say about that?' And in this way he gradually seduces her with the tricks that are used to frighten children and to reassure children. ²⁵ On the second and third nights, when she is a little more trusting, he works her with his hand ²⁶ and kisses her on every part of her body.

²⁷ When he has placed his hand on her thighs and succeeded in caressing them, he moves his hand upward in stages and caresses her even where her thighs join her torso. If she restrains him from caressing her, he unsettles her by saying, 'What wrong am I doing?' and continues doing it until she has become used to it. And when he has succeeded in this, he touches her hidden places. ²⁸ Then he loosens her waistband, unties its knot, puts aside her clothes, and caresses her where her thighs join her torso. And all of these things he does under other pretexts. Then he penetrates her and gives her sexual pleasure. But he should not break his vow before the right time.

---

²⁸ Within the three nights, he does these things but does not break his vows. He penetrates her from the fourth day on, and gives her sexual pleasure without upsetting her.

²⁹ He teaches her, demonstrates his love for her, and describes the wishes that he had in the past. He promises to do, in the future, whatever is to her liking. He breaks down her anxiety about her co-wives. Gradually, in time, when she is no longer a virgin, he makes advances to her without unsettling her. That is how he wins the girl's trust.

³⁰ And there are verses about this:

> A man who answers a young girl's true feelings
> in this way subdues her by a stratagem;
> and so she falls in love with him
> and begins to trust him.

³¹ A man achieves success with virgins when
> he rubs them neither too much the right way*
> nor too much the wrong way;
> and so he conquers midway in between.

³² If a man knows how to win a virgin's trust,
> awakening her love for him,
> he increases women's respect for him
> and becomes dear to them.

³³ But if a man neglects a virgin
> because he thinks, 'She is too bashful',
> she despises him as a beast,*
> for she thinks, 'He does not understand my intentions.'

³⁴ Or if a man who does not understand
> a virgin's true feelings makes advances to her,
> even by force, she experiences, all at once,
> fear, trembling, anxiety, and hatred.

³⁵ If she does not experience the pleasures of love

---

²⁹ He teaches her the sixty-four techniques.

³¹ If he rubs her the right way too much, this establishes the path for the future, too, and from this obstacle to his own wishes he fails to achieve his object. If, however, he rubs her the wrong way too much, from that moment all her passion cools, and how can he achieve his object?

³⁵ She does not know the pleasures of love if he neglects her, thinking, 'She is too bashful', but he pollutes her with anxiety if he forces his advances upon her. Then she hates all men, thinking, 'They are all just like him', or, because she does not experience the pleasures of love, she leaves him for some other man.

or if he pollutes her with anxiety,
she becomes a man-hater or,
hated,* she leaves him for another man.

people who shouldn't court a virgin

CHAPTER THREE

[26]   *Making Advances to a Young Girl*

¹But a man who has good qualities but no money, or who has indifferent qualities but no opportunities, or who has money but is a neighbour, or a man who is dependent on his mother, father, and brothers, or who is regarded as a child and welcomed as a guest, should not court a virgin, because he will not get her. ²From childhood on, however, all by himself he may make her fall in love with him. ³A man in such circumstances, living as a child with the family of his mother's brother in the South under humiliating arrangements, separated from his mother and father, may win the daughter of his mother's brother even if her wealth raises her so far above him as to make her unattainable, even if she has already been given to another man. ⁴He may also set his sights on another girl outside the family. ⁵Ghotakamukha says, 'Since making such a girl fall in love in this way achieves religious aims, it is to be praised.'

⁶He gathers flowers with her, strings beads, plays house, puts on puppet shows, and prepares things to eat and drink, all in a manner appropriate to their familiarity and their age. ⁷And with her and

---

¹ A man of indifferent qualities does have qualities such as good looks and a good nature, but lacks a noble birth or money and therefore lacks social status. The neighbour who lives next to the woman's house does not get her, because of all the quarrels that arise about the boundaries between the two properties and because his money makes him arrogant.

² If she has fallen in love with him, she will marry him by herself in the love-match wedding that consists of nothing but desire.

³ In the South one can marry the daughter of one's maternal uncle.

⁴ A girl outside the family would be someone other than the daughter of the mother's brother, and not related to the man's parents at all.

⁷ The game of the middle finger consists of grabbing the middle finger when it is hidden by the other fingers; in the game of six pebbles, a

qualified servants and women servants, he plays the games of that region that are right for her, such as dice, board games, the games of the fist, of the little finger, of the middle finger; and the game of grabbing six pebbles. ⁸And with her girlfriends he plays other, livelier local games, such as 'eyes shut tight', 'the start', 'the line of salt', 'striking the wind', 'heaps of wheat', and 'finger-tips'.*

⁹He wins the inalienable love of the girl whom he thinks she trusts, and learns all about her intimate girlfriends. ¹⁰He treats the girl's foster-sister* with the greatest love and consideration, for, if she likes him, even if she recognizes his intentions she does not warn anyone against him but works to unite him with the girl. Even if she is not asked, she can be a kind of teacher, ¹¹for even if she does not recognize his intentions, she advertises his good qualities because of her love for him, so that the woman he wants falls in love with him. ¹²When the woman he wants is eager to have something, he finds out about it and gets it for her. ¹³Playthings that she has not had before, that the other girls seldom get, he produces for her with no apparent effort. ¹⁴For example, he shows her a ball with many streaks in different colours close together, one after another; and then dolls made of string, wood, horn, and ivory, and things made of beeswax, flour, and clay. ¹⁵And he demonstrates for her the kitchenware used to cook food. ¹⁶Within the range of his powers, he sends her, secretly, two little penises* carved in wood, and a man and a woman joined together; goats and sheep, and little houses for the families of gods, all made of clay, bamboo, and wood; cages for parrots, cuckoos,

---

person cups his hand and throws six small stones up into the air and catches them on the back of his hand.

⁸ In 'eyes shut tight', one person closes his eyes and the others hide; then he opens his eyes, and whomever he finds has to hide his eyes. 'The start' is a game played with dark fruits. In 'striking the wind', they stretch out their arms like wings and whirl around like a wheel. In 'heaps of wheat', they hide a gold coin in one of many piles of rice; then they mix all the piles together and divide them again into portions; each person chooses one portion and looks for the coin in it, and if he does not find it he has to give that portion to someone else. In 'finger-tips', one person closes his eyes and the others tap him on the forehead and ask, 'Who just hit you?' Other games might be 'leap-frog', 'one-foot', and so forth.

love-birds, quails, pheasants, and partridges; water-pots in various forms; mechanical toys; lutes; oysters; cosmetics such as red lac, red arsenic, yellow arsenic, red mercury sulphide, and black collyrium; sandalwood paste and saffron; and, in the course of time, areca nuts and betel leaves for betel. And openly he gives her more public things. He works hard to ensure that she will regard him as someone who will fulfil all of her wishes. [17] Secretly he strives to see her, and thus starts a conversation. [18] He announces that the reason for his secret gifts to her is his fear of her parents, and, 'because another man may want to have one of those gifts'. [19] As her love for him grows, if she has a mind for storytelling he charms her by telling stories that have meaning for her and that steal her heart. [20] If marvellous things can impress her, he astonishes her by performing magic tricks. If she is curious about the fine arts, he impresses her by his skill in them; if she is fond of singing, he captivates her ear with songs. On the full moon night in the rainy season, on the eighth day of the waning half of the month in autumn, and on the full moon night in winter; at celebrations, festivals, eclipses, or homecomings, he impresses her with various sorts of coloured chaplets, ear ornaments, and rare pearls, and with gifts of clothing, rings, and jewellery, as long as he thinks that this will not make trouble for her.

[21] If the girl's foster-sister has had some experience of men and so knows that he is different from other men, he teaches her the sixty-four techniques.* [22] And by teaching them to the foster-sister he demonstrates to the woman he wants his own skill in giving sexual pleasure. [23] He dresses richly and makes sure that she has an unobstructed view of him; he finds out if she has erotic feelings for him by observing her gestures and signals. [24] For it is commonly said:

---

[17] He starts a conversation through the mouth of someone else who arranges the secret meeting.

[19] He tells her stories connected with her, such as the story of Shakuntala, the king's wife.

[20] The fine arts are the ones that begin with cutting leaves into shape. He can see her when the moon is in the constellation of the Gemini, or of the Deer's Head, or of the Pleiades.*

[21] He thinks, 'The daughter of the girl's nurse should know that I am different from other men, if she has already made love. Otherwise, how could she know the difference?'

'Young women desire right from the start a man whom they know well and see all the time, but, even when they desire him, they do not make advances.'

That is how a man makes advances to a young girl.

[27]   *Interpreting her Gestures and Signals*

That's sick!

[25] Let us now talk about those gestures and signals.

[26] She does not look at him face to face. When he looks at her, she acts embarrassed. She reveals the splendid parts of her body, under some pretext. She looks at the man when he is otherwise distracted, cannot see her, or has gone past her. [27] When questioned about something, she replies by smiling, lowering her head, and mumbling indistinctly, with unclear meaning, very softly. She delights in staying near him for a long time. When she is some distance from him, she speaks to her attendants in an altered tone of voice, hoping that he will look at her. And she does not leave that place. [28] When she sees something or other, she laughs and begins to tell a story about it in order to stay there for a while. She kisses and hugs a child on her lap. She paints the auspicious dot on the forehead of her servant woman. With her attendants as an audience, she imitates gracefully this and that mannerism of his. [29] She confides in his friends, pays attention to their advice and follows it. She befriends his attendants, talks with them, and plays dice with them. And she instructs them in their own duties as if she were in charge of them. When one of them tells another stories about the man, she listens very carefully.

[30] Encouraged by her foster-sister, the girl enters the man's house. Placing the foster-sister between them, she offers to play dice with him, or some other game, or just to chat. When she is not dressed up she avoids letting him see her. When he asks her for her ear-ornament or ring or garland, she takes it off her body, very slowly, and puts it in his friend's hand. Anything that he gives her she wears all the time. When there is talk of another suitor, she becomes dejected and will have nothing to do with people of that suitor's faction.

[31] There are two verses about this:

---

[27] She does this only when the man questions her.

When a man sees these gestures and signals
full of erotic feeling,
he starts thinking of various ways
to make love with that virgin.
³²A man wins a young girl by children's games,
a woman in the prime of youth, by the arts,
and a mature, affectionate woman,
by winning over the people she trusts.*

Interesting

CHAPTER FOUR

[28]   *The Advances that a Man Makes on his Own*

¹When he has seen a virgin's gestures and signals, he uses some method to make advances to her. ²During a game of dice or some other game, he disagrees with her and takes her hand, with a meaningful expression on his face. ³He follows the rules for the embraces that have been described, beginning with the 'touching' embrace.* ⁴He cuts a leaf into the shape of an embracing couple and shows it to her to suggest his own intentions, ⁵and, from time to time, he shows her other shapes of this sort. ⁶When they are playing in the water, he dives underwater at some distance from her, comes up close to her, touches her, and dives underwater again right there. ⁷In games like 'new leaves',* he confesses his special erotic feelings, ⁸and he tells her about his suffering, without explaining it, ⁹and about an erotic

---

³² These are the arts of love.

¹ These are methods for a man who has no helper. There are also some for a man with a helper. These methods are of two sorts, public and intimate. First he describes the public ones.

⁴ He shows her a couple of geese and so forth, to suggest his own intentions, the sexual act.

⁷ In the course of these local games, he confesses his feelings by such things as cutting shapes in leaves, just described.

⁸ He says, 'I do not know what has caused this agony in my mind.' And even if he does not explain it, he talks about it more and more, making it seem the most important thing.

⁹ He says, 'In my dream, I made love to a woman who looked just like you.'

dream, pretending that it was about another woman. [10] At a theatrical spectacle or in a group of her people he sits down near her and finds some excuse to touch her. [11] He presses his foot against her foot as if to use it as a footrest. [12] Then he touches her toes, one by one, little by little, [13] and presses the tips of her toenails with his big toe. [14] If he succeeds in this, he wants more, step by step. [15] And he keeps doing it so that she eventually tolerates it.

[16] When she is washing his feet, he presses her fingers by using his toes as a pincer. [17] Whenever he gives her anything or receives anything from her, he invests it with erotic feeling. [18] When he has washed out his mouth, he sprinkles her with the water. [19] When the two of them are seated in a deserted or dark place, he makes her let him do what he wants, or when they are lying down in the same place. [20] There he lets her know his true feelings, without distressing her. [21] 'I have something to tell you in private', he says, and there he demonstrates his feelings without speaking (as we will describe in the discussion of other men's wives). [22] But if he knows her feelings, by faking an illness he gets her to come to his own home to bring him news. [23] When she comes to him, he gets her to rub his head; and he takes her hand and places it, feelingly, on his eyes and forehead. [24] Under the pretext of preparing medicines, he charges her with something to do, [25] saying, 'You must do this, for no one but a virgin can do it.' And when she leaves, he lets her go only after getting her to promise to return. [26] He uses this method for three nights and three twilights. [27] When she comes to him, he stretches out their conversation in order to see her again and again. [28] Even with other women present, he makes more and more advances to her to win her trust (though he does not tell her with words). [29] 'For', says Ghotakamukha, 'even a man whose feelings have gone far does not

---

[14] He wants to climb her like a staircase, to touch her between the legs, on the thighs, on the flanks, and so forth, one after the other.

[16] Now he describes the intimate methods.

[17] He does this by touching her with his nails.

[20] On a seat or a bed, he tells her with his facial expressions but not with words, because of his fear that she will reject him.

[23] He says, 'I have such a headache; do rub it with your hand.'

[29] Even a man who has inspired exceptional trust does not succeed, because virgins expect to be wooed many times over.

succeed with virgins by remaining indifferent.' ³⁰But only when he thinks that he has succeeded quite well with her does he start to make advances. ³¹It is commonly said: 'In the evening, at night, and in darkness, women's fears are muted, they resolve to make love, they are full of passion, and they will not refuse a man. Therefore this is the time to have them.'

³²But if there are no advances that a man can make on his own, he gets her girlfriend or foster-sister—who knows his purpose and is close to the girl but does not tell her his purpose—to bring the girl to his arms. Then he makes advances to her as has been described above. ³³Or he can get one of his own servant women to make friends with her at the very start. ³⁴At a sacrifice, a wedding, a pageant, a festival, a disaster, in the crowd engaged in watching a theatrical spectacle, and here and there, he sees her gestures and signals,* tests her feelings for him, gets her alone and makes advances to her. ³⁵Vatsyayana says: Women who have revealed their feelings and who are propositioned at the right time and place never turn away. Those are the advances that a man makes on his own.

[29] *The Advances that a Virgin Makes to the Man She Wants*

³⁶A virgin may have good qualities but only modest opportunities; or she may come from a good family but have no money and therefore not be sought by the men who are her peers; or she may have been separated from her mother and father, or live in the family of her relatives. When such a virgin reaches the prime of her youth, all by herself, she tries to get married.* ³⁷With a child-like love she makes advances to a good-looking, strong young man of good qualities. ³⁸Or if there is someone of whom she thinks, 'Disregarding the opinions of his mother and father, this man will fall for me all by himself, because his flesh is weak', she takes possession of him by doing him favours that please him and by seeing him all the time. ³⁹Her mother, with her girlfriends and foster-sisters, keeps her in his sight. ⁴⁰With flowers, perfumes, and betel in her hand she stays near him in deserted places at odd times. In demonstrating her skill in the fine arts, or in massaging him or scratching his head, she shows how experienced she is. She tells stories that are tuned to the nature of the man she wants, and she behaves as has

been described in the discussion of making advances to a young girl.*

⁴¹Scholars say: 'Not even when she is very close to him should she herself make advances to a man. For a young woman who makes advances to a man herself destroys her luck in love.' ⁴²But she goes along with his advances, ⁴³and when he embraces her she betrays no emotional excitement. She receives his signals blandly, as if she did not understand them. Only when he forces her does she let him grasp her mouth. ⁴⁴When he begs her to imagine his sexual arousal, only with great difficulty can she bear any touching of the hidden places.* ⁴⁵And even when he begs her, she is not very open with him, because time is uncertain and changeable. ⁴⁶But when she thinks, 'He is in love with me and will not turn away', only then does she urge the man who is making advances to her to free her from her state of childhood. ⁴⁷And when she has lost her virginity, she reveals this to the people she trusts. Those are the advances that a virgin makes to the man she wants.

[30]   *The Advances that Win a Virgin*

⁴⁸And there are verses about this:

> But a virgin who is pursued
> chooses to marry the man who, she thinks,
> will support her and give her pleasure,
> who will do what she likes and is in her power.
> ⁴⁹When greed for money makes a virgin
> marry a man without considering
> his good qualities, his appearance, or his experience,
> or even the rivalries among his other wives,

---

⁴¹ When she is very close to him, she is in the power of *kama*.

⁴² She goes along with it so that he does not turn away from her.

⁴⁴ When the man begs her to arouse him by placing her hand on his own hidden place, then only with difficulty will she touch the man's hidden place.

⁴⁵ She reveals neither her feelings nor the parts of her body.

⁴⁶ She thinks, 'He will not abandon me.' She urges him to free her by marrying her with the love-match wedding and then by taking her maidenhead.

⁵⁰ then she will not entice a man who has good qualities,
　a strong man who is in her power,
　who seeks her with all his might
　and makes advances to her with various methods.
⁵¹ Better even a poor man in her power,
　even a man without good qualities, who supports himself alone,
　than a husband who has many people to support,
　even if he has good qualities.
⁵² The wives of rich men are generally many and headstrong,
　and even though they have superficial enjoyments,
　their pleasure, too, is superficial,
　for they have no intimate trust.
⁵³ But if a man who is of low birth
　makes advances, or a greybeard,
　or a man inclined to travel abroad,
　he is not fit for union.
⁵⁴ Nor is a man fit for union
　who makes advances on a whim,
　or who is addicted to dishonest gambling,
　or who has a wife and children.
⁵⁵ One wooer should be wooed
　among suitors who have the same good qualities:
　this suitor is the best
　because his very nature is love.

CHAPTER FIVE

[31]　　　　　*Devious Devices for Weddings*

¹ When it is virtually impossible for a man to see a virgin alone, he insinuates himself into intimacy* with her foster-sister by giving her pleasing things and doing favours for her. ² Pretending not even to

---

⁵² Their superficial enjoyments come from material possessions like houses. But they do not have the intimate trust, the inner pleasure that comes from sexual ecstasy.

¹ He lures the foster-sister who has already been with a man, in order to send her into the other woman's presence as his authorized envoy.

know the man, the foster-sister gets the girl to fall in love with him because of his good qualities. She describes mostly the man's qualities that are pleasing to the girl, [3] and she emphasizes the faults of the other suitors that especially conflict with the girl's desires, [4] with her parents' greed and lack of understanding of good qualities, and with the fickleness of her relatives. [5] And she tells the girl stories about other virgins of equal caste, such as Shakuntala, who found a husband by their own resolve and made love with great joy,* [6] while women in illustrious families are likely to be oppressed by co-wives, hated, miserable, and rejected. [7] She describes what the future would be like with him; [8] she describes the unblemished happiness and the man's love for his one and only wife. [9] To a girl who wants him, she gives reasons that dispel her fear of danger, anxiety, and embarrassment. [10] She performs all the functions of a messenger. [11] By saying, 'The man will take you by force, as if you knew nothing about it', she gets her to say, 'Yes, that would be entirely acceptable.'

---

[4] She says, 'Your parents are greedy and do not understand good qualities, for they throw out a man who does have good qualities and are trying to round up a rich man who has no good qualities.'

[5] If the girl thinks, 'He is not right for me', the foster-sister tells her about women who chose by their own resolve, not according to their parents' wish. Kaushika saw the celestial nymph Menaka, whom Indra had sent to him to pose an obstacle to the ascetic power he was generating through his yogic praxis; his passion was ignited and he desired her. She took his semen and right then and there gave birth to a maiden whom she abandoned in the wilderness; then she returned to the sky. The great sage Kanva saw the maiden in the midst of a flock of *shakunta* birds and in pity took her to his hermitage and brought her up, naming her, because of the circumstances, Shakuntala. In time she grew to the prime of her youth, and when she saw King Dushyanta, who had come there on a hunt, by her own resolve she gave him her hand in marriage. Other virgins, too, became the wives of kings.

[6] A greedy father may give a girl in marriage into an illustrious family.

[8] If he has only one wife, there will be none of the misery brought by co-wives.

[9] Thinking, 'She does want him, but she sees his faults', she dispels her fear of ruin, her anxious fear of parents and elders, and her embarrassment toward the people around her.

[11] 'If he takes you by force, it will not be your fault.'

¹² When the girl has been won over and waits for him in the place of assignation, the man marries her by taking consecrated fire from the house of a Brahmin who knows the Veda, spreading sacred grass on the ground, making an offering of oblations in accordance with the ritual texts, and circumambulating the fire three times. ¹³ Only then does he inform her mother and her father,* ¹⁴ because the scholars' rule says, 'Weddings witnessed by the consecrated fire cannot be revoked.' ¹⁵ And after he has taken her maidenhead, he gradually informs his own people. ¹⁶ Then he gets her relatives to give her to him, in order to wipe out the stain on the family honour and out of fear of reprisals. ¹⁷ Immediately, he wins over her relatives with endearing gifts and by his love. ¹⁸ That is how he carries out a love-match wedding.*

¹⁹ If he is not winning her over, he enlists the help of another girl of good family, who moves freely between both houses, who is affectionate and was in the past intimate, and he has her bring the girl with her to an accessible place on some pretext. ²⁰ Then he brings the fire from the house of a Brahmin who knows the Veda, and so forth, just the same as above. ²¹ If a wedding is to take place soon, he makes the girl's mother regret it because of the faults in the other groom that he brings to her attention, ²² and then, with the mother's permission, the man is brought to a neighbour's house at night, and he brings the fire from the house of a Brahmin who knows the Veda, and so forth, just the same as above. ²³ Or the girl may have a brother of the same age as the man, who is addicted to courtesans and to the wives of other men; the man wins his love by doing him endearing favours and giving him help in difficult affairs, for a very long time. In the end, he confides his intentions to him. ²⁴ For in general, young men will even give up their lives for the sake of contemporaries of the same character, vices, and age. Therefore, the brother is the one that he gets to bring her to an accessible place on some pretext, and so forth, just the same as above.

---

¹⁶ Her relatives think, 'If the king hears that the man has done this, then he will have him punished.'

¹⁹ The man buys, with money, the help of a woman who is affectionate toward him and was connected with him in the past because their parents were friends.*

²² He uses money to enlist the neighbour's help.

²⁵ And on festivals such as the eighth day of the waning half of the month in autumn, her foster-sister gives her an intoxicating drink and, on the pretext of something that she herself has to do, brings her to the man in an accessible place. There, when the drink has made her unconscious, he takes her maidenhead, and so forth, just the same as above. → WTF?

²⁶ Or when she is sleeping alone (because he has kept her foster-sister away), while she is unconscious, he takes her maidenhead, and so forth, just the same as above.*

²⁷ Or when the man finds out that she has gone to another village or to a park, he comes there with a strong force of helpers and frightens off or murders the guards, and carries off the virgin.* Those are the devious devices for weddings.

²⁸ With regard to maintaining religion,
each form of wedding is better than the one that follows it;
but each time the preceding one is not possible,
the following one should be used.*

²⁹ For since mutual love is the fruit
of wedding rites, therefore even
the love-match wedding, though of middling rank,
is respected as a means to a good end.

³⁰ Indeed, the love-match wedding is regarded
as the best of all, because it gives pleasure
and costs little trouble and no formal courtship,
and because its essence is mutual love.

There a hierarchy of actions can follow. ▽

---

²⁵ The wedding in the manner of the Ghouls involves taking a girl who is sleeping or drunk. A pretext might be saying, 'I forgot my ring when I came here; let us go there.' This takes place when the moon is in the constellation of the Deer's Head.

²⁶ Here he does not bring the fire and so forth, because there is no *dharma*.

²⁷ The use of force distinguishes the wedding of the Ogres.

²⁸ The Brahma wedding is better than the love-match wedding, which is better than the wedding of the Demons, the Demons better than the Ghouls, and the Ghouls better than the Ogres.

END OF BOOK THREE

BOOK FOUR · WIVES

CHAPTER ONE

[32]   *The Life of an Only Wife*

[1] An only wife, with deep, intimate trust, treats her husband like a god and always acts in ways compatible with him. [2] Following his thinking, she takes on herself his cares about the household. [3] She keeps the house clean and heart-warming to look at, with well-polished surfaces, all sorts of floral arrangements, and smooth and shiny floors, and she makes sure that offerings are made three times a day and that the gods in the family shrine are properly honoured. [4] For, Gonardiya says,* 'Nothing holds the heart of householders like this.' [5] She treats the man's older relatives, servants, sisters, and sisters' husbands according to their merits.

[6] In well-weeded plots of ground she sees to the planting of beds of herbs and green vegetables, and clumps of sugar-cane, and patches of cumin-seed and caraway, mustard seed, parsley, soy-beans, and bay-trees; [7] and musk rose, gooseberry, white-flowered Indian jasmine, Spanish jasmine, red amaranth, Arabian jasmine, East Indian rose bay, Adam's apple, China rose, and other flowers, as well as other plants that make a great display, such as Indian lemon grass, beard-grass, and scurvy grass. And in the orchard she makes charming plots of open ground [8] and has a well dug, or a pool or a pond, in the middle of it. [9] She does not have a close relationship with any woman who is a beggar, a religious mendicant, a Buddhist nun, promiscuous, a juggler, a fortune-teller, or a magician who uses love-sorcery worked with roots. [10] In preparing meals she finds out, 'This is what he likes, this is what he hates, this is good for him, this is bad for him.'

---

4 He quotes Gonardiya out of respect, since he was the author of the book on this subject.

5 The older relatives are her father-in-law and so forth.

6 She plants herbs such as coriander and ginger, and vegetables such as beets.

7 The open ground is to walk on.

¹¹ When she hears his voice outside as he approaches the house, she stands ready in the centre of the house and says, 'What should be done?' ¹² Pushing aside the female servant, she herself washes his feet. ¹³ She does not let the man see her alone when she is not wearing make-up and jewellery. ¹⁴ If he has spent too much or spent the wrong amount, she tells him in private. ¹⁵ Only with his permission does she go to a betrothal, a wedding, or a sacrifice, or get together with her girlfriends, or visit the gods. ¹⁶ In any game, she follows his lead. ¹⁷ She lies down after him, gets up before him, and never wakes him up when he is asleep. ¹⁸ She keeps the kitchen well guarded and well lit. ¹⁹ Mildly offended by the man's infidelities,* she does not accuse him too much, ²⁰ but she scolds him with abusive language when he is alone or among friends. She does not, however, use love-sorcery worked with roots,* ²¹ for, Gonardiya says, 'Nothing destroys trust like that.' ²² She refrains from bad language, nasty looks, talking while avoiding his gaze, standing at the doorway or gazing from it, chatting in the park, and lingering in deserted places. ²³ She guards against her own sweat, dirty teeth, and bad body odour, for these cool his passion. ²⁴ When she goes to him to make love, she wears gorgeous jewellery, a variety of flowers and scented oils, and a dress dazzling with many different tints. ²⁵ Her everyday dress is made of delicate, smooth, thin silk, with a modest amount of jewellery, good perfume but not too much of scented oils, and flowers both white and of other colours. ²⁶ When the man fasts or follows a vow, she herself also undertakes this for her own purpose; if he tries to stop her, she refutes his arguments, saying, 'I am not going to be thwarted in this matter.'

²⁷ When the price is right, at the right time, she buys household goods made of clay, bamboo, wood, leather, and iron. ²⁸ She lays in a stock of salt and oil as well as hard-to-get perfumes, spices, and medicines, and keeps them hidden within the house. ²⁹ And she buys, and sows at the proper season, the seeds of all sorts of edible plants,

---

¹³ His passion for her may cool if he does not see her with her body well dressed.

¹⁴ If he has spent wrongly,* he will be taken for a poor man. He would be embarrassed if she told him in the company of other people.

¹⁹ She says, 'Do not do it again', but not too much, lest he be humiliated.

²⁶ She does this in order to demonstrate her devotion to him.

such as radishes, arrowroot, ginger, wormwood, mangoes, melons, cucumbers, eggplants, pumpkins, squashes, round yams, trumpet-flowers, horse-eye beans, sesame, sandalwood, glory-tree, garlic, and onions. [30] She does not tell other people about her own assets or about her husband's counsels. [31] She surpasses all the women of her group in her skill, her dazzling appearance, her cooking, her pride, and her services. [32] She calculates the year's income and adjusts the expenditure to it. [33] She makes butter from the milk left over from meals, and also from sesame oil and molasses. She spins threads from cotton balls and then weaves cloth with those threads. She collects string-bags, cords, ropes, and bark-fibres; she oversees the grinding and pounding; when rice is boiled, she makes use, afterwards, of the water, the froth, the husks, the uncooked kernels, and the coals. She knows the servants' wages and maintenance. She sees to the tilling of the fields, the care of the cattle, and the upkeep of the carriages. She looks after the rams, cocks, quails, parrots, pheasants, cuckoos, peacocks, monkeys, and deer. And she prepares the daily portions of income and expenditures.

[34] She collects the man's discarded, worn-out clothes, both many-coloured and pure white, and gives them as a favour to servants who have done good work, and as gifts that bestow honour, or she uses them for something else. [35] She sees to the stocking and use of pots of wines and liquors, and to selling and buying them, and she keeps track of the income and expenditure from them. [36] She welcomes and honours the man's friends in the proper way, with gifts of garlands, scented oils, and betel. [37] She serves her father-in-law and mother-in-law, remaining dependent on them; she does not answer back to them, but makes brief, never harsh conversation, not laughing too loud, and treats those who are dear and not dear to them as if they were dear and not dear to her. [38] She is moderate in her enjoyments. [39] She is considerate to servants, [40] but never gives anything to anyone without telling the man. [41] She instructs each servant in the limits of his own work and honours him on festival days. That is the life of an only wife.

---

[31] The services are those that she does for her husband.
[33] She uses the water and the froth for drinks for the women servants, the husks to plug holes, the uncooked kernels to feed the poultry, and the coals to make iron pots.

[33]   *Her Behaviour during his Absence*

⁴²When he is away on a journey, she wears only jewellery that has religious meaning and power, devotes herself to fasts dedicated to the gods, waits for news, and manages the household. ⁴³She sleeps at the feet of older relatives and their people, and accomplishes her tasks with their approval. She goes to great pains to acquire and look after things that the man wants. ⁴⁴She spends the usual amount on undertakings for daily tasks and special occasions. She also sets her mind on accomplishing those undertakings that he has begun. ⁴⁵She does not go to the family of her own relatives except on occasions of disaster or celebration. And even there she is chaperoned by the man's servants, she does not stay too long, and she does not change out of the clothing that she wears when the man is absent. ⁴⁶She fasts with the permission of older relatives. She increases capital and decreases expenditures as much as possible, by authorizing buying and selling to be accomplished by incorruptible servants carrying out orders.

⁴⁷When he returns, she appears to him first in her ordinary clothes, and she honours the gods and brings gifts. That is her life during his absence.

⁴⁸And there are two verses about this:

> An only wife who wishes for her man's welfare
> adapts herself to his behaviour,
> whether she is a woman of good family,
> a second-hand woman, or even a courtesan.
> Women of good behaviour
> achieve the goals of religion, power, and pleasure,
> a firm position, and
> a husband without a co-wife.

---

⁴³ She makes her bed near her mother-in-law and her mother-in-law's people, for the sake of her own purity.

⁴⁴ The daily tasks including managing food and drink, and the special occasions would include celebrating the birth of a child. The tasks that the man has begun might be establishing a temple to the gods, or a park.

⁴⁷ Her ordinary clothes would be those that she wears during his absence.

CHAPTER TWO

[64]   *The Senior Wife*

¹If his wife is frigid or promiscuous or unlucky in love, or if she continually fails to bear a child or gives birth only to daughters, or if the man is fickle, he supplants her with a co-wife.* ²Therefore, from the very start, a woman tries to avoid this by making known her devotion, good character, and cleverness. And if she does not have children, she herself is the one to urge him to take a co-wife. ³And when she is being supplanted, by applying all her powers she establishes her own position as higher.

⁴She looks upon the newly arrived woman as a sister. Making an extraordinary effort, she helps her dress and make herself up in the evening, and she makes sure that the man knows about this. She pays no attention if the other woman becomes hostile or haughty as a result of her luck in love. ⁵She disregards it if the other woman makes a mistake with her husband. Then, if she thinks, 'This is a mistake that she herself will also mend', she advises her carefully about it. ⁶But she reveals further particulars about it to the man, privately.

⁷She treats the other woman's children in no special way,* treats her servants with great sympathy and her girlfriends with affection. She does not care too much for her own relatives, and makes an extra fuss over the other woman's relatives. ⁸But if she is supplanted by many co-wives, she allies herself with the one just below her. ⁹She provokes quarrels between the woman whom the man wishes to promote to the favourite and the woman who used to be lucky in

---

³ She establishes herself higher than the co-wife.

⁴ She has to make an effort, because she does not want to do this; to demonstrate her affection, she makes it known to the man by means of a female servant.

⁵ For she thinks, 'This mistake may make her unlucky in love.'

⁶ She reveals details that the man has not seen, to make affection grow between her and him.

⁷ This is how a woman with no children acts toward a woman who has children.

love, ¹⁰ a woman for whom she then shows sympathy. ¹¹ By uniting the other co-wives, without actually getting into the argument herself she maligns the one he wants to promote to the favourite. ¹² But she encourages the other woman to quarrel with the man, egging her on by taking her side. ¹³ And she makes the quarrel grow. ¹⁴ Or, if she notes that the quarrel is dying down, she herself fans the flames. ¹⁵ But if she realizes, 'The man even now inclines to her', then she herself makes peace between them. That is the life of the senior wife.

[35]   *The Junior Wife*

¹⁶ The junior wife, however, regards her co-wife like a mother. ¹⁷ She does not even give anything to her relatives without the other woman's knowledge. ¹⁸ She reports her own experiences to her. ¹⁹ With her permission, she sleeps with the husband. ²⁰ She never reports to any other woman what the other woman says. ²¹ She has more regard for the other woman's children than for her own. ²² But privately, she serves the husband more. ²³ And she does not tell him how she herself suffers from the hostility of the co-wives. ²⁴ She tries to get some special secret token of her husband's esteem, ²⁵ and she says, 'I will live on this, as if it were food to last me on a journey.' ²⁶ But she never talks in public about that, either in boast or in passion, ²⁷ for a woman who betrays a secret wins her husband's loathing. ²⁸ Gonardiya says, 'Out of fear of the senior wife, she seeks only a secret love-token.'

²⁹ If the senior wife is unlucky in love and has no children, the junior wife pities her and urges the man to pity her. ³⁰ But if the junior wife is able to dislodge the senior wife, she assumes the role of the only wife. That is the life of the junior wife.

---

¹⁰ She feigns sympathy for the woman who is the object of the quarrel and covertly encourages her to keep the quarrel going.

²² She serves him more in bed, so that he will love her more than he loves the other women.

²³ Since the man would not trust it if she told it herself, she lets someone else tell it.

²⁴ The token is special because it is more than the other wives have.

[36]   *The Second-hand Woman*

³¹ A second-hand woman, however, is a widow who is tormented by the weakness of the senses and so finds, again, a man who enjoys life and is well endowed with good qualities.* ³² But the followers of Babhravya say, 'Since she may at will go away again from him too, thinking, "He is *not* well endowed with good qualities", she will then want yet another man.' ³³ It is in search of physical pleasure that she tries, again, to find yet another man. ³⁴ Gonardiya says, 'Complete pleasure comes from men's endowments and capacity for enjoyments; therefore one man differs from another.'* ³⁵ Vatsyayana says: It is because his mind is compatible with hers.

³⁶ With her relatives, she gets the man to provide sufficient funds to cover the cost of such things as drinking parties, picnics, faith offerings, and gifts to honour friends. ³⁷ Or she may pay for his jewellery and her own out of her own capital. ³⁸ There is no rule about love-gifts. ³⁹ If she leaves the man of her own accord, she gives back everything he has given her except for his love-gifts. But if he throws her out, she does not give anything back. ⁴⁰ She takes over his house as if she were the woman in charge, ⁴¹ but she acts with affection to women of good families, ⁴² with consideration to the servants, always joking, and with great respect for his friends. In the arts,* she has skill and greater knowledge. ⁴³ When there are occasions for a quarrel,

---

³⁴ The man who is well-endowed and brings enjoyments is different from the man who is poorly endowed and lacks the capacity for enjoyments. But a woman who walks out again and again becomes a special kind of courtesan.

³⁵ Even if he is well-endowed and brings enjoyments, if his mind is not compatible she will not find complete pleasure. And so this man and the other are different. Thus V shows that, by this criterion, she will not go on to yet another man.

³⁹ She leaves him of her own accord when it is his fault.

⁴² Her knowledge is greater than the man's.

⁴³ There is an occasion for her quarrel if there have been frequent breaks between them, if he has an affair with a loose woman, if he stays away for two nights, or if he does not sleep with her when it is her turn.

she herself scolds the man. [44] She practises the sixty-four arts of love in private. And she herself does favours for the co-wives. She gives jewellery to their children and makes little ornaments for them, and clothing, with care, but she expects those children to serve her as if she were their master. She gives even more things to his entourage and his crowd of friends. And she is always in the mood for company, for drinking parties, picnics, festivals, and amusements. That is the life of the second-hand woman.

[37]   *The Wife Unlucky in Love* = Servants

[45] But a woman who is unlucky in love and oppressed by rivalry with her co-wives seeks support from the wife who seems to be chosen most often by their husband. She shows that chosen wife the knowledge of the arts that can be revealed. Because she is unlucky in love, she has no secrets.* [46] She performs the functions of a nurse for the man's children. [47] She wins over his friends and then gets them to tell him about her devotion to him. [48] She leads the way in religious duties and in vows and fasts. [49] She is considerate to the servants and has no more regard for herself than for them. [50] In bed, she requites the man's passion in a way that suits him. [51] She does not scold him or show him any contrariness. [52] She restores his desire for any woman with whom he may have quarrelled. [53] If he desires some woman who must remain concealed, she brings the other woman to him and hides her. [54] She takes pains to make the man regard her as a chaste and undeceiving wife. That is the life of the wife unlucky in love.*

⟶ No other possible explanation.

[44] In private, in bed with the man, she practises the arts beginning with 'embracing' and ending with 'a man's sexual strokes'.

[45] The arts that can be revealed are the fine arts, such as cutting leaves into shapes. Her skill is a means of dispelling her husband's lack of love for her.

[50] Whatever way he wants to make love, even if she does not want to, she should do it that way, in order to bring him to satisfaction.

[51] She does not say, 'You do not love me any more.' She does not show him contrariness by hiding any part of her body.

[52] She thinks, 'By this device I will get him to incline to me.'

[53] The woman who must be concealed may be another man's wife.

[38]   *Women of the Harem*

⁵⁵ The life of the women of the harem, too, can be surmised from the preceding sections.

⁵⁶ The woman chamberlain or bodyguard* brings their garlands, scented oils, and clothes to the king, saying, 'The queens have sent these.' ⁵⁷ The king takes these and gives them back to the queens as a gift, like the leftovers* of a deity. ⁵⁸ In the afternoon, he goes, carefully dressed, to see, all together, all the women of the harem, who are also well dressed. ⁵⁹ He chats and jokes with them, giving to each one the place and honour due to the time she has served in the harem and her worth. ⁶⁰ Immediately after that, he sees, in exactly the same way, the second-hand women, ⁶¹ and then the courtesans and the dancing girls who belong to the harem. ⁶² Their places are in the inner rooms assigned to them.

⁶³ Now, when the king arises from his afternoon siesta, the women attendants who keep track of the roster come to him followed by the servants of the woman whose turn it is to spend the night with the king, of the woman who has been passed over on her night, and of the woman who is in her fertile season. And they present the king with scented oils, each marked with the stamp of the woman's seal ring, and tell him whose turn it is to sleep with him that night and who is in her fertile season. ⁶⁴ Whichever one among these oils the king takes, he announces that the woman who owns it will sleep with him that night.

⁶⁵ At festivals, and at concerts and plays, all of the women of the harem are appropriately honoured and served with drinks. ⁶⁶ They do not go out, nor do women from outside enter, except for those whose purity is well known. And so the work is carried out undisturbed. Those are the women of the harem.

---

⁶² The queens are in the centre rooms. In quarters outside these rooms are the second-hand women; outside these, the courtesans; and further out, the dancing girls.

⁶⁶ The work of making love should be their one concern.

A Man's Management of Many Women

⁶⁷ And there are verses about this:
>   But a man who has collected many wives
>   must treat them equally.
>   He should not treat them with contempt,
>   nor put up with their deceptions.

⁶⁸ Whatever sort of love-play one woman favours,
>   or whatever peculiarity her body may have,
>   or whatever reproach she lets slip in pillow talk—
>   he must not tell that to the other women.

⁶⁹ He should never give women their head
>   in a cause against a co-wife,
>   and if one woman begins to slander another in this way,
>   he should charge her herself with those faults.

⁷⁰ He should keep his women happy,
>   one by confiding in her privately,
>   another by honouring her in public,
>   yet another with gifts as tokens of his esteem.

⁷¹ He should enchant each one individually,
>   with picnics, luxuries, gifts,
>   honours to her family, and with
>   the pleasures of love in bed.

⁷² A young woman who controls her temper
>   and behaves according to the textbook
>   puts her husband in her power
>   and lords it over her co-wives.

---

⁶⁷ He must not put up with their infidelities, or else, if these deceptions are tolerated, they will do it again.

⁷⁰ The one who is shy, he pleases by confiding in her privately; the one concerned about her status among the co-wives, by honouring her in public; the one who is proud, by giving her gifts as tokens of his esteem.

⁷¹ Picnics are for the woman who likes that sort of thing; luxuries for the one who is frivolous and extravagant; honours to her family are for the one who is always thinking about doing something for her relatives; and pleasure in bed is for the one who loves to make love.

END OF BOOK FOUR

CHAPTER ONE

[39] *haracteristic Natures of Women and Men*

[1] The reasons for having affairs with the wives of other men have already been discussed. [2] A man must consider, from the very beginning, whether such women can be won, and without disaster, and whether they are eligible for sex, and what their future will be, and how they behave. [3] For when a man sees that his desire is progressing from one stage to the next stage, then, in order to ward off these fatal blows to his own body, he should make advances to other men's wives. [4] Now, there are ten stages of desire, [5] and their signs are: love at first sight, the attachment of the mind and heart, the stimulation of the imagination, broken sleep, weight loss, revulsion against sensual objects, the loss of all sense of shame, madness, loss of consciousness, and death. [6] Scholars say: 'In considering an affair with another man's wife, a young woman's bearing and telltale signs are the basis on which to judge her character, honesty, purity, accessibility, and the fierceness of her sexual energy.' [7] Vatsyayana says: Because relying on a woman's bearing and telltale signs is fallible, a man should understand a woman's conduct from her gestures and signals.

[8] Gonikaputra says, 'A woman desires any attractive man she sees, and, in the same way, a man desires a woman. But, after some consideration, the matter goes no farther.' [9] A woman is different in this regard: [10] A woman does not consider religion or the violation of religion; she just desires. But consideration of some other factor keeps her from making advances. [11] And by her very nature she resists a man who makes advances to her, even if she desires to respond. [12] If he makes advances to her again and again, however, she gives in. [13] A

---

[1] Thus V reminds the reader of the reasons, apart from pleasure and children, that have been explained in the discussion of the types of women who can be lovers [1.5.4–31].

man, by contrast, considers the stability of religion and the conventions of noble people and turns back even when he desires. [14] And even when he is pursued he does not give in, because he is aware of these considerations. [15] He makes advances for no special reason, and even when he has made his advances, he does not make them again. And he becomes indifferent toward her when she has given in. [16] It is commonly said: 'A man scorns a woman who is easy to get, but desires a woman who is hard to get.'

[40]   *Causes of Resistance*   → An extensive list

[17] Here are the causes of a woman's resistance: [18] love for her husband, [19] regard for her children, [20] the fact that she is past her prime, [21] or overwhelmed by unhappiness, [22] or unable to get away; [23] or she gets angry and thinks, 'He is propositioning me in an insulting way'; [24] or she cannot imagine being with him, thinking, 'He is inscrutable'; [25] or she fears, 'He will soon go away. There is no future in it; his thoughts are attached to someone else'; [26] or she is nervous, thinking, 'He does not conceal his signals'; [27] or she thinks, 'His affection is all for his friends, and his regard is only for them'; [28] or she fears, 'His advances are just a tease'; [29] or she is diffident, thinking, 'How glamorous he is'; [30] or if she is a 'doe' she fears, 'His sexual energy is too fierce', or

---

[15] He makes advances for no special reason other than pleasure.

[19] She thinks, 'My child is still suckling at my breast.'

[20] An overripe woman is ashamed to be forced to show her body to strange men.

[21] The death of someone she loved, for example, turns her away even if she has begun to want someone.

[22] Because her husband is always near her, she does not see how to get away to make love.

[24] She thinks, 'His mind is difficult to grasp', and because she does not understand him well, her mind and heart do not imagine him.

[25] She thinks, 'Sex with him will not be a long-term prospect.'

[26] She thinks, 'He will make me the laughing-stock of society.'

[27] She thinks, 'He does what his friends tell him to do; he has nothing but scorn for me.'

[28] She thinks, 'His advances are all hollow, without any true motive.'

[30] She is of dull sexual energy, and fears that he is a 'stallion'.

'He is too strong';* ³¹or she becomes shy when she thinks, 'He is a man-about-town, accomplished in all the arts';* ³²or she feels, 'He has always treated me just as a friend'; ³³or she cannot bear him, thinking, 'He does not know the right time and place', ³⁴or she does not respect him, thinking, 'He is an object of contempt'; ³⁵or she despises him when she thinks, 'Even though I have given him signals, he does not understand'; ³⁶or if she is an 'elephant cow' she thinks, 'He is a "hare", of dull sexual energy'; ³⁷or she feels sympathy for him and thinks, 'I would not want anything unpleasant to happen to him because of me'; ³⁸or she becomes depressed when she sees her own shortcomings, ³⁹or afraid when she thinks, 'If I am discovered, my own people will throw me out'; ⁴⁰or scornful, thinking, 'He has grey hair'; ⁴¹or she worries, 'My husband has employed him to test me'; ⁴²or she has regard for religion.*

⁴³A man should eliminate, from the very beginning, whichever of these causes for rejection he detects in his own situation. ⁴⁴If it is connected with her nobility, he excites more passion. ⁴⁵If it is a matter of apparent impossibility, he shows her ways to manage it. ⁴⁶If

---

³¹ A country girl or an unsophisticated girl would be shy of such a man.

³⁴ She thinks, 'Because he is so low, one of my girlfriends or some other person will look down on me.'

³⁷ She thinks, 'Something bad may happen either to his body or to his money, if he makes love to me.'

³⁸ She notices a disease in her body, for example, or a bad smell.

⁴² There actually are a few women who have regard for religion and the violation of religion.

⁴⁴ Love for her husband, regard for her children, the fact that she is past her prime or overwhelmed by unhappiness, and regard for religion [5.1.18–21, 42]—these are causes inherent in the woman, connected with her nobility, and he can counteract this tendency by making her passion for him grow.*

⁴⁵ If she is unable to find an opportunity to get away, or thinks, 'I would not want anything unpleasant to happen to him', or if she sees her own shortcomings [5.1.22, 37, 38], he shows her how to manage it.

⁴⁶ If she thinks, 'He is inscrutable', or, 'He is a man-about-town, accomplished in all the arts', or 'He has always treated me just as a friend', or 'My husband has employed him to test me' [5.1.24, 31, 32, 41]—these are causes inherent in him, exciting her respect. But when he becomes very intimate, her awe of him trickles away.

the problem is her respect for him, he becomes very intimate with her. ⁴⁷ If it stems from her contempt, he demonstrates his extraordinary pride and his erudition. ⁴⁸ If it comes from his contempt, he prostrates himself before her. ⁴⁹ If she is afraid, he reassures her.

[41]   *Men who are Successful with Women*

⁵⁰ The following men are generally successful with women: a man who knows the *Kamasutra*, a good storyteller, a man who has been close to the woman from childhood, a man in the prime of youth, a man who can gain a woman's trust by engaging her in such things as games, a man who carries out her commands, a good conversationalist, a man who does what the woman likes, a man who used to be the messenger of another man, a man who knows a woman's vulnerable spots,* a man who is sought by a woman of the highest class, a man secretly involved with the woman's girlfriend, a man famous for his luck in love, a man who grew up with the woman, a sexy next-door neighbour, a sexy servant, the husband of her foster-sister, a newly engaged man, a generous man who loves picnics and theatrical plays, a man so strong and hot that people call him a bull, an impetuous man, a brave man, a man who surpasses her husband in learning, good looks, good qualities, and enjoyments, a man who dresses well and lives well.

---

⁴⁷ If she fears, 'His advances are just a tease'; or thinks, 'He does not know the right time and place', or, 'He is an object of contempt', or 'He does not understand', or 'He has grey hair' [5.1.28, 33–35, 40]—these are causes inherent in him, exciting her contempt. His pride, and his demonstration of his knowledge of the texts and the arts, washes away the contempt.

⁴⁸ If she thinks, 'He is propositioning me in an insulting way', or, 'His face cannot keep a secret', or, 'His affection is all for his friends' [5.1.23, 26, 27]—these are causes inherent in him, exciting her contempt. He prostrates himself when he is making advances in a place where they are entirely alone.

⁴⁹ If she thinks, 'How glamorous he is', 'His sexual energy is too fierce', 'He is a "hare", of dull sexual energy', or 'If I am discovered, my own people will throw me out' [5.1.29, 30, 36, 39]—these are causes inherent in her, exciting her fear.

⁵⁰ The impetuous man acts quickly, without thinking a lot about it; he just waits for a word from the woman.

[42]   *Women who can be Won without Effort*

⁵¹ Just as a man judges his chances of success from considering his own qualities, so he should judge them from considering the woman's qualities, too.* ⁵² The following are women who can be had without any effort, who can be had merely by making advances:* a woman who stands at the door; a woman who looks out from her rooftop porch onto the main street; a woman who hangs about the house of the young man who is her neighbour; a woman who stares constantly; a woman who, when someone looks at her, looks sideways; a woman who has been supplanted by a co-wife for no cause; a woman who hates her husband; a woman who is hated; a woman who lacks restraint; a woman who has no children; ⁵³ a woman who has always lived in the house of her relatives; a woman whose children have died; a woman who is fond of society; a woman who shows her love; the wife of an actor;* a young woman whose husband has died; a poor woman fond of enjoying herself; the wife of the oldest of several brothers; a very proud woman who has an inadequate husband; a woman who is proud of her skills and distressed by her husband's foolishness, lack of distinction, or greediness; ⁵⁴ a woman

---

⁵² She stands at the door, hoping to see men. Supplanted for no cause, because she is not promiscuous or anything of that sort, she cannot bear that and seeks another man. Both a woman who hates her husband, even if he has good qualities, and a woman who is hated by her husband, are fickle. The woman who is unrestrained toward the things that should be restrained, by her very nature goes astray. The woman who has no children sees no children coming from her husband and goes to other men.

⁵³ The woman raised in the house of her relatives shatters her good behaviour as soon as she becomes independent. The woman whose children have died goes to other men because she thinks, 'Whatever child is born to my husband, that child dies', or simply because she has no children. The wife of an actor, or of a dancer or mime artist, is usually a courtesan; a wife who has many young brothers-in-law is usually given some experience by them.

⁵⁴ When he failed to get her, she married another man, but he can win her now, because of her former love for him. A woman who takes sides can be won by the man whose side she takes. A woman whose husband

who, when she was a virgin, was courted by a man who made a great effort but somehow did not get her and now woos her again; a woman whose intelligence, nature, wisdom, perception, and personality are similar to those of the would-be lover; a woman who is by nature given to taking sides; a woman who has been dishonoured by her husband when she has done nothing wrong; a woman who is put down by women whose beauty and so forth are the same as hers; a woman whose husband travels a lot; the wife of a man who is jealous, putrid, too pure, impotent, a procrastinator, unmanly, a hunchback, a dwarf, deformed, a jeweller, a villager, bad-smelling, sick, or old.

[55] And there are two verses about this:

> Longing* springs from one's own nature
> but there are ways to make it grow.
> When intelligence has washed away anxiety,
> longing becomes unwavering and undying.
> [56] A man who knows his own chances of success
> and discerns women's telltale signs
> cuts away the causes of their resistance
> and succeeds with women.

---

travels a lot is broken down by celibacy; how could she not desire other men? The wife of a man who is jealous, without cause, is sooner or later carried off by voluptuaries. If a man does not clean his body, his wife turns away from him because he is so putrid, so foul. 'Too pure' is the name of a specific caste, whose women are generally courtesans. A procrastinator is a man who decides to accomplish some task but does not actually begin it at that time. A jeweller's wife is always going to the market, where she gets a bad reputation. A villager's wife is easily won by the man-about-town. A man whose body smells bad makes her nervous. An old man is no longer capable of sex.

[55] 'A woman desires any attractive man she sees' [5.1.8], but she may become anxious if she cannot see a way of devising some means by which they can make love. When she sees the means, however, she is no longer anxious.

CHAPTER TWO

[43]   *Ways of Becoming Intimate*

¹Scholars say: 'A man can win virgins more easily through his own advances than through a female messenger, but he can win the wives of other men, who are in a more delicate situation, more easily through a female messenger than on his own.' ²Vatsyayana says: In all instances, if it is within the realm of his powers, the man's own action is more effective, but if this is difficult or impossible to do, then he should employ a female messenger. ³It is commonly said: 'Women who are acting rashly for the first time, and who converse without restraint, can be seduced by a man on his own; women who are the opposite, by a messenger.'

⁴But when the man makes advances by himself he must achieve intimacy from the very start. ⁵He sees her on a natural or contrived occasion. ⁶A natural occasion might occur near his own house, and a contrived one near the house of a friend, relative, minister of state, or doctor, at a wedding, sacrifice, festival, disaster, picnic, or other such occasion. ⁷When she sees him, he gazes at her constantly, sending signals, smoothing down his hair, snapping his nails, jingling his jewellery, chewing on his lower lip, and making various other pretences. When she is looking he talks with his friends* about her under the pretext of discussing other matters; he displays his generosity and fondness for enjoyments. Seated on the lap of a friend, he shifts the position of his arms and legs, yawns, raises one eyebrow, speaks slowly, and listens to the woman's words. He carries on, with a child or another adult, a conversation that seems to be about something else but has a double meaning, about her; thus he himself conveys his wish for her. Under a pretext, but intending no one but

---

³ Women who act rashly shatter their good character; if they speak freely with the man, what need is there for a messenger for them? But women of the opposite sort have often shattered their good character and converse with restraint. Now, the pursuit of a woman who is acting rashly for the first time is forbidden, even in order 'to ward off fatal blows to the body' [5.1.3]. But knowing that a man cannot pursue a woman by himself without achieving intimacy, V describes the causes of intimacy.

⁵ He sees her only after he has sent a messenger.

her, he kisses and embraces a child, gives him betel with his tongue, caresses the child's chin with his index finger, all of this done in a manner appropriate to the circumstances and the opportunity. ⁸He fondles a child on her lap, gives him toys and takes them away again. And out of the intimacy gained by this means he strikes up a conversation with her, and making himself agreeable to someone who is able to talk with her, he uses that person to establish some reason for coming and going. And within her hearing, but without looking at her at all, he talks about the *Kamasutra*.

⁹As he grows more intimate with her, he places in her hands something for her to keep temporarily for him and something else for her to keep for a long time, and every day, at any moment, he withdraws some small part of it—perfumes or areca nuts. ¹⁰Then he arranges for her to meet his own wives and engage in confidential conversations, sitting together by themselves. ¹¹This is so that he can see her all the time and get her to trust him. ¹²When she desires something from the goldsmith, jeweller, basket-maker, dyer in indigo or saffron, and so forth, he himself, together with his own servants, takes the trouble to obtain these things for her. ¹³And while he is accomplishing that business, he can see her for a long time, and people will know about it. ¹⁴And that transaction will lead to others, each connected with the one before. ¹⁵Whenever she wants something done, or wants some object or something requiring a certain skill, he shows her that he himself has the plan, the resources, the experience, the means, and the intelligence for it. ¹⁶He converses with her and her entourage about past events, the things that people have done, and ways of testing the quality of material things. ¹⁷In the course of doing this, he makes bets about such things and appoints her the umpire for these bets. ¹⁸But if he disagrees with her, he says, 'How amazing!'* Those are the ways of becoming intimate.

[44]   *Making Advances*

¹⁹When she has become intimate with him and revealed her gestures and signals to him, he makes advances to her with the methods that are used on a virgin.* Generally the advances in that case are rather subtle, because virgins have not yet made love. But he makes advances to other women in the very same way, though quite blatantly,

because these women have made love. ²⁰ When he has understood her signals and uncovered her favourable feelings for him, he uses her possessions as they share one another's objects of enjoyment. ²¹ In the course of this sharing, they exchange precious perfumes, upper garments, flowers, and also rings. When she takes betel from his hand as he prepares to go to a social gathering, he asks for a flower from her hair. ²² In doing this, he gives her, with signals, a precious, desirable perfume, in a container marked with the traces of his own nails and teeth. ²³ He whittles away her nervousness by making more and more advances to her. ²⁴ By degrees, he goes with her to a place where they are alone together, embraces her, kisses her, takes betel from her, and after giving it to her exchanges things with her and caresses her in her hidden places. Those are the advances.

²⁵ A man should never pursue one woman in a place where he is pursuing another. ²⁶ If a woman who has had an affair with him in the past lives there, he should placate her with loving conciliations. ²⁷ And there are two verses about this:

> The man should not mount any woman,
> even if she is very ready to be taken,
> in a place where the husband
> has been seen to stray toward another woman.
> ²⁸ A wise man, aware of his own security,
> will not even think about a woman
> who is worried, well-guarded, afraid,
> or with her mother-in-law.

---

²⁰ He himself uses the woman's things and gets her to use his.

²² When the man gives her the perfume by the hand of another person, he marks its container with his teeth and nails; when he gives it himself, he gives it with signals.

²⁴ He caresses her armpits and the places where her thighs join her torso, but not her sexual organ.

²⁵ He should not pursue two women in the same house.

²⁷ Even if she is very easy to get, he should not make love to a woman in a house where the woman's husband has been seen to make love to another woman.

²⁸ A man who decides, 'I am not able to do it in this case', will not even think about a woman who is worried about her lover, well-guarded by men with weapons, afraid of her husband, or supervised by her mother-in-law.

they understand one another's signals.
²⁵ If a man sees, through a woman's replies,
that she has grasped and accepted his signals,
then, with no further hesitation,
he makes advances to her.
²⁶ If a woman immediately reveals
her feelings through her signals,
he can make advances to her
quickly, right at first sight.
²⁷ If a woman is given slippery signals
but returns a candid answer, he realizes,
'She, too, can be won in a moment',
for she longs ardently for sexual pleasure.
²⁸ This subtle method has been prescribed
for a woman who is firm, not bold,
and who takes care to make tests.
Candid women can simply be won.

CHAPTER FOUR

[46]   *The Duties of a Female Messenger*

¹ If a woman has revealed her gestures and signals but lets him see her only at infrequent intervals and has not done this before, he seduces her by means of a female messenger. ² The messenger gets access to the woman through her good character and then charms her by showing her little stories in pictures painted on a cloth, teaching her ways to become lucky in love, gossiping about people, reciting stories told by the poets and stories about men who have seduced other men's wives, and praising her beauty, intelligence, skill, and good

---

²⁵ He does not worry, 'Will I win her, or not?' There are two kinds of women, candid and not candid. To show that this rule does not apply to the ones who are candid, he says the next verse.

²⁷ She receives signals that are not candid, but she signals a candid answer.

²⁸ Of the two types of women just mentioned, candid women 'can be had merely by making advances' [5.1.52].

character. ³The messenger inspires regret in the woman by saying, 'How could a girl like you have a husband like that?' ⁴And she says, 'You are lucky in love, but he is not fit even to be your servant.' ⁵And in the woman's presence, when true feelings are being revealed, she speaks relentlessly of the husband's dull sexual energy, jealousy, dishonesty, ingratitude, disinclination for enjoyment, stinginess, fickleness, and other things hidden in him. ⁶When she notices that a particular flaw disturbs the woman, that is the one she insists upon. ⁷If the woman is a 'doe', then it is not a flaw for him to be a 'hare', ⁸and similar arguments can be made for a 'mare' or an 'elephant cow'.

⁹Gonikaputra says: 'When he has won the woman's trust in this way, if this is her first rash act or if she has a delicate nature, he seduces her through a female messenger.'* ¹⁰The messenger tells the woman about the man's accomplishments, how well he suits her, his sexual moves.* ¹¹And as the woman reveals more and more of her true feelings, the messenger talks about the real purpose of her mission in a devious manner, with the following argument: ¹²'Listen, you are lucky in love, but this is an extraordinary thing. That man over there, the son of such a good family, is a lover who fell madly in love with you at first sight. Since he is very delicate by nature, and has never been afflicted like this before, by anyone else, he is suffering terribly, burning up. It is therefore quite possible that he will even die of this today.' That is how she describes him. ¹³If she succeeds in this, on the next day she tells her stories again, marking the favourable response in the woman's speech, face, and eyes.

¹⁴As the woman listens, the messenger tells her well-known,

---

³ 'A husband like that' is ugly and so forth.

⁷ But it is a flaw if he is a 'stallion'.

⁸ For a 'mare' or 'elephant cow', there is a no flaw if he is a 'bull' or a 'stallion'.

¹⁰ There are three kinds of sexual moves, at the beginning, middle, and end of love-making.

¹² 'Even though other women are in love with him, when he saw you . . .'

¹⁴ (1) Ahalya* was the wife of Gotama; the king of the gods fell in love with her and she desired him. (2) The fire-priest instructed a woman in the fire ritual. Agni, the god of fire, so desired her that he took on a form and arose out of the fire altar. When she became pregnant, her

relevant stories, about Ahalya, Avimaraka, Shakuntala, and others. [15] She speaks of the man's sexual powers, his knowledge of the sixty-four arts, and his luck in love, and she describes how he has made love secretly with some praiseworthy woman, which may or may not have happened in the past. [16] She notes the woman's signals, [17] and when she sees her smile, she converses with her, [18] and invites her to sit down. [19] She asks her, 'Where have you been?' 'Where did you sleep? Eat?' 'Where did you spend time?' or 'What did you do?' [20] She reveals herself to her when they are alone together. [21] She gets her to tell little stories. [22] She sighs and yawns, thoughtfully. [23] She gives her love-gifts. [24] She remembers her at sacrifices and festivals. [25] She lets the woman go only after she has promised to let the messenger see her again.

[26] The woman keeps the conversation going by saying to the

---

father-in-law, fearing a stain on the family, abandoned her in the forest. She gave birth to a son, whom the general of the Shabaras raised as his own child. That son, in his childhood, played among the herds of sheep and goats and wandered around with them. By drinking their milk he became very strong, so strong that, even though he was just a little child, he killed goats and sheep with his bare hands. And for that reason, the general gave him the appropriate name of Avimaraka ['Sheep-killer']. When he reached the prime of his youth, one day an elephant attacked the daughter of a king who was sojourning in the forest, and he killed the elephant and saved her. After that she fell in love with him and of her own will gave him her hand in marriage. These stories are relevant to a discussion of the seduction of other men's wives.

[15] The sixty-four techniques are those of Panchala, singing and so forth.* She says, 'He has such luck in love that he was desired even by a man.' Even if it did not happen it has become as if it had happened.

[19] For she thinks, 'Through this device she will say something connected with the man.'

[20] For she thinks, 'She will tell some secret.'

[21] For she thinks, 'Perhaps she will tell a story about the man, in order to talk about fickleness.'

[23] She gives her bangles or upper garments.

[24] She remembers her, saying, 'Why did you not come today?'

[26] The messenger has pursued the conversation by saying, 'Your face, even just hearing someone mention your name, makes him happy.'

messenger, 'You speak so well, but why are you telling me these terrible things?' [27] The woman lists the man's faults, his dishonesty and fickleness. [28] She herself does not tell how she saw him before or spoke with him, but she longs for the messenger to talk about it. [29] When the messenger is telling her about the man's wishes, she laughs scornfully but does not scorn him.

[30] When the messenger has understood the woman's signals she strengthens her resolve with recollections of the man. [31] But if the woman is not familiar with him, the messenger snares her with stories about his good qualities and stories about his love for her.

[32] Auddalaki says: 'Two people who have not become familiar with one another and have not sent one another signals have no use for a messenger.' [33] The followers of Babhravya say: 'Two people who have sent one another signals, even if they are not familiar with one another, can use a messenger.' [34] Gonikaputra says: 'Two people who are familiar with one another, even if they have not sent one another signals, can use a messenger.' [35] Vatsyayana says: Even two people who have not sent one another signals and are not familiar with one another can use a messenger, because of their confidence in the messenger.

[36] To such women, the messenger shows gifts that the man has sent, gifts that steal the heart, such as betel, perfumed oils, a garland, a ring, or a garment. [37] These bear the traces of the man's nails and teeth, and various other marks, as his possessions. [38] On the garment he draws, in saffron, hands cupped together in supplication. [39] The messenger shows the woman leaves cut into shapes with the forms of various intentions, and ear ornaments and chaplets with letters written on leaves concealed within them, [40] letters in which he tells of his own wishes. And she gets the woman to send back gifts in return. [41] When two people have accepted one another's gifts in this way, their meeting depends on their confidence in the female messenger.

[42] The followers of Babhravya say: 'This meeting can take place on the occasion of visiting the gods, at a festival, playing in a park, bathing or swimming, at a wedding, a sacrifice, disaster, or festival,

---

[36] Such women are not familiar with the man.

[38] The cupped hands are intended to give rise to the impression, 'This man is intent on nothing but propitiating you in this way.'

the spectacle of a house on fire, the commotion after a robbery, the invasion of the countryside by an army, at theatrical spectacles, or in various sorts of activities.'* [43] Gonikaputra says, 'A meeting is easy to arrange in the houses of a girlfriend, a beggar woman, a Buddhist nun, or a female ascetic.' [44] Vatsyayana says: But in the woman's own house, where he knows the exits and entrances and where it is possible to devise in advance counter-measures against potential dangers, his arrival and departure are secured even at an unpredictable time, and the meeting is reliable and easy to arrange.

[45] The types of female messengers are the fully authorized messenger, the messenger with limited authority, the letter carrier, the messenger acting for herself, the foolish messenger, the wife as messenger, the mute messenger, and the wind messenger.

[46] The fully authorized messenger understands the goal that is in the minds of both the man and the woman and then by her own intelligence undertakes to bring it about. [47] She is generally used by a man and a woman who are familiar with one another and have spoken together. [48] She may be employed by the woman even if the couple are not familiar with one another and have not spoken together; [49] or she may be employed, out of erotic curiosity, by two people who are suited to and appropriate for one another, even though they are not familiar with one another.

[50] The messenger with limited authority knows just one part of the task and one part of the courtship, and completes the rest. [51] She is used by two people who have sent one another signals but have seen one another only at long intervals.

[52] The letter carrier just brings communications. [53] She reports the time and place of the meeting for two people who are familiar with one another and whose feelings are deep.

[54] The messenger acting for herself is sent as a messenger by another woman, but she herself seduces the man and, pretending not to know that she is seducing him, tells him how she dreamed about

---

44 But they should not meet in the house of someone such as a woman friend, because their arrival and departure are not secure, since she is not always at home.

54 She says, 'You have even called your wife by my name! It would be all right to address her in this way if she were beautiful.' She gives him something: such as betel, a chaplet, or areca nuts, to declare her passion.

enjoying passionate sex with him; or she reproaches him for calling his wife by the wrong name,* and reviles his wife. Under this pretext, she expresses her own jealousy. Or she gives him something marked by her nails and teeth and says, 'I decided to give this first of all to you.' And when they are alone together she asks him, 'Who is lovelier, your wife or I?' [55] He sees the messenger and receives her in a secluded place. [56] A woman is also a messenger acting for herself if she makes an agreement with another woman under the pretext of serving as her messenger, but by means of carrying that woman's messages wins the man for herself and ruins that woman's chances. [57] The man, too, is sometimes said to play that role and woo for himself when he is the messenger for another man.

[58] The woman gets the confidence of the man's naïve wife,* enters in unhindered, and asks her about the man's doings. She teaches the wife tricks. She dresses her up in a way that sends signals to him. She gets her angry with him and says, 'This is how you must act.' And she herself makes the traces of nails and teeth on the wife. Through that means, the woman signals to the man. She, the wife, is the foolish messenger, and [59] he uses her to get the woman's replies.

[60] Or the man gets his own foolish wife to get together with the woman to gain her confidence, and he uses her to send signals. He even has his wife talk to the woman about his skill and experience. She is the wife as messenger, and he uses her to get the woman's signals.

[61] Or he sends a young servant girl who knows nothing about wickedness on a project that is not at all wicked. But in the process he secretes a written message or the traces of his nails or of his teeth in a garland or an ear ornament. She is the mute messenger, and he uses her to ask for the woman's replies.

[62] A woman who is a neutral bystander may transmit a statement that bears the identifying mark of a previously arranged matter, that

---

[55] The man makes advances to her, if he wants to make love with her.

[58] She sends signals in order to indicate her own desires. She gets the wife angry, in order to show that she, too, is jealous, saying, 'This man is fickle and is attached to another woman. How is it that you do not get angry?' She marks the wife with the traces of nails and teeth to announce her own longing to make love. The wife is the foolish messenger, because she does not understand the purpose of a messenger.

another person could not grasp, or that has both a common meaning and a special double meaning. She is the wind messenger, and he uses her to ask for the woman's replies. Those are the types of female messengers.

⁶³ And there are verses about this:

> A widow, a fortune-teller, a servant girl,
> a beggar woman, and a woman artist
> quickly enter a woman's confidence
> and understand the duties of a messenger.

⁶⁴ She inspires hatred of the husband,
> describes his sexual charms,
> and reveals the various enjoyments of sex,
> that other women, too, have had.*

⁶⁵ And she describes the man's love for the woman,
> and, again, his skill in love-making,
> and tells how he is sought by great women,
> and remains constant.

⁶⁶ The messenger, through her skill with words,
> can take even an unintended meaning
> uttered by mistake
> and twist it right around.

---

⁶⁴ She inspires hatred by praising his good looks and so forth, as has been said: 'She inspires regret' [5.4.3]. And she describes his sexual charms, as has been said: 'She tells about the man's accomplishments, how well he suits her, his sexual moves' [5.4.10]. She reveals the enjoyments of sex, as has been said: 'She speaks of the man's sexual powers, his knowledge of the sixty-four arts, and his luck in love' [5.4.15]. She describes these not just in front of the woman herself, but in front of her friends, too.

⁶⁵ She says, 'Listen, you are lucky in love, but this is an extraordinary thing' [5.4.12]. As has been said: 'She describes how he has made love secretly with some praiseworthy woman, which happened or did not happen in the past' [5.4.15]. She describes his constancy toward the woman.

CHAPTER FIVE

[47]   *The Sex Life of a Man in Power*

> [1] Kings and ministers of state
>   do not enter into other men's homes,
>   for the whole populace sees what they do
>   and imitates it.
> [2] The three worlds* watch the sun rise
>   and so they too rise;
>   then they watch the sun moving
>   and they too start to act.

[3] Therefore, because it is impossible and because they would be blamed, such men do nothing frivolous. [4] But when they cannot help doing it, they employ stratagems. [5] A young village headman, or a king's officer, or the son of the superintendent of farming, can win village women just with a word, and then libertines call these women adulteresses. [6] Sex with these women takes place when they are engaged in such activities as doing chores, filling granaries, bringing things in and out of houses, cleaning house, working in the field, purchasing cotton, wool, flax, linen, and bark, spinning thread, and buying, selling, and exchanging goods. [7] And in the same manner, the man in charge of the cow-herds may take the women of the cow-herds; [8] the man in charge of threads* may take widows, women who have no man to protect them, and wandering women ascetics; [9] the city police-chief may take the women who roam about begging, for he knows where they are vulnerable, because of his own night-roamings; [10] and the man in charge of the market may take the women who buy and sell.

[11] On occasions such as the eighth day of the waning half of the month in autumn, the full-moon night in winter, and the spring festival, the women of market-towns, cities, and mountain villages generally attend the parties of the women of the harem in the home of the man in power. [12] There, when the drinking party is over, the women of the city go individually, each according to her intimacy with the women of the harem, to the houses devoted to enjoyments, where they sit and tell stories and are honoured and given drinks; and they go home by evening.

¹³ On such an occasion, a royal servant girl, who has already become acquainted with the woman whom the man wants, is sent there and talks with her. ¹⁴ She enlists her by showing her lovely things. ¹⁵ Even before this, when the woman was still in her own home, the royal servant had said to her, 'While we are all at the party there, I will show you the lovely things that are in the king's mansion.' And then, at that time, she enlists the woman, saying, 'I will show you, outside, a floor inlaid with coral.' ¹⁶ And there is a floor made of jewels, and a grove of trees, a vineyard, bath-houses and a rooftop porch, secret passages in the palace walls, paintings, tame deer, mechanical contrivances, cages of birds, tigers, and lions, all the things that she had described before. ¹⁷ And when they are alone together, she tells the woman that the man in power is in love with her, ¹⁸ and she describes his expertise in making love. ¹⁹ She gets the woman to agree and not to tell anyone about their plan.

²⁰ If she does not agree, the man in power comes to her himself, conciliates her with courtesies, makes love with her, reunites her with the servant girl, and then dismisses her lovingly. ²¹ And he accustoms the woman's husband to receiving favours and after that has that man's wives brought into the harem all the time, to get him accustomed to it. Then, on this occasion, a royal servant girl is sent, and so forth, just as before.

²² Or, a woman of the harem becomes friendly with the woman the man wants by sending her own servant woman to her. And when the friendship has progressed, she invites the woman to come and see her, under some pretext. When the woman has entered, and has been honoured and given drinks, a royal servant girl is sent, and so forth, just as before.

²³ Or, if the woman the man wants is famous for a particular skill, a woman of the harem should treat her with courtesies and invite her to demonstrate that skill. When the woman has entered, a royal servant girl is sent, and so forth, just as before.

²⁴ Or, a beggar woman says to the wife of a man who has lost all his money or is frightened, 'This woman of the harem, who has won

---

¹³ The king sends her to a woman to whom he wishes to make love.
²⁰ The man makes love to her with the sexual act that suits her.
²⁴ The man may be frightened of the king's court.

over the king so that he does what she says, listens to my words. Because I am compassionate by nature, I will approach her and get her to let you enter. And she will reverse your husband's great loss of fortune.' When the woman agrees, the woman of the harem lets her enter two or three times and dispels the woman's fears. And when the woman hears that she has nothing to be afraid of, she is overjoyed. Then a royal servant girl is sent, and so forth, just as before. ²⁵ This last stratagem is also prescribed for the wives of men who are seeking employment, oppressed by ministers of state, seized by force, weak in practical skills, dissatisfied with their own possessions, hoping to become friends with the king, striving for a rank among the royal families, harassed by their relatives, wishing to harass their relatives, informants, and others embroiled in specific enterprises.

²⁶ Or, if the woman the man wants is already intimate with another man, he has her seized, makes her into a servant girl, and gradually introduces her into the harem. ²⁷ Or he has her husband slandered by a spy, saying, 'He is an enemy of the king', and then seizes the woman as the man's wife, and by this means has her enter the harem.

Those are the secret methods.* They are generally used by the king's sons.

²⁸ But the man in power should not enter another man's home in this way. ²⁹ 'For when Abhira, the Kotta king, went to another man's home, a washerman employed by the king's brother killed him. And the superintendent of horses killed Jayasena the king of Varanasi.' So it is said.

³⁰ Open sexual affairs may be pursued according to the custom of the region. ³¹ It is said of the people of Andhra that the virgins of the

---

²⁶ He makes her into a servant girl because a woman who has been publicly ruined is a kind of courtesan. First he makes her into a common woman and then he introduces her into the harem gradually, not violently or right away, so that no one will think, 'He did this by a trick.'

²⁷ This pair of methods is to be used on women who have not abandoned their families. They are used by the king's sons, but not by the king.

²⁹ In Gurjurat there is a place named Kotta, whose king, named Abhira, went to another man's house in order to sleep with the wife of Vasumitra, the head warrior. There, a guard employed by his brother, who deserved the kingdom, killed him. Jayasena the king of Varanasi had gone into another man's house to make love with that man's wife.

countryside, on the tenth day after they have been given in marriage, take some gift suited for the purpose and enter the harem. As soon as the king has enjoyed them, they are dismissed. [32] It is said of the people of Vatsagulma, that the women in the harems of men in power under state ministers go to the king at night to serve him. [33] In Vidarbha, the women of the harem invite the beautiful women of the countryside to stay with them for a month or half a month, under the pretext of friendship. [34] In the far West, a man will give his own wives, if they are good-looking, to kings and ministers of state as a kind of love-gift. [35] And in Surashtra, the women of the city and the women of the countryside, in groups or one by one, enter the royal court in order to serve the king in his erotic games.

[36] And there are two verses about this:

> These and many other devices
> for seducing other men's wives
> were put into circulation by kings,
> and are employed in region after region.*

> [37] But a king who takes pleasure in the welfare of his people*
> should absolutely not use these devices.
> A man who suppresses the band of six enemies within him
> conquers the earth too.

CHAPTER SIX

[48]   *The Life of the Women of the Harem*

[1] The women of the harem cannot meet men, because they are carefully guarded; and since they have only one husband shared by many women in common, they are not satisfied. Therefore they give pleasure to one another with the following techniques. [2] They dress up a

---

[33] But the real purpose is sex.

[37] The six enemies are desire, anger, greed, pride, intoxication, and joy.

[2] By imagining a man, they experience a heightened emotion that gives extreme satisfaction. These things have a form just like the male sexual organ: the bulbs of arrowroot, plantain, and so forth; the roots of coconut palms, breadfruit, and so forth; and the fruits of the bottle-gourd cucumber, and so forth.

foster-sister or girlfriend or servant girl like a man and relieve their desire with dildos or with bulbs, roots, or fruits that have that form. ³ They lie on statues of men that have distinct* sexual characteristics. ⁴ Kings, too, if they are sympathetic to their women even when their passion does not stir, make use of dildos until they achieve their goal, so that in one night they can even go to many women. But when the woman he loves has her turn to sleep with him or is in her fertile season, then the man acts out of desire. Those are the Oriental customs. (⁵ With the very same technique that women use, men, too, if they cannot get any sexual action, are said to relieve their desire in things other than the vagina, in creatures other than the human species, in statues of women, and by simple masturbation.*)

⁶ The women of the harem generally get their women servants to bring in men-about-town dressed as women. ⁷ Their foster-sisters, too, if they are intimate with the women on the inside, may make an effort to accost these men, showing them what a future there is in it. ⁸ They describe how easy it is to enter, the place where they can get out, the spaciousness of the building, the carelessness of the guards, and the irregularities of the entourage. ⁹ They should not, however,

---

³ These statues have indistinct sexual characteristics because they do not have beards yet; they have the bodies of men but the appearance of women.

⁴ They strap on an artificial instrument made of wood to achieve their satisfaction. This is known as the technique for the harem.

⁵ Men who cannot get a woman relieve their desires in a thigh or hand, and so forth, moving it back and forth; or in a sheep, mare, and so forth; or simply by using their hand to churn their instrument with a 'lion's pounce', as it is said:

Sitting with legs stretched out at right angles to one another,
propping yourself up with your two hands planted
on the ground between them, rub it between your arms;
that is the way you do the 'lion's pounce'.

someone should object, 'It goes against religion to shed your
the wrong places', you reply, 'What about wet-dreams? The
iation and restoration for that applies to this case.'
of a false representation would be saying that the harem is
when it is not. This might corrupt what has not been
ut people in danger.

use false representations to get people to enter, for this would be a serious mistake.

[10] Vatsyayana says: A man-about-town, however, should not enter a harem even if it is easy to get into, because this usually ends in disaster. [11] But if he has considered, with an eye to the rewards, all the factors—if the harem has an exit and is deeply hidden by thick woods, the wall enclosing the harem is long and divided up, the guards are few and careless, and the king is away—and if he has been invited many times, and he has worked out a way over the wall, and the women have shown him the way to do it, he may enter. [12] And within the realm of possibility, he should come out every day.

[13] He gets close to the guards on the outside through some pretext. [14] He represents himself as attached to a servant girl who works inside and who knows his real purposes. And he reveals to the women who go inside the harem his sorrow at not being with that girl, and he gets them to do the whole job of a messenger. [15] He finds out who the king's spies are. [16] If, however, the female messenger cannot find a way for him to get in, but the woman he wants has sent him signals, he stations himself where she can see him. [17] Even at that very spot, however, he makes some pretext to the guards about his servant girl. [18] When the woman's gaze is fixed on him, he sends messages to her with his gestures and signals. [19] Where her gaze falls, there he places a portrait of her, and fragments of songs with double meanings, and little toys with special marks on them, and a ring marked with an impression. [20] He perceives her answer to his question. And then he strives to enter.

[21] He finds out where she goes all the time and he hides himself right there, ahead of time. [22] Or he disguises himself as a guard and enters at a time that she appoints. [23] Or he goes in and out clothed in a bedspread or a cloak. [24] Or he makes his shadow and his

---

[13] He says, 'Through such and such a connection, you are my brother or my sister's husband!' He becomes friendly with them, so that they will be slack in guarding against him.

[14] He fakes the sorrow of failing to be with the servant girl.

[19] He leaves a ring with his name on it, marked by the traces of his nails and teeth.

[24] Some people make the body disappear, but not the shadow. But only those who make both disappear are not seen.

body disappear by means of the magic trick of the 'pocket-no pocket'.* ²⁵ The technique for this is: He cooks the heart of a mongoose, the fruits of a fenugreek plant and a long gourd, and snake eyes, over a fire that does not smoke. Then he rubs into this the same measure of the collyrium used as eye make-up. When he has smeared his eyes with this, he can move about without a shadow or a body. ²⁶ And on the nights of the full moon, he can move about by the light of many lamps, or by a subterranean passage.

²⁷ And there is this verse about this:

Also when things are carried out,
and when things to drink are brought in
for festivals and drinking parties, and there is a lot of
confused activity among the maidservants;
and when there is a move from one house to another,
and a changing of the guard,
and an outing to a park or a festival,
and when they return from the festival;
and when the king has gone away on a journey
that will last for a long time—
that is usually when young men enter
and also when they leave.

²⁸ The women of the harem, knowing
one another's purposes and sharing a single purpose,
may make the rest of the women, too,
defect to their side.
Therefore, by getting them to corrupt one another
and to remain resolute in accomplishing their single purpose,
he immediately becomes safe from being betrayed
and enjoys the fruits that he desires.

²⁹ Among the people of the far West, women who have business in the royal court are the ones who bring likely looking men into the harem, because they are not very well guarded. ³⁰ The Abhira women get what they want from the guards of the harem themselves, the ones

---

²⁶ In these ways, he can enter everywhere and abduct anyone.

²⁸ They know one another's secrets and think, 'What one of us wants to do, all of us should arrange to do together.' They make the others defect so that they too will be in the same situation. Their single purpose is shattering their fidelity.

who call themselves Warriors. ³¹ The Vatsagulma women bring in, together with errand girls, the sons of men-about-town dressed in the girls' clothing. ³² The Vidarbha women use their own sons, who move freely in and out of the harem, each excepting the son she gave birth to. ³³ The women who rule their own country use their own kinsmen and relatives, who enter the harem in the same way, but no other men. ³⁴ The women of Gauda use Brahmins, friends, servants, attendants, and houseboys. ³⁵ The women of Sindh use doormen, artisans, and any other men of that sort who are not prevented from entering the harem. ³⁶ The men of the Himalayas boldly bribe the guard with money and enter *en masse*. ³⁷ In Vanga, Anga, and Kalinga, the Brahmins of the city, under the pretext of bringing flowers, go to the harem with the king's full knowledge. They chat with the women from behind a curtain. Once they have met like that, they get together. ³⁸ In the East, nine or ten women *en masse* conceal one young man at a time. That is how a man can seduce other men's women. That is the life of the women of the harem.*

Always want more

[49]   *The Guarding of Wives*

³⁹ For these very reasons a man should guard his own wives. ⁴⁰ Scholars say: 'Guards stationed in the harem should be proved pure by the trial of desire.' ⁴¹ Gonikaputra says: 'But fear or power may make them let the women use another man; therefore guards should be proved pure by the trials of desire, fear, and power.'* ⁴² Vatsyayana says: Religion prevents treachery. But a man will abandon even religion because of fear. Therefore guards should be proved pure by the trial of religion and fear.

⁴³ The followers of Babhravya say: 'To find out about his own wives' purity or impurity, a man should test them through charming women who have deeply hidden their own involuntary signals and who will report what other people say.' ⁴⁴ But Vatsyayana says: Because corrupt people can succeed among young women, a man should not set in motion, without a reason, the corruption of a person who is not corrupt.

FEAR

---

³⁸ They conceal a young man who is capable of the sexual act.
⁴⁴ Corrupt people cause ruin.

⁴⁵ The things that ruin women are as follows: too much socializing, not enough restraint,* independence from her husband, un-restrained access to men, separation from her husband during his absence, living abroad, the loss of her means of subsistence, close contact with loose women, and her husband's jealousy.

⁴⁶ A man who knows texts and considers, from the text,
  the devices whose telltale signs are detailed
  in the discussion of the seduction of other men's wives,
  is never deceived by his own wives.

⁴⁷ But he himself should never seduce other men's wives,
  because these techniques show only one of the two sides
  of each case, because the dangers are clearly visible,
  and because it goes against both religion and power.

⁴⁸ This book was undertaken in order
  to guard wives, for the benefit of men;
  its arrangements should not be learned
  in order to corrupt the people.

END OF BOOK FIVE

BOOK SIX · COURTESANS

[Who is this directed to?]

CHAPTER ONE

[50]   *Deciding on a Friend, an Eligible Lover,*
and an Ineligible Lover

[1] Courtesans find sexual pleasure and a natural way of making a living in their sexual relations with men. [2] Doing it for sexual pleasure is natural, and for gain is artificial, [3] but she makes the artificial, too, appear natural, [4] because men trust women who are driven by desire. [5] In order to demonstrate that it is natural, she betrays no greed. [6] And in order to make the future secure, she does not get money from him by objectionable methods.

[7] She is always well dressed as she looks out on the main street, easily seen but not too much exposed, because she is just like something for sale. [8] She makes friends with people through whom she can attract the man, cut him off from other women, ward off losses and rebound from them, get money, and avoid being treated with contempt by her lovers. [9] These friends are policemen, officers of the courts, fortune-tellers, bold men, heroes, men who know the same things as she knows, men who have a grasp of the arts,* libertines, panders, clowns, garland-makers, perfumers, wine-merchants, washermen, barbers, beggars, and whichever other men can be used to accomplish her goals.

---

[4] Men become attached to a woman who lets them think, 'She is in love with me', but not to women who are driven by money.

[9] Policemen and officers of the courts ward off her losses and get money for her. Fortune-tellers bring men to her and urge them on by saying, 'If you make love with this woman, your fortunes will flourish.' Bold men and heroes ward off her losses and get money for her. Men who know the same things love her and get money for her. Men who have a grasp of the arts learn the arts from the woman and publicize them, which brings lovers to her. The panders and the others bring in money through their own work and bring lovers to her through their free access to the houses of other men.

[10]Lovers who are eligible just for the sake of money are these: an independent man, a man who has just come of age, a rich man, a man whose source of income is transparent, an official, a man who obtains wealth without difficulty, a jealous rival, a man with a steady income, a man who believes he is lucky in love, a braggart, an impotent man, a man who wants to be known as a real man, a man who competes with his equals, a man generous by nature, a man who has influence with a king or a minister of state, a fatalist,* a man who

---

[10] These lovers are for money and not for love, but their money can be used for sexual pleasure and fame. An independent man is not dependent on his elders. A man who has just come of age is not too old. When she wants something from a man whose source of income is not in public view, because it comes from some other region, even when he gives her money, it is a useless gift. An official can give her money derived from whatever money he officiates over. A man whose wealth comes easily, either through an inheritance or by finding some treasure or through a favour from the king, gives it away easily, too. A jealous rival gives her a lot of money in competition with another lover. A tax-collector or usurer has a steady income. A man who believes he is lucky in love, although he is unlucky in love, does not want people to think that he is unlucky in love, and so he gives the woman a lot of money in the course of getting her away from another man. An impotent man, a non-man, gives her a lot of money in order to proclaim his virility. A man who wants people to think he is a real man gives her a lot of money when she asks for it. When two men equal in family, knowledge, wealth, or age are rivals, each thinks, 'That man who is my equal gave a lot to that courtesan; I will give her more.' Such a lover keeps spending more, like a mare who always wants to be in front. If a man has the ear of a king or minister of state, even if he himself does not give her anything, he can get the king or minister to give her something, by saying, 'This is the woman I love.' A fatalist thinks, 'My fortune is drying up because my good luck is drying up, not because it is spent on pleasures', and so he gives her a lot of money. A man who transgresses his gurus' words gives her a lot even though he is doing wrong. A rich only son is never restrained by his parents even if he gives her a lot, because they do not want him to go anywhere else. A man whose sexual desire is concealed thinks, 'People must not find out', but since he is tormented by desire, he gives her a lot. A hero makes friends and makes money. A doctor, even if he does not give the courtesan money, gives, in fact, by healing her when she is ill.

despises wealth, a man who transgresses the instructions of his elders, a man who sets an example for his siblings, a rich only son, a man who wears the sign of a religious order, a man who conceals his sexual desire, a hero, and a doctor.

[11]But men who are rich only in love and fame are eligible lovers because of their good qualities. [12]The man's good qualities are these: he is born of a great family, learned, knowledgeable about all customs, a poet, a skilled storyteller, eloquent, resolute, skilled in the various crafts, concerned for his elders. He has ambition, great endurance, and loyalty, is generous but not envious, and loving to his friends. He is fond of crowds, salons, theatrical performances, parties, and all kinds of games. He is free of disease, sound of limb, full of the breath of life, like a bull, friendly. He does not drink wine. He attracts women and flirts with them but is not in their power. He has an independent income, is not coarse, prone to anger, or nervous.

[13]The woman's qualities, on the other hand, are these: the woman is beautiful, young, with auspicious marks, sweet, in love with good qualities but not with money, by nature inclined to love and sex, with

---

[12] The man's good qualities are described here in keeping with the statement above [at 1.5.28]: 'We will explain the good qualities and lack of good qualities in both [kinds of lovers] in the discussion of courtesans.' V calls him 'the man' here, and not 'the lover', to apply more generally; he also gives him other names, such as 'suitor' in his relationship to a virgin, 'successful suitor' in his relationship to a second-hand woman, 'paramour' in his relationship to the wife of another man, and 'lover' in his relationship to a courtesan. The man is learned, in logic and so forth. He knows all customs, even the customs of heretics. He composes poems in Sanskrit and other languages. He is skilled in crafts such as sketching. He does services for those who are mature in knowledge or in years. It is said: 'The qualities of a man of endurance are heroism, indignation, speed, and cleverness.' A Brahmin who does not drink makes a lot of profits. A 'bull' is sexually potent. The man flirts by glossing over the flaws in the condition of the women's bodies.

[13] Here, too, V says 'the woman', not 'the courtesan'. Auspicious marks indicate that she will have the good fortune to be loved. A woman inclined to love and sex is fond of both external foreplay and the sexual act. When a woman with a steady mind decides, 'This has to be done', she does it. A woman true to one type has one consistent form, not a deceptive one.

a steady mind, true to one type,* a seeker of special things, never living in a greedy way, and fond of salons and the arts. [14] The following are the common qualities that the woman has, in addition: intelligence, good character, good behaviour, honesty, gratitude, the ability to see far and long, no habit of interrupting or contradicting, a knowledge of the right time and place, and urbanity.* And she is free from depression, excessive laughter, malignant gossip, verbal abuse, anger, greed, dullness, and fickleness. She speaks only when spoken to and is skilled in the *Kamasutra* and its ancillary sciences.

[15] The inverses of these qualities are the faults. [16] These are not eligible lovers: A man wasting away, sick, with worms in his faeces* or 'crow's-mouth', in love with his wife, coarse in speech, miserly, or pitiless; a man whom the elders have thrown out, a thief, or a hypocrite; a man who is addicted to love-sorcery done with roots, who does not care about honour or dishonour, who can be bought for money even by people he hates, or is shameless.

[17] Scholars say: 'The reasons for taking a lover are passion, fear,

---

[15] The inverse of the common qualities are such faults as birth from a bad family and so forth, ugliness and so forth, stupidity and so forth.* And if he has these, a lover is not a lover.

[16] A man wasting away is suffering from tuberculosis ('the royal sickness'). Worms in the faeces is a condition generally called 'faeces-flies', in which worms appear in the opening from which faeces are excreted; when semen infected with the disease through contact with the faeces enters a woman, she gets a fever. Crow's-mouth is a foul-smelling mouth; or else it means that, just as a crow puts things both pure and impure into his mouth, so this man desires women without reflecting about it, and becomes ineligible for sex. A man who loves his wife does not give the courtesan money because he never becomes attached to anyone else. A man who can be bought even by people he hates is so greedy that he surely will not give her money.

[17] These are the reasons: passion, which sometimes arises naturally, by itself; fear of death, like the fear that afflicted Rambha because of Ravana, who said to her, 'If you do not satisfy my desire, I will kill you'; gain, getting land and so forth; rivalry, like that between the two women, Devadatta and Anangasena, who fought over Muladeva; curiosity, which arises when one hears that a man is debauched and wonders, 'Is he, really?'; exhaustion, for sex revivifies; religion, which is served by sex with a learned Brahmin who has nothing; compassion, taking pity

gain, rivalry, revenge against an act of hostility, curiosity, partiality, exhaustion, religion, fame, compassion, the words of a friend, diffidence, resemblance to someone loved, wealth, allaying passion, a shared caste, living in a house together, continuity, and the future.' [18] Vatsyayana says: Gain, warding off losses, and love are the reasons. [19] Gain, however, should not be thwarted by love, since gain is the chief concern. [20] But the relative weight of fear and so forth* should be tested. That is how to decide on a friend, an eligible lover, an ineligible lover, and the reasons for taking a lover.

[51]   *Getting a Lover*

[21] Even when a lover propositions her, she does not accept him immediately, for men scorn what is easy to get. [22] In order to find out the lover's true feelings she sends him servants with masseurs, singers, and clowns, or people devoted to him. [23] If they are not available, she sends the libertine and so forth. From them she finds out if the man is pure or impure, passionate or not passionate, attached to her or not attached, generous or not generous. [24] And

---

on someone who says, 'I will die if you will not make love with me'; the words of a friend, who says, 'Someone to whom I owe a favour has arrived; do, please, sleep with him tonight'; diffidence toward someone who has the status of an elder; allaying passion, for an excessive volume of semen* is dispelled by sex with any man.

[18] The author here is saying: This is a matter either of practical calculation or of abstract theory. Healing, friendship, dispelling sorrow, and cultivating the arts are matters of practical calculation; while gain, warding off losses, and love are theoretical, for everything can be subsumed under them. The category of gain includes rivalry, curiosity, partiality, exhaustion, religion, fame, the words of a friend, and allaying passion. The category of warding off losses includes fear, hostility, and compassion. All the rest [passion, diffidence, resemblance to someone loved, a shared caste, living in a house together, continuity, and the future] are subsumed under love.

[21] And so there is a common saying:

He scorns the woman easy to get,
and desires the woman hard to get.

But when he has propositioned her over and over, she may accept him.

when she has found out about him, she offers him her love through the mediation of the pander.

²⁵ Under the pretext of a quail-fight, cock-fight, or ram-fight, or of hearing a parrot or a mynah talk, or of a theatrical spectacle or some art, the libertine brings the man to her home, ²⁶ or her to his. ²⁷ When the man arrives, she gives him a love-gift, something that will arouse his love or erotic curiosity, saying, 'This is for you alone, and no one else, to enjoy.' ²⁸ She charms him through whatever sort of conversation pleases him and through courtesies. ²⁹ When he has gone, she immediately sends after him a servant girl to joke with him and to give him a small gift. ³⁰ Or she herself goes, with the libertine, under some pretext. That is how to get a lover.

³¹ And there are verses about this:

>When a man comes to her
>she gives him, with love,
>betel and garlands and carefully prepared fragrant oils,
>and she engages him in conversation about the arts.
>³² She gives him things out of affection
>and exchanges things with him;
>and of her own accord
>she lets him know that she wants to make love.
>³³ Through love-gifts, hints,
>and courtesies with just one meaning,
>she becomes intimate with her lover, and after that
>she gets him to love her.

---

²⁵ The art might be singing.

²⁸ The conversation could be about poetry or about art. Giving him liquor, betel, and so forth are courtesies.

³³ The pander and the others drop hints by saying, 'Why don't you sleep here?' These courtesies make direct suggestions about nothing but sex.

to what he has said, if he is devoted to her. ²⁹ ~~She is attentive to all his stories, except when they are about another wife.~~ ³⁰ When he sighs, yawns, stumbles, or falls, she wishes him health; ³¹ when he sneezes, cries out, or is startled, she exclaims, 'Live!'* ³² If she becomes depressed, she pretends to be ill or to have the morbid longings that pregnant women have. ³³ She does not praise another man for his good qualities, ³⁴ nor blame another man for the flaws that he has in common with her man.

³⁵ ~~She keeps anything he has given her.~~ ³⁶ When there has been a false* accusation of infidelity or some misfortune has occurred, she wears no jewellery and refuses to eat. ³⁷ And she grieves in unity with him. ³⁸ She chooses to leave the region with him and to be ransomed from the king. ³⁹ She can live a long life only because she has him. ⁴⁰ When he gets money, or achieves something he wants, or improves his physical strength, she makes an offering to her personal deity, as

---

²⁹ In order to express her jealousy and anger, she does not respond to a story about another wife.

³² When she is depressed because she has heard something unpleasant about the man and he asks her the cause of her depression, she says, 'I have had this illness for a long time; it is an old enemy that afflicts me.'

³³ Or else he will think, 'She is attached to another man.'

³⁶ As long as he thinks, 'She has been unfaithful', for that entire period, in order to prove him wrong, she demonstrates the torment of her body by acting exhausted, anointing her limbs with oil, fasting, and so forth. A misfortune might be the death of the man's son or brother and so forth, or his falling ill or getting a fever.

³⁷ She laments, saying, 'How can this have happened to you when you have done nothing wrong?' In this way she shows him, 'I too am miserable because of this misery.'

³⁸ She says, 'My mother is truly perverse. Take me away from her and bring me to another country, where I can live independently.' And if she is bound to the king, she gets him to like this idea: 'Ransom me from the hands of the king, or else he will have me brought back when I have run away.'

³⁹ 'Otherwise I will die at any moment', she says.

⁴⁰ He gets back his physical strength after an illness. She says, 'Formerly, I asked the Goddess to fulfil my hopes for getting money and so forth, and that is why these wishes have been fulfilled; now I must make the offering to her.'

she had promised in advance. [41] She always takes care to dress well and wear jewellery, and takes little food. [42] She mentions his name and his lineage in her songs; when she is weary, she lays his hand on her breast and forehead, and she falls asleep in the pleasure that she experiences in that. [43] She sits on his lap and goes to sleep there, and when he gets up and moves away from her, she goes after him. [44] She wants to have a child by him, and does not want to live longer than he.

[45] When they are alone together, she does not speak of things that he does not know. [46] She restrains him from making a vow or fasting, by saying, 'It is my fault.' But if this is not possible, then she too takes on that role. [47] If there is a quarrel, she says, 'Even he cannot decide the matter.'* [48] She herself looks upon what is his and what is hers as indistinguishable. [49] She does not go to parties and so forth without him.

[50] She is proud of wearing leftover garlands and eating leftover food. [51] She admires his lineage, character, artistic skill, caste, knowledge, class, wealth, homeland, friends, good qualities, age, and sweetness. [52] She urges him to sing, and so forth, if he knows how. [53] She goes to him with no regard for danger, cold, heat, or rain. [54] On the occasion of making funeral offerings for reincarnation in other bodies she says, 'And let him alone be mine!'* [55] She does what he wants with regard to his wishes, tastes, feelings, and character. [56] She is suspicious of love-sorcery worked with roots. [57] She always argues with her mother about going to him, [58] and if her mother

---

[43] When he goes to a friend's house, or to see a deity, then she thinks, 'I cannot be separated from him for even a moment', and she herself follows him.

[44] She says, 'I am in my fertile period, and so you should not sleep anywhere else!' and 'If my death comes before his, it would be a blessing.'

[46] She takes the same vow.

[47] If there is a quarrel with someone about a fine point of meaning in some matter, she says, 'If anyone can do it, he is the one.'

[50] She says, 'Give me your leftover garlands and so forth. And when you are invited somewhere and do not take me with you, always send me what you do not eat.'

[56] When he says, 'You are always using love-sorcery to put me in your power, so that I will be totally submissive to you', she replies, 'No! I would never do anything like that!'

[58] Her mother forces her to go to another lover.

forces her to go elsewhere, then she longs for poison, fasting to death, a sword, or a rope. [59] And she convinces the man of this, through her secret agents, or she herself makes him grasp her situation. [60] But she does not argue about money, [61] and she does nothing without her mother.

[62] When he goes on a journey, she makes him swear to return quickly. [63] And when he is away, she makes a vow to abstain from washing and she refuses to wear jewellery, except for jewellery with religious meaning and power. Or she wears one conch-shell bangle. [64] She remembers things that happened in the past, goes to fortune-tellers and oracles who channel supernatural voices, and envies the constellations, the moon, the sun, and the stars. [65] When she has a dream-vision of what she longs for, she says, 'May I be united with him!' [66] If she is disturbed by a dream of what she does not long for, she performs the ritual to set it at peace.

[67] When he is coming home, she performs a ritual to honour the god Kama, [68] makes offerings to the deities, [69] brings out a full pot* with her girlfriends, [70] and performs a ritual to honour the crows.* [71] And right after he comes to her for the first time, she does this very same thing, without the ritual to honour the crows.

[72] To a man who is attached to her she says that she will follow him

---

[59] She convinces him that it is all her mother's fault alone, not hers. Her position is that the lives of courtesans are despicable, because their mothers, thirsting for money, make them abandon a man they are fond of and join them with some other man.

[61] In the end, when her mother tells her even what to eat, she does not disobey.

[64] She envies them, thinking, 'They are being rewarded for their merit, for my lover sees them; I must have no merit, for he does not see me.'

[65] If she sees an auspicious dream that is true, she tells her people about it in the morning. If she has a false dream, she tells them she did not have a dream. If her lover is in another region and has some wish that is not fulfilled, she knows of this by these various dreams.

[66] If she thinks, 'Something unwished-for has happened to him', she summons the Brahmins.

[70] She says, 'I am fulfilling the promise I made when I said, "If my beloved comes back to me, I will give you a ball of rice."'

[72] She says, 'When you have gone to heaven, it will not be possible for me to live.'

even beyond death.* [73] The signs of his being attached to her are that he trusts her with his true feelings, lives in the same way as she does, carries out her plans, is without suspicion, and has no concern for money matters.

[74] All of this has been said to give an example taken from the teachings of Dattaka. What remains unsaid is what a person learns from the experience of the world and from the nature of men. [75] And there are two verses about this:

> Because of the subtlety and excessive greed of women
> and the impossibility of knowing their nature,
> the signs of their desire are hard to know,
> even for those who are its object.

[76] Women desire and they become indifferent,
> they arouse love and they abandon;
> even when they are extracting all the money,
> they are not really known.

CHAPTER THREE

[53]   *Ways to Get Money from Him*

[1] She has both natural and contrived ways of getting money from a man who is attached to her. [2] Scholars have said about this: 'She should not use contrived means for this, if she can obtain it naturally or get even more through inventiveness.' [3] Vatsyayana says: He will give double the agreed amount when it is embellished through a contrived means.

[4] She contrives the following pretexts to get money from him: She gets money in order to take from merchants, on credit against future payment, such things as jewellery, cooked food, raw ingredients, drinks, garlands, garments, and perfumes.* [5] She praises his wealth to his face. [6] She pretends to need money for such things as vows, trees, parks, temples, pools, gardens, festivals, and love-gifts. [7] She says that

---

[3] She will get double what would come to her through natural means and discussion, and without deductions.

[4] He gives her the money but she does not actually get the things.

[7] She says this so that he thinks, 'She was robbed coming to my side', and gives her other jewellery.

her jewellery was stolen by guards or thieves, as a result of her going to him, ⁸ that her property in the house was lost through fire, someone breaking through a wall, or carelessness, ⁹ and so was some jewellery that the owner has asked to have back, and the man's jewellery. And she lets him know, through spies, about the expenses she has incurred in order to go to him. ¹⁰ She incurs debts for his sake, and she quarrels with her mother about the expenses that he has caused her.

¹¹ She no longer goes to parties given by friends, because she has no presents for them. ¹² And the valuable present that these friends previously brought her, which she had mentioned previously, now must be reciprocated. ¹³ She abruptly ceases her usual activities. ¹⁴ She engages artisans on the man's behalf. ¹⁵ She does favours for a physician and a minister of state for the sake of a particular project. ¹⁶ When disasters befall friends who have done her favours, she helps

---

⁸ She reports to him, 'Through carelessness, a fire broke out and burnt up my property.' She herself must not set a fire, however, because then through her fault many lives might be lost. Or thieves, or people who pretend to be thieves, dig an opening in a wall to rob the house. She says, 'Through my carelessness, or my mother's, things were lost in the house.'

⁹ Someone else had hidden jewellery there, for some reason, and now has asked to have it back; and the man had left his own jewellery there. But now that he learns that it has been destroyed by fire, of course he gives her money, and does not ask for his own jewellery. In front of the man, spies brought in by servants sent by the man say, 'To come to you, she spent these funds on rum, betel, and so forth.'

¹² She says, 'These friends brought valuable presents to me at my festival.' She had mentioned them to him before the friends' party had taken place. For when she asks for them in advance he gives them at the time of the affair, and if he does not give them, she certainly does not go to him then.

¹³ She abruptly ceases her daily care of her body, so that he thinks, 'Now she is not even able to care for her body', and gives her money.

¹⁴ She says, 'This excellent artisan demands a lot to do the work, and I do not have it, but if you give it, the work will be done; if not, I will have it done when I have the money.'

¹⁶ These favours were done for the man, and those for whom the favours have been done will do favours for the man if disasters—of human origin or acts of gods—befall him.

them out. ¹⁷ She carries out home improvements. She outfits the son of a girlfriend on a ceremonial occasion. There are the longings that a pregnant woman has for special food. She is ill. She cheers up an unhappy friend. ¹⁸ She sells a part of her jewellery for the man's sake. ¹⁹ She shows a merchant the jewellery that she always uses, or the household goods and cooking utensils, in order to sell them. ²⁰ When there is a pooling of similar household goods with those of rival courtesans de luxe, she takes the special ones. ²¹ She does not forget former kindnesses, and she speaks warmly of them in public. ²² Through spies, she makes sure that he hears about the abundant gains made by rival courtesans de luxe. ²³ Then, in the man's presence, she describes to those women her own even greater gains, whether or not this is so, with an air of embarrassment. ²⁴ She openly refuses men with whom she has had former connections, when they try to get her to come back to them again by offering her abundant gains. ²⁵ She remarks on the generosity of the man's rivals. ²⁶ And if

---

¹⁷ The pregnant woman is her girlfriend. The courtesan says to the man, 'Because of the death of a son (or whatever) of a friend of yours, I am so unhappy. Seeing this, you should cheer me up.' With this sort of pretext she manages the home improvements and so forth.

¹⁹ In the presence of the lover, the woman shows the jewellery and so forth to a merchant with whom she has a prior understanding, so that the man thinks, 'She must have nothing left at all, if she is trying to sell the things she uses all the time', and so he gives her money.

²⁰ Here V cites the teaching of Dattaka—'When there is a pooling of similar household goods, she takes the special ones'—and adds a phrase to clarify it: 'with rival courtesans de luxe.' Because the goods are similar, they accidentally get exchanged, and so that this should not happen again, in the presence of her lover she takes from the hand of the merchant, from time to time, some goods that are superior in both size and quality, so that the lover will give her money to pay for it. Generally, courtesans of the same class borrow one another's household goods as the need arises.

²¹ She praises them in his presence, so that he says, 'The kindness that I did has not come to naught here', and he gives her money again.

²³ She does this so that he too becomes ashamed, and gives her money.

²⁴ She does this so that he hears about this, says, 'She loves me', and gives her money.

²⁶ Thinking, 'He will not come back to this house', she gets a child to

she thinks, 'He will not come back', she begs like a child. Those are the ways to get money.

[54]   *Signs that his Passion is Cooling*

²⁷ She always knows when his passion is cooling, from the changes in his natural feelings and the look of his face. ²⁸ He gives her too little or too much. ²⁹ He is close with those who are against her. ³⁰ He pretends to do one thing and does something else. ³¹ He abruptly stops doing what he usually does. ³² He forgets his promises, or keeps them in the wrong way. ³³ He speaks with his own people through signs. ³⁴ He sleeps somewhere else, making the excuse that he has to do something for a friend. ³⁵ He talks secretly with the servant of a woman who was previously his mistress.

³⁶ Before he realizes it, she finds some pretext and gets her hands on his valuables.* ³⁷ A creditor takes them from her hands by force. ³⁸ If he argues about this, he can be sued in court. Those are the signs that his passion is cooling.

[55]   *Ways to Get Rid of Him*

³⁹ If a man is attached to her and has done favours for her in the past, even if he now yields but little fruit, she keeps him around by lying.

---

    request, 'Give this to me'. Or else it means that she abandons her shame, like a child, and begs him.

²⁹   He makes friends with those in the faction opposed to the woman.

³¹   He does not give her what he has been giving her every day.

³³   He does not communicate with them with words, for he thinks, 'She must not hear this.'

³⁴   He sleeps somewhere other than inside the woman's house.

³⁶   She does this before he realizes, 'My passion for her is cooling'.

³⁷   She had taken the man's money from this creditor, who had had it as a debt; and by a previous agreement, the creditor took it back by over-powering her by force.

³⁸   If the man argues, 'But this is mine; why are you taking it?' the creditor sues him in court. And if he does not argue, the goal is achieved.

³⁹   She deceives him, because he is still attached to her. But even if he has previously done her many favours, she gets rid of him if he wants another woman.

40 But if he has nothing left at all and no resources to do anything about it, she gets rid of him by some contrivance, without any consideration, and gets support from another man. **41** She does for him what he does not want, and she does repeatedly what he has criticized. She curls her lip and stamps on the ground with her foot. She talks about things he does not know about. She shows no amazement, but only contempt, for the things he does know about. She punctures his pride. She has affairs with men who are superior to him. She ignores him. She criticizes men who have the same faults. And she stalls when they are alone together. **42** She is upset by the things he does for her when they are making love. She does not offer him her mouth. She keeps him away from between her legs. She is disgusted by wounds made by nails or teeth. When he tries to hug her, she repels him by making a 'needle' with her arms. Her limbs remain motionless. She crosses her thighs. She wants only to sleep. When she sees that he is exhausted, she urges him on. She laughs at him when he cannot do it, and she shows no pleasure when he can. When she notices that he is aroused, even in the daytime, she goes out to be with a crowd.

43 She intentionally distorts the meaning of what he says. She laughs when he has not made a joke, and when he has made a joke, she laughs about something else. When he is talking, she looks at her entourage with sidelong glances and slaps them. And when she has interrupted his story, she tells other stories. She talks in public about the bad habits and vices that he cannot give up. Through a servant

---

40 If someone should remark, 'How can she just throw him out, when he has given her sexual pleasure and profit?' V replies, 'She gets support from another man', and this man gives her both pleasure and profit.

42 She crosses her two arms, places her hands on her own shoulders, and puts her two arms together to make a needle. When he tries to make love, with some difficulty, and she sees that he is exhausted, she urges him to go on, but does not help him out by offering to play the part of the man [2.8.1]. There actually is a kind of sexual donkey who makes love in the daytime even though it is forbidden. When she realizes, from his gestures and signals, that he wants to make love, she goes out.

girl, she insults him where he is vulnerable. [44] She does not see him when he comes to her. She asks for things that should not be asked for. And at the end, the release* happens of itself. That is Dattaka's view of the liaison.

[45] And there are two verses about this:

The work of a courtesan is to test lovers and then join with them,
to enchant the man she joins,
to get money from the man she has enchanted,
and at the end to release him.
[46] A courtesan who manages a liaison
according to this method
is not cheated by her lovers
but makes piles of money.

CHAPTER FOUR

[56]   *Getting Back Together with an Ex-lover*

[1] When she is getting rid of her present lover after she has squeezed all the money out of him, she may get together with a man who was previously her lover. [2] If he still has money or has made money, and still loves her, she can get together with him. [3] If he has gone elsewhere, she must find out about him; he may belong in any of the six possible categories, according to the circumstances:

[4] [a] He left her of his own accord and he left the other woman, too, of his own accord.

[5] [b] He left both her and the other woman because they got rid of him.

[6] [c] He left her of his own accord and he left the other woman because she got rid of him.

----

[44] It was Dattaka who set forth the rules for the relationship between the lover and the courtesan, up to this point; I did not invent it. For it was he who decided, through the commission of the courtesans, to make this condensation. But it was Babhravya who set forth in a useful form what I am going to tell now, about getting back together with an ex-lover and so forth.

⁷[*d*] He left her of his own accord and stayed with the other woman.

⁸[*e*] He left her because she got rid of him and he left the other woman of his own accord.

⁹[*f*] He left her because she got rid of him and he stayed with the other woman.

¹⁰[*a*] If a man who left both her and the other woman of his own accord tries to talk her into taking him back, she should not take him back, because he has a fickle mind and has scorned the qualities of both women.

¹¹[*b*] A man who left both her and the other woman because they got rid of him has a constant mind. If the other woman got rid of him, even though he has money, because she could get a lot of money from another man, the courtesan may take him back, thinking, 'Since that woman insulted him, he will give me a lot of money out of spite.' ¹²But if she rejected him because he has no money or is stingy, he is not a good prospect.*

¹³[*c*] If he left her of his own accord and left the other woman because she got rid of him, and if he gives her more than he did the first time, then he is fit for a liaison.

¹⁴[*d*] If a man who left her of his own accord, and stayed with the other woman, tries to talk her into taking him back, she must find out about him. ¹⁵She may think, 'He went away because he was looking for something special, and now he wants to come back from her to me because he did not see that special something; and if he comes back because he wants to know me better, he will give me a lot of money, because of his love for me. Or, because he has seen her faults and now sees that I have most of the good qualities, being a man who recognizes good qualities, he will give me the most money.' ¹⁶But if she realizes, 'He is a child, whose gaze never rests in a single place, or a man who generally breaks agreements, or someone who does anything he can do, as fickle in his passion as turmeric is in its colour',* then she either will or will not get back together with him.

---

¹⁵ 'He was looking for some special kind of sex, which he did not see in that woman, because she lacked sophistication. He wants to come back from her to me, because he has seen that special something in me.'

[17] [e] If a man who left her because she got rid of him, and left the other woman of his own accord, tries to talk her into taking him back, she must find out about him: [18] 'If he comes back because he loves me, he will give me a lot of money. Since that other woman did not please him, my good qualities will win him over. [19] Or since, in the past, I got rid of him for no cause, now he wants to cultivate me and vent his hatred on me. Or he wants to get my confidence and get back, in retaliation, the wealth that I took away from him when he was courting me. Or he wants to get revenge by breaking me away from my present lover and then abandoning me.' A man that has such unpleasant ways of thinking is not one to get back together with. [20] Time will reveal if he changes his way of thinking.

[21] [f] A man who left her because she got rid of him, and stayed with the other woman, and tries to talk her into taking him back, has been covered by this last case. [22] Among those who try to talk her into taking them back, the one who stayed with the other woman is the one that she herself tries to talk herself into taking back: [23] 'I got rid of this man for a false reason, and he went elsewhere, and now I should make an effort to bring him back.' [24] Or, 'Once he hears from me, he will break away from her [25] and he will stop her income.' [26] Or, 'He has now come into some money; he is living in a bigger house; he has an administrative job. He has separated from his wives. He has freed himself from those on whom he was dependent. He has split with his father or brother.' [27] Or, 'If I get together with him, I will get the wealthy lover whom he is now keeping away from me.' [28] Or, 'His wife has treated me with contempt; I will get him to leave her.'* [29] Or, 'His friend is in love with my co-wife, who hates me; I will use him to get his friend to break away from her.' [30] Or, 'I will make trouble

---

[27] 'He is keeping him away from me now, because of his friendship with him.'

[28] 'When I had broken with him, he went back to his own wife. And I will treat her with contempt because of this, and by getting back together with him I will get him to leave her, and so I will get revenge for this insult.'

[29] 'The friend of my ex-lover has power and possessions, and he is in love with my present or former co-wife, who wishes to harm me. By means of the ex-lover, I will get that friend to break away, so that she will have no profit and will have to do favours for me.'

[30] 'He left me to go elsewhere, and he also left her to go elsewhere.'

for him by making him appear light-minded, because of his fickleness.'

[31] The libertine and the others explain to him that the woman got rid of him before because her mother was so evil-minded, and she herself was powerless, even though she was in love with him; [32] and that, although she sleeps with her present lover, she has no desire, and she hates him. [33] They try to get him back by playing upon his memories of her and his former love for her, [34] and they say, 'She vividly remembers what you did for her.' That is how to get back together with an ex-lover.

[35] Scholars say: 'Between two lovers, one who had an affair with her in the past and one who did not, the one who had an affair with her in the past is better. For she knows his character and has seen his passion, and he serves her well.' [36] Vatsyayana says: A man who had an affair with her in the past does not give her very much money, because all the money has already been squeezed out of him, and it is hard to get his trust again; but a man who did not have an affair with her in the past easily falls in love with her. [37] Nevertheless, there are exceptions according to the nature of the man.

[38] And there are verses about this:

She may wish to get back together again
to break another woman away from the lover,
or the lover from another woman,
and to hurt, again, the lover who stays with another woman.
[39] When a man is too deeply attached to her,
he fears that she will make love with another man
and he disregards her lies.
And, because of his fear, he gives her a lot.

---

[34] They mention what he did for her, by giving money or warding off losses, to show that she is grateful.

[38] 'Breaking another woman away from the lover' refers to the situations in which 'his wife has treated me with contempt' [28] or 'his friend is in love with my co-wife, who hates me.' [29]. 'Hurting the lover who stays with another woman' refers to the situation in which 'he will stop her income' [25]. 'Breaking the ex-lover away from another woman' states a reason for staying with the ex-lover.

⁴⁰ She welcomes the man who is not attached* to her
and scorns the man who is attached to her.
And if a messenger should come from another man
who is very experienced,
⁴¹ a woman stalls for time with her former lover,
when he is trying to talk her into taking him back:
she makes sure that the connection is unbroken,
and does not give up the man who is attached to her.
⁴² But a woman may talk with a man who is attached to her
and in her power and then, nevertheless, go elsewhere.
And when she has taken the money from him, too,
she enchants just the man who is attached to her.
⁴³ A clever woman gets back together with an ex-lover
only after she has tested, at the start,
the future outlook, the gain,
the abundant love, and the friendship.

CHAPTER FIVE

[57]   *Weighing Different Kinds of Profits*

¹ If she has a multitude of lovers and can make a lot of money every day, she need not confine herself to a single lover. ² Taking into account the place, the time, and the conditions, and her own qualities

---

⁴⁰ The man who is not attached to her is an ex-lover who is still very much
in love with her; she welcomes him because his feelings for her are
known. The man who is attached to her is not in love with her, and so
she treats him with contempt. Another man, who is very clever, gives
her a great deal of money, saying, 'Do not make a connection with
another man.'

⁴¹ Although he uses the more general term, 'a woman', he is referring only
to a courtesan in this section. She does not make love with the man
right then, or else there might be a break from her present, attached,
profitable lover. And the previously intimate ex-lover is willing to wait
for another time, because he loves her so much and has hope.

⁴² She enchants just the man who is attached to her because she loves him
for having stayed; she does not make any connection with the other
man.

and luck in love, and whether she is charging more or less than other women, she establishes the price of a night. ³She also sends messengers to her lover, and she herself summons men with whom he has some connection. ⁴She may go two, three, or even four times to a single lover in order to take extraordinary profits, and then she establishes a liaison.

⁵Scholars say: 'When she has several lovers at once, however, who offer equal opportunities for profit, the obvious choice is the one who gives her whatever she wants.'* ⁶Vatsyayana says: The one who gives gold is best, because gold cannot be taken back again and can buy everything that is needed. ⁷Of gold, silver, copper, bronze, iron, furniture, utensils, bedding, blankets, special clothing, perfumed articles, sharp spices, dishes, ghee, sesame oil, grain, and the species of cattle, each should be chosen rather than the one that follows. ⁸When the things are the same, or of the same quality, the choice should be made on the basis of a friend's advice, temporary needs, future needs, the lover's qualities, and love.

⁹Scholars say: 'Between a lover who is in love and another who is generous, the obvious choice is the generous one.' ¹⁰Vatsyayana says: But it is possible to cultivate generosity in a man who is in love. ¹¹For even a greedy man, if he is in love, spends generously, but a generous man cannot be made to fall in love through mere persistence.

¹²Scholars say: 'In this case [of a man in love versus a generous man], too, between a wealthy man and one who is not wealthy, the choice is the wealthy man; and between a generous man and a man who does what she needs to have done at the moment, the clear choice is the man who does what she needs to have.' ¹³Vatsyayana says: But the man who does what she needs to have done, when he has done it once, thinks that he has given satisfaction. A generous man, however, has no regard for the past. ¹⁴In this case [of a generous man versus a man who does what she needs], too, the choice is for the man who takes care of future needs.

¹⁵Scholars say: 'Between a grateful man and a generous man, the

---

⁸ The woman chooses on the basis of her own love and the man's love for her.

¹³ Because he is generous, he does not consider the past and say, 'I already gave money to her, and I will not give it again.'

clear choice is the generous man.' [16] But even when she has pleased a generous man for a long time, when he sees one false move or believes unjust slander by a rival courtesan de luxe, he has no regard for the trouble she went to in the past. [17] For in general, generous men are dignified, straightforward, and thoughtless. [18] Vatsyayana says: A grateful man has regard for the trouble she has taken in the past and his passion does not suddenly cool toward her. And since his character has been tested and proven, he is not susceptible to unjust slander.* [19] In this case [of a generous man versus a grateful man], too, the choice is for the man who takes care of future needs.

[20] Scholars say: 'Between a friend's advice and getting money, the clear choice is for getting money.' [21] Vatsyayana says: Money will be gained in the future, too; but a friend whose advice is once disregarded may become offended. [22] In this case [of a friend's advice versus getting money], too, the choice is for the man who takes care of temporary needs. [23] In this case, she brings the friend around by showing what she needs to have done, saying, 'I will take your advice for what is going to happen tomorrow', and then she still keeps the money for her temporary needs.

[24] Scholars say: 'Between getting money and warding off losses, the clear choice is getting money.' [25] Vatsyayana says: Money gained has a limit; loss, however, once it breaks out, continues to move in directions that no one can predict. [26] In this case [of getting money versus warding off losses], too, the choice must be made with regard to the relative weight of each factor. [27] This means that the choice is for a loss warded off rather than a doubtful gain.

[28] The top courtesans de luxe spend their excess profits by building temples, pools, and gardens; setting up raised mounds and fire altars;

---

[16] A false move is an infidelity committed by the woman.

[17] Because they are dignified, they do not disregard a false move. Because they are straightforward, they accept unjust slander, such as, 'That woman is always making false moves.' Because they are thoughtless, they have no regard for the pains a woman takes on their behalf.

[18] He does not accept unjust slander.

[26] A heavy gain outweighs a light loss, and a heavy loss outweighs a light gain.

[28] Mediation is given through the hand of another person, since a Brahmin cannot receive a gift from a courtesan.

giving thousands of cows to Brahmins through the mediation of people worthy to receive them; bringing and offering articles of worship to the gods, or providing money sufficient to spend on that worship. [29] Those who live on their beauty spend their excess profits by getting jewellery for all their limbs, decorating their houses elegantly, and glorifying the furnishings of their houses with expensive household goods and servants. [30] Servant women who carry pots of water spend their excess profits by having spotless clothes to wear all the time, buying food and drink to stave off hunger, using perfumed things and betel all the time, and wearing jewellery that is partly made of gold. [31] Scholars say: 'This example of the top courtesans de luxe also applies to the excess profit of all of them, even the middle and lowest ones.' [32] Vatsyayana says: This is not a real livelihood, because the profit is not constant, depending as it does on place, time, ability, power, love, and people's customs.

[33] If she desires to keep a lover from going elsewhere, or if she desires to get a man away from some woman to whom he is attached, or if she wants to separate another woman from her gains, or if she thinks that by taking up with a man who is not eligible she will improve her own position, prosperity, future, and her sex appeal; or if she desires to get the man to help her ward off a loss; or if she wishes to betray another man who is attached to her, because she regards his former favours as if they had never been done; or if she simply wants love; then she will even take just a very small profit from a man of good intentions. [34] She will not, however, take anything at all if she is thinking of the future and seeks refuge with him in the hope of warding off a loss.

[35] But if she thinks, 'I will abandon him and take up a liaison with someone else'; 'He will go'; 'He will get together with his wives'; or, 'He will lose his money'; 'His supervisor or his master or father will come and work on him like an elephant goad'; or, 'He will lose his position'; or, 'He is fickle', then she wants to make her profits from him in the present moment. [36] If she thinks, 'He will get the favour that the ruler promised him'; 'He will obtain an administrative post

---

[29] Those who live on their beauty do not know the arts.
[31] The middle and lowest are the women who live on their beauty and the women who carry water pots.

or position'; or, 'The time for him to get his livelihood is coming near; his ship will come in; his landholding or grain will ripen'; 'What is done for him is not lost; he always keeps his word', then she wants him for the future, or she engages him in a liaison.

³⁷ And there are verses about this:

> For both future and present purposes,
> she should avoid, at a great distance,
> men who have amassed their wealth with difficulty
> and men who are the cruel favourites of the king.

³⁸ She should make every effort to captivate
> men whom it is disastrous to avoid
> and prosperous to seek,
> and she should use every pretext to get close to them.

³⁹ And she should seek out, even by spending her own money,
> those who think on a large scale and have great energy,
> those who, in a good mood, will give her money
> even for some small matter, and without counting it.

CHAPTER SIX

[58] *Calculating Gains and Losses, Consequences,
and Doubts*

¹ Losses result even from gains that are being amassed, and so do other consequences and doubts. ² All of these come from weakness of mind; from excesses of passion, of self-importance, of duplicity, of honesty, of confidence, and of anger; and from carelessness, recklessness, and the workings of fate. ³ Their results are the failure to reap the fruits from expenditures that have been made; lack of a future; blockage of money that is supposed to come in; disappearance of what has been gained; development of a harsh temperament; sexual vulnerability; injury to the body; hair-loss; collapse; and mutilation of the limbs. ⁴ Therefore, from the very start one should try to root out these causes and pay attention to the factors that increase gains.

⁵ The three gains are money, religious merit, and pleasure, ⁶ and the three losses are loss of money, loss of religious merit, and hatred. ⁷ The production of something from something else, when these

three gains are being amassed, is a consequence. [8]'Is it to be or not to be?' is a pure doubt about the uncertainty of achieving an object. [9]'Will this happen or that?' is a mixed doubt. [10]Two goals achieved when a single goal was being pursued make a two-sided result, [11]and something produced by a group is a group result. We will be referring to these. [12]The form of the three gains has been discussed. The three losses are precisely the opposite of them.*

[13]A gain that has the consequence of further gain occurs when she has a lover of the highest class and openly gets money from him but also becomes acceptable, sexually accessible, and sought after by other men, and gets a future. [14]A gain that has no consequence occurs when she goes from one lover to another merely for profit.

[15]A gain that has the consequence of a loss occurs when a man attached to her gives her money from someone else, which cuts off her future and puts an end to her money; or when she has a lover who is low or hated by everyone, which destroys her future. [16]A loss that has the consequence of a gain occurs when, by spending her own money, she takes as a lover a hero or minister of state or a powerful man who is greedy; even though this liaison is fruitless, it brings a future with it and is undertaken in order to prevent some disaster or to allay some factor that might be greatly destructive of her gains.

[17]A loss that has no consequences occurs when she gratifies, even by spending her own money, a miser who thinks he is lucky in love, or an ungrateful man who by his very nature cheats, and in the end this is fruitless. [18]A loss that has the consequence of further loss occurs when she gratifies in that very way just such a man who is a favourite of the king, rich in cruelty and power, and in the end this is fruitless, but when she gets rid of him that also does her harm.

[19]The consequences for religious merit and pleasure can be calculated in the same way, [20]and each can be combined with

---

[12] The gains have been discussed in the passage about the three aims of human life [1.1.2].

[15] Because of his own lack of funds, the man who is attached to a woman gives her money that he took from another man and should give back to him, so that people say, 'She is living with a robber.'

[20] There are twenty-four combinations of consequences: each of the six—gain, loss, religious merit, violation of religion, pleasure, and hatred—coupled with four of the others.

one of the others in the appropriate way. Those are the consequences.

²¹ The doubt about money is, 'Will he give it or not, even if he is fully satisfied?' ²² The doubt about religious merit is, 'Will I serve religion or not, by throwing out a man from whom no more money can be taken, once all the money has been squeezed out of him and he is no longer fruitful?' ²³ The doubt about pleasure is, 'Will there be pleasure or not, if I go to a servant or some other low man whom I find attractive?'

²⁴ The doubt about loss is, 'If I do not go to a powerful but low man, will that cause me a loss or not?' ²⁵ The doubt about the violation of religion is, 'If I abandon a man who is attached to me but is absolutely fruitless, and he goes to the world of his ancestors, does that violate religion or not?' ²⁶ The doubt about hatred is, 'Will my passion cool or not toward a man whom I do not find attractive and who hesitates even to speak of passion?' Those are the pure doubts.

²⁷ Now for the mixed doubts. ²⁸ The doubt is: 'Will gain or loss result from gratifying a newcomer whose character is unknown or a newly arrived man who is powerful because he has the protection of a favourite?' ²⁹ The doubt is: 'Will I serve religion or violate it if I go, on the sympathetic advice of a friend, to a Brahmin who knows the Veda, or to a man who is under a vow of chastity or consecrated for a sacrifice, or a man who has taken a vow or who wears the sign of a religious order, if he has seen me and conceived a passion for me and wants to die?' ³⁰ The doubt is: 'Will pleasure or hatred result if I go to a man without knowing if he has or does not have good qualities, because people have not yet tested him?' ³¹ Each can be combined with one of the others. This ends the discussion of the mixed doubts.

³² These are the two-sided results, according to Auddalaki: 'A two-sided gain occurs when she goes to another man and gain comes, also, from the man who is attached to her, out of rivalry. ³³ A two-sided loss occurs when she spends her own money on a fruitless liaison with another man, and the man who is attached to her, unable to put up with that, takes back the money he had given her. ³⁴ A

---

²⁶ He hesitates to say, 'There will be no pleasure', because he is tormented by passion. But he is not even attractive to her.

²⁹ He wants to die because he has reached the final stage of desire.

two-sided doubt about gain occurs when she has gone to another man and worries, "Will there be gain in this or not?" and "Will the man who is attached to me also give something, out of rivalry, or not?" 35 A two-sided doubt about loss occurs when she has gone to a man at her own expense: "Will my former lover, in his frustration and anger, do me harm or not?" and, "Will the man who is attached to me, unable to put up with it, take back the money he had given me or not?"'

36 But the followers of Babhravya say: 37 'A two-sided gain occurs when gain comes both from the man she goes to and from the man who is attached to her to whom she does not go. 38 A two-sided loss occurs when she spends her money fruitlessly on going to another man and cannot recoup her loss of money from the man she does not go to. 39 A two-sided doubt about gain occurs when she has gone to another man, and she wonders: "Will he give me money without my incurring expenses or not?" and "Will the man who is attached to me and to whom I have not gone give me money or not?" 40 A two-sided doubt about loss occurs when she has gone to another man at her own expense, and she wonders: "Will my former lover, frustrated, demonstrate his powers or not?" and, "Will the one I do not go to become angry and cause me a loss or not?"'

41 Six mixed results are produced by combining these: gain on one side and loss on the other; gain on one side and doubt about gain on the other; gain on one side and doubt about loss on the other. 42 Considering among these, together with her helpers, she acts in such a way as to maximize gain, even when there is doubt about gain, or to cut her losses significantly. 43 She treats religious merit and pleasure

---

40 She does not go to the man who is attached to her.

43 Two-sided results for religious merit occur when [6.6.29] she goes to the Brahmin who is going to die, for religious merit comes both from the fact that she is serving a Brahmin and that he is otherwise going to die of his love for her. Two-sided results for the violation of religion occur when [29] she goes to the man under a vow of chastity, both because he breaks his vow and because he is unwilling. Two-sided doubts about religious merit arise when [38] she goes to another man who has no money, and she worries, 'Will religious merit be served or not?' and [22] the man who is attached to her can give her nothing, because she has squeezed all the money out of him, and she worries,

in this same way: they can be combined, one with another, and paired with their opposites. Those are the two-sided results.

[44] When a group of voluptuaries keep one woman for all of them, that is a group liaison. [45] When she gets together with first one of them and then another, she gets money from them one by one, through their rivalry. [46] At occasions such as the spring festival, she announces, through her mother: 'My daughter "will go tonight to the man who does this or that for me."' [47] And from going to them in a way that causes rivalry, she targets what she needs: [48] gain from one and gain from all of them, loss from one and loss from all, gain from half and gain from all, loss from half and loss from all. Those are the group results.

[49] Doubt about gain and doubt about loss can be calculated as above. And religious merit and pleasure can be combined with them in the same way. Those are the gains and losses, consequences, and doubts.

Types of Courtesans

[50] The servant woman who carries water, the servant girl, the promiscuous woman, the loose woman, the dancer, the artist, the openly

---

'Will religious merit come from this or not?' Two-sided doubts about the violation of religion arise when [29] she goes to another man from a religious order and makes him break his vow, and she wonders, 'Will religion be violated or not?' and [29] the man attached to her, who has taken a vow, intends to give her a lot of money, and she wonders, 'Will religion be violated or not?'

Two-sided results for pleasure occur when [23] she goes to another attractive man and also [32–4] satisfies her desire with the attractive man who is attached to her. Two-sided results for hatred occur when [26] her passion cools both from going to another unattractive man and from going to the unattractive man attached to her. Two-sided doubts about pleasure arise when [30] she goes to another man, without knowing if he has good qualities or not, and she wonders, 'Will pleasure result or not?' and [33] the man attached to her is unrequited and she wonders, 'Will pleasure result or not?' Two-sided doubts about hatred arise when [26] she goes to another man and wonders, 'Will my passion toward this man cool or not, since he hesitates to talk about dispelling passion?' and [26] 'Will my passion cool or not toward the man attached to me, to whom I feel the same way?'

ruined woman, the woman who lives on her beauty, and the courtesan de luxe: those are the types of courtesans. [51] And all of them must choose appropriate lovers and helpers and consider the ways to please them, ways to get money from them, to get rid of them and to get back together with them, the consequences of various profits, the consequences from and doubts about gain and loss. That is all about courtesans.

[52] And there are two verses about this:

Since men want sexual pleasure
and women, too, want sexual pleasure,
therefore union with women
is the main subject of this text.

[53] There are women who care most of all for passion,
and there are also women who care most of all for money;
passion was described earlier,
and the practices of courtesans in this book about courtesans.

---

[53] Of the two kinds of women, the earlier parts of this text—about virgins, sex, wives, and other men's wives—are about women who care most of all about passion.

NO PASSION

END OF BOOK SIX

These women have passion

CHAPTER ONE

[59]   *Making Luck in Love*

[1] The *Kamasutra* has now been told in full. [2] But a person who has not obtained the object of desire through the methods it describes may have recourse to these secret recipes. [3] Beauty, good qualities, the right age, and generosity—these make you lucky in love. [4] But an ointment made of the leaves of the East Indian rose bay, wild ginger, and the Indian plum can also make you lucky in love. [5] So can an ointment made of these substances, finely ground up and mixed with myrobalan oil, all prepared in a human skull. [6] And so can eye make-up made with oil prepared from hogweed, the mauve savannah-flower, the yellow silk-cotton flower, red amaranth, and blue lotus leaves, [7] or garlands coated with the same materials. [8] You become lucky in love if you lick a powder made of the dried filaments of white lotuses, blue lotuses, and rose chestnuts, mixed with honey and clarified butter, [9] or if you coat yourself with an ointment made of these substances together with the leaves of the East Indian rose bay, Indian plum, and cinnamon bay-tree. [10] Holding a gold-plated peacock's eye or hyena's eye in your right hand makes you lucky in love. [11] You may also use, in the very same way, an amulet made from a jujube-berry and one made from a conch-shell, employing the methods of the *Atharva Veda*.

[12] When a master sees that a servant girl has reached the ripeness

---

[4] Spread this ointment on your body.

[6] Use the leaves of the blue lotus and the roots of all the others.

[10] Cover it with leaves of pure gold.

[11] Have them gold-plated and hold them in your hand.

[12] As the common saying goes: 'For what is hard to get becomes precious and sought after.' And as the poet says:
   'There are two kinds of marriages to a courtesan,
   one brought about by the gods and the other by human effort.
   The divine variety is caused by Kama's bow,
   and the other kind by the lover.'

of her youth with a knowledge of magic and a skill in applying it, he keeps her away from any other man for just one year. When her lovers have become ardent out of sheer perversity, since she has been kept from them, he gives the girl to the one who, out of rivalry with the others, gives a lot of money. That is a way to increase luck in love. [13] When a courtesan de luxe sees that her own daughter has reached the ripeness of her youth, she protects her by inviting lovers whose intelligence, character, and beauty are similar to the girl's, and she makes this agreement: 'Whoever gives such and such can take her hand in marriage.' [14] And, seemingly without her mother's knowledge, the daughter inspires love, to excess, in the rich sons of the men-about-town. [15] She manages to see them here or there in the course of enjoying the arts, or in music-halls, or at the home of a beggar woman. [16] And when they give the money that has been stipulated, the mother offers the daughter's hand in marriage. [17] But if the mother does not get that amount of money, she may even supplement it with a part of her own money and say to her daughter, 'He gave this.' [18] Or she may get him to marry the girl and then take her virginity. [19] Or, if she has secretly united the girl with these men, while she herself pretends to know nothing about it, she then reports it to judges whom she knows.

[20] But if the daughter has already lost her virginity with a girlfriend or a servant girl, and if she thoroughly understands the *Kamasutra* and is well grounded in the techniques that can only be done with practice, and she is secure in her age and in her ability to make her own luck in love, then the courtesans de luxe let her go. Those are

[14] She wants the men to think, 'She is so much in love with us that, even though she is well-guarded, she will come to us without letting her mother know.'

[18] If her own daughter has been married through a wedding in the manner of the gods, she gets him to take her virginity through one of the means described above [3.5.15, 25–6]. The distinction made here is between the man who takes her hand in marriage and then takes her virginity [7.1.18] and the man who gives money as described above [7.1.16] and then takes her virginity.

[19] When she has secretly joined her own daughter with an attractive man who has taken her virginity, she says, 'I did not give permission for this.'

[20] They take her virginity by using a finger.

the Oriental practices.* [21] The marriage is without infidelity for the duration of a year. From then on, she is free to indulge her desires. [22] Even after that year, if the man who married her invites her, she must go to him for that night even if she loses money by doing so. Those are the ways in which a courtesan marries and increases her luck in love. [23] All of this also applies to the daughters of women who make their living on the stage. [24] But those women can give their daughter to a man who does them special favours on a musical instrument. That is how to make luck in love.

[60]   *Putting Someone in your Power*

[25] If you coat your penis with an ointment made with powdered white thorn-apple, black pepper, and long pepper, mixed with honey, you put your sexual partner in your power. [26] If you make a powder by pulverizing leaves scattered by the wind, garlands left over from corpses, and peacocks' bones, it puts someone in your power.* [27] If you pulverize a female 'circle-maker' buzzard that died a natural death, and mix the powder with honey and gooseberry, it puts someone in your power.* [28] If you cut the knotty roots of the milkwort and milk-hedge plants into pieces, coat them with a powder of red arsenic and sulphur, dry and pulverize the mixture seven times, mix it with honey, and spread it on your penis, you put your sexual partner in your power. [29] If you burn the same powder at night, you can make the moon, viewed through the smoke, appear golden. [30] If you mix the same powder with monkey shit and scatter the mixture over a virgin, she will not be given to another man.

――――――――

[22] She loses the money she would get from another man who is her present lover.

[23] These women are dancers and so forth.

[24] The musical instrument accompanies dancing, singing, and so forth.

[25] Do this in such a way that the woman you want does not realize, 'A man with something spread on his penis is making love to me.'

[26] Sprinkle the powder made of these materials on the head of women and on the two feet of men. This 'peacock' is not the bird called the peacock but a kind of pheasant.

[29] This is a way to amaze someone when the occasion arises.

[30] Use a monkey with a red face.

³¹ They say that if you hollow out the trunk of a rosewood tree and keep in it, for six months, a mixture of orris roots and mango-oil, and then take it out and keep it for another six months, the ointment, which the gods are fond of, puts someone in your power. ³² They say that if you take thin sticks from the heart of a cashew tree and place them for six months in a tree hollowed out in the same way, they develop the perfume of acacia flowers. The ointment made from them, which the demigods* are fond of, puts someone in your power. ³³ They say that if you mix panic-seed* and East Indian rose bay, coat them with mango-oil, and keep them in a hollowed-out rose chestnut tree for six months, the ointment, which the semi-serpents are fond of, puts someone in your power. ³⁴ They say that if you coat a camel's bone with the juice of a marigold* and burn it, and keep the resulting ointment in a hollow shank-bone and mix it with antimony, using a stick made of camel-bone, the resulting pure collyrium works on the eyes and puts someone in your power. ³⁵ You can also make salves for the eyes in this way using the bones of hawks, vultures, and peacocks.

[61]   *Stimulants for Virility*

³⁶ If you drink milk infused with kidney beans, pepper, and sugar-cane, and mixed with sugar, you become as virile as a bull. ³⁷ If you drink milk prepared with the testicles of a ram or billy goat, and mixed with sugar, it gives you the virility of a bull. ³⁸ So does drinking milk prepared with cock's-head root, dates, and horse-eye bean, ³⁹ or milk prepared with almond seeds, sugar-cane root, and cock's-head root. ⁴⁰ Scholars say: 'If you make a cake by grinding up some water chestnuts, kysoor root, and licorice, together with dates and

---

³³ Use the flowers of the panic-seed plant.

³⁴ The shank-bone is a camel's. You break it into pieces the size of grains of rice, dip it thirty-seven times, and then burn it. Mix it with equal parts of antimony. It affects vision by dispelling darkness and so forth.

³⁶ Boil the first three ingredients in cow's-milk. When it cools, add the sugar and drink it.

³⁷ Boil it.

⁴⁰ 'Endless' means many.

jujubes, adding clarified butter and milk sweetened with sugar, and cooking it over a slow fire, and you eat it until you are satisfied, you can make love with endless women.' [41] Scholars say: 'If you wash a bean and a lotus with milk, soften them with warm clarified butter, take them out, make them into a rice-pudding with milk from a cow who has a grown calf, and eat it with honey and butter, you can make love with endless women.' [42] Scholars say: 'If you make a cake out of cock's-head root, horse-eye bean, sugar, honey, butter, and wheat, and eat it until you are satisfied, you can make love with endless women.' [43] If you make a rice-pudding with rice that has been prepared with the juice from a sparrow's egg, pour honey and butter on it, and eat it until you are satisfied, you can—and so forth as above.* [44] If you skin sesame seeds and prepare them with the juice from a sparrow's egg, add the fruits of water chestnuts, kysoor root, and horse-eye beans, together with wheat-meal and bean-meal, and milk with sugar, butter, and cooked barley, then bake a cake and devour it until you are satisfied, you can—and so forth, as above. [45] Scholars say: 'Butter, honey, sugar, licorice, in quantities of eight parts of each to one part of wine-palm hemp and one hundred and twenty-eight parts milk: this six-part nectar of immortality is ritually pure, bestows virility and long life, and keeps the juices flowing.'* [46] Scholars say: 'A dish made of asparagus, "dog's-fang" prickly-fruit, and molasses, with a decoction of long-pepper and honey, cooked in cow's milk with goat's butter, and eaten every day at the beginning of the spring,* is a food that is ritually pure, bestows virility and long life, and keeps the juices flowing.' [47] Scholars say: 'A dish made of asparagus, "dog's-fang" prickly-fruit, and the crushed fruits of the flax plant, cooked with four times as much water until it reaches the right consistency, and then eaten early every day at the beginning of spring, is a food that is ritually pure, bestows virility and long life, and keeps the juices flowing.' [48] Scholars say: 'Rise early every day and eat four ounces* of a dish made of barley-meal cooked with an exactly equal quantity of powdered "dog's-fang" prickly-fruit, a dish that is ritually pure, bestows virility and long life, and keeps the juices flowing.'

---

[43] A young man who eats this will have an enormous capacity for sex.

⁴⁹ You can learn the techniques that compel love
   from the Veda of Long-Life and from the Veda,*
   from people who know the magic recipes and spells,
   and from other qualified people.
⁵⁰ You should not use techniques
   that are doubtful, dangerous for the body,
   obtained by killing living creatures,
   or made of impure substances.
⁵¹ A man who has amassed inner powers
   obeys rules that educated people follow
   and that Brahmins and well-wishing friends
   recommend.

CHAPTER TWO

[62]   *Rekindling Exhausted Passion*

¹ If you are unable to pleasure a woman of fierce sexual energy, have
recourse to devices. ² As you begin to make love, caress her with your
hand between her legs and enter her only when she has become wet.
That is a way of kindling passion.* ³ Oral sex kindles the passion of a
man who is of dull sexual energy, past his prime, too fat, or
exhausted from love-making. ⁴ Or use sex tools,* ⁵ made of gold,

---

⁴⁹ The Veda meant here is the *Atharva Veda*. The qualified people are
   those who are adept at the spells and can be trusted.

¹ If he cannot give her a sexual climax because he has no passion left, he
   resorts to contrivances.

² Even if a man of dull sexual energy begins to make love because his
   penis is hard, nevertheless from the start he massages her between the
   legs with his hand in the 'elephant trunk' technique [2.8.19]. And he
   enters a woman of fierce sexual energy only when she has become wet
   after he has massaged her with his hand, because this inspires passion
   for as long a time as the woman desires.

³ A man whose passion has arisen but who does not start to make love,
   because his penis is not hard, may kindle his passion with oral sex,
   which gives rise to the delight of ejaculation. For the penis of an old
   man or a fat man stands up only with difficulty.

silver, copper, iron, ivory, or buffalo horn, [6]or ones made of tin or lead, which are soft, cool the semen, and produce a violent* effect during the sexual act. Those are the techniques of the followers of Babhravya. [7]Vatsyayana says: ~~The ones made of wood more closely resemble the original.~~

[8]The inside should be the size of the penis, and it should be thick, with raised bumps on the outside to make it rough. [9]Two of these make a 'wraparound',* [10]and three or more, up to the full length of the penis, make a 'little topknot'. [11]When you twine around one single string of beads as much as the size allows, it is a 'single topknot'. [12]A device fastened around the hips, with a mouth and hole at both ends and huge, rough cups over the testicles, used with force appropriate to the size, is a 'coat of mail' or a 'little net'. [13]In the absence of these, attach to your hips, with a string, a cucumber, lotus stalk, or bamboo section, well greased with sesamum oil and decoctions; or use a smooth garland of wood, knotted and strung with many gooseberry kernels. Those are the unpierced techniques.

[14]~~But they say that a man whose penis has not been pierced does not experience real sex.~~ [15]And so the people of the South pierce a

---

[6] These tools are cool to the touch at the time of penetration, but during the sexual act they have the effect of sexual violence. The ones made of wood are just the opposite.

[7] A certain woman may be fond of one particular thing, and so it is good to use ones made of wood, too.

[8] It should be as wide as the erect penis, hollowed out inside, and fastened securely on the erect penis, like a second surface.

[9] Two bracelets can be joined in a special way in three or four places.

[11] Wrap around a string of beads made of something such as lead, as much as the circumference of the penis will allow.

[12] It has a mouth at one end through which the penis enters and a slit on both sides for the string that ties it to the hips. It has rough, raised dots all over it. It is called a 'coat of mail' because it covers the entire penis. Both the 'coat of mail' and the 'little net' should be used with consideration of the length and circumference of the penis to which it is attached.*

[13] Take the wooden garland and wind it around the penis so that it fits very tightly.

GROSS

boy's penis just like his ears. ¹⁶A young man has it cut with a knife and then stands in water as long as the blood flows. ¹⁷To keep the opening clear, he has sexual intercourse that very night, continuously.* ¹⁸Then, after an interval of one day, he cleans the opening with astringent decoctions. ¹⁹He enlarges it by putting larger and larger spears of reeds and ivory-tree wood in it, ²⁰and he cleans it with a piece of sugar-cane coated with honey. ²¹After that, he enlarges it by inserting a tube of lead with a protruding knot on the end, ²²and he lubricates it with the oil of the marking-nut. Those are the techniques of piercing. ²³He inserts into the enlarged opening sex tools made in various shapes: ²⁴the 'round', the 'round on one side', the 'little mortar', the 'little blossom', the 'thorny', the 'heron's bone', the 'little elephant's tusk', the 'eight circles', the 'spinning top', the 'water chestnut', or others according to the method and the act. They must be able to bear a lot of use, and may be soft or rough* according to individual preferences. That is how to rekindle exhausted passion, the sixty-second section.

---

¹⁶ Someone skilled pulls back the foreskin to expose the glans, holds it back, and then cuts through the glans sideways so that there is an opening on both sides. Standing in the water stops the bleeding.

¹⁷ To keep the opening from closing up, he couples many times, because this produces an obstacle to the sense of self and so dispels the pain.

¹⁸ He cleans the wound.

²¹ He uses lead because it expands; and the lead knot, wrapped as if by a palm leaf, soon enlarges the opening.

²² He lubricates the opening in order to insert things in it.

²⁴ The 'round' one has a little trough in the middle, in which a leather thong is attached; the 'round on one side' has, on the other side, a trough like an elongated eight-day old sliver of moon, in which a leather thong is attached; the 'little mortar' is narrow in the middle, where a leather thong is attached. Both the 'little blossom' and 'the thorny' should be inserted lengthwise; 'the eight circles' and 'the spinning top' should be inserted on an angle. Other objects may be used, too, and any means that give sexual pleasure. Attaching a leather thong to some of them prevents any harm from resulting from the act. As for individual preferences, one must determine the roughness of the vagina, according to its smooth, medium, or extremely rough quality, and choose a device of appropriate roughness; and, similarly, one must determine the softness of the vagina, and find devices appropriate to that softness.

[63] *Methods of Increasing the Size of the Male Organ*

²⁵ Rub your penis with the bristles of insects* born in trees, then massage it with oil for ten nights, then rub it again and massage it again. When it swells up as the result of this treatment, lie down on a cot with your face down and let your penis hang down from a hole in the cot. ²⁶ Then you may assuage the pain with cool astringents and, by stages, finish the treatment. ²⁷ This swelling, which lasts for a lifetime, is the one that voluptuaries call 'prickled'.

²⁸ You can make an enlargement that lasts for a month by rubbing your penis with, one at a time, the juices of ground cherry, sweet potato, water leeches, fruits of the nightshade, fresh buffalo butter, 'elephant's ear' teak tree leaves, and heliotrope. ²⁹ You can make an enlargement that lasts for six months by rubbing it with those astringents when they have been cooked in oil, ³⁰ or by cooking in oil, over a slow fire, the seeds of pomegranates, cucumbers, and gritty cucumbers, and the juice of the fruits of the nightshade, and then rubbing or bathing your penis with this mixture. ³¹ You learn these various techniques from qualified people. Those are the methods of increasing the size of the male organ.

[64]   *Unusual Techniques*

³² Any woman whom you sprinkle with powdered thorns of milk-hedge, mixed with hogweed, monkey-shit, and the roots of the glory lily, cannot desire any other man. ³³ If a man makes love with a woman whose vagina has been rubbed with a mixture of powdered rue, kinka oil plants, marigolds, iron, and ants, together with a decoction of the juices of the fruits of rattan and Java plum, his passion for her vanishes.* ³⁴ If a man makes love with a woman who

---

²⁵ Do not use anything else that comes from trees, just these insects. Hold the creatures with tweezers and press the stings hard against the sides of the penis. Let the penis hang down from the hole in the bed to make it longer.

²⁶ When it has reached the size you want, use the cooling astringents, or else both the swelling and the pain will go on increasing.

³³ The minute that he touches her, his penis will not stand up.

has bathed in buffalo buttermilk mixed with powdered dung-beetles, mint, and ants, his passion for her vanishes. ³⁵ An ointment, or a garland, made from the flowers of wild jasmine, hog-plum, and Java plum, makes someone unlucky in love. ³⁶ An ointment made of the white flowers of the 'cuckoo's-eye' caper bush makes an 'elephant-cow' contract tightly for one night. ³⁷ An ointment made of powdered white lotus, blue lotus, 'morningstar' tree blossoms, rose dammar blossoms, and marjoram, makes a 'doe' open wide.*

³⁸ If you prepare gooseberries with the sap of milkwort, fly agaric mushroom, and bowstring hemp, together with fruits of the kinka oil plant, it turns the hair on the head white. ³⁹ Bathing the hair on the head in an infusion of the roots of the henna plant, the ivory tree, the 'kohl-black' flower, butterfly grass, and 'smooth leaf' ebony, makes it grow. ⁴⁰ If you rub it with this same mixture, combined with well-cooked oil, it makes it black and gradually restores it.* ⁴¹ If a lip has been reddened with lac and you rub it seven times with the sweat from the testicles of a white horse, it becomes white. ⁴² Such things as henna can restore the colour. ⁴³ A woman falls under the power of a man when she hears the sound of him playing a flute that has been coated with a decoction of mint, wild ginger, East Indian rose bay, Indian plum tree, cedar wood, and prickly pear. ⁴⁴ Food prepared with the fruit of a thorn-apple tree makes anyone who eats it insane, ⁴⁵ and well-aged molasses restores that person. ⁴⁶ If you coat your hand with the shit of a peacock that has eaten yellow arsenic and red arsenic, whatever object you touch becomes invisible. ⁴⁷ If you mix water with oil and with the ashes of charcoal and grass, it takes on the colour of milk. ⁴⁸ Iron pots turn to copper if you coat them with ground black myrobalan, hog-plum, heart seed, and panic-seed. ⁴⁹ If you fill a lamp with the oil of heart seed and panic-seed, and make its wick out of silk and the sloughed skin of a serpent, and place long strips of wood beside it, they appear to be serpents. ⁵⁰ You become famous and live a long life if you drink the milk of a white cow who has a white calf, ⁵¹ or if you receive the blessings of respected

---

³⁷ It opens her wide for one night.

⁴³ Coat the flute by washing it, many times, inside and out, with water in which the herbs have been steeped.

Brahmins.

52 By combining earlier texts
and following their methods,
Vatsyayana composed this *Kamasutra*,
with great effort, in a condensed form.

53 A man who knows its real meaning
sees religion, power, and pleasure,
his own convictions, and the ways of the world
for what they are, and he is not driven by passion.

Contradicts pg 160

54 The unusual techniques employed to increase passion,
which have been described as this particular book required,
are strongly restricted right here in this verse,
right after it.*

55 For the statement that 'There is a text for this'
does not justify a practice. People should realize
that the contents of the texts apply in general,
but each actual practice is for one particular region.

56 Vatsyayana learned and thought about
the meanings of the *sutras* of Babhravya's followers,
and then he made this *Kamasutra*,
following the rules.

57 He made this work in chastity and in the highest meditation,
for the sake of worldly life;
he did not compose it
for the sake of passion.

Page 45

58 A man who knows the real meaning of this text
guards the state of his own religion, power, and pleasure
as it operates in the world, and he becomes
a man who has truly conquered his senses.

59 The man who is well-taught and expert in this text
pays attention to religion and power;

---

54 They are forbidden for the particular places and people who are
strongly cautioned against them.

55 This was said earlier [at 2.9.41].

56 He learned them from gurus and thought about them with his own
intelligence.

he does not indulge himself too much in passion,
and so he succeeds when he plays the part of a lover.

END OF BOOK SEVEN

END OF THE *KAMASUTRA*

APPENDIX

EXCERPTS FROM DEVADATTA SHASTRI'S COMMENTARY

Shastri provides essays on some of the central topics of the *Kamasutra*, as well as summarizing essays at the end of several chapters. Here are some examples of each.

1.1.17 On reflection, it appears that all of human life is permeated by sexuality. That is why the Vedas and the Upanishads, too, give examples of sex between man and woman. The ten sections on sleeping together in the *Rig Veda* correspond to various types of sex discussed in the *Kamasutra*. The text does not deal with an improper subject or science. From a spiritual viewpoint, too, the universe in all its variety is essentially sexual. The chief component of sex is attraction and of attraction, sex. Attraction toward respected elders appears in the form of faith, devotion, and other pure sentiments. Among equals, the same attraction appears as friendship and comradeship. Toward inferiors, attraction takes the form of compassion and kindness, towards children, parental affection. The same sexuality is manifested as maternal sentiment in the mother's heart, as lust in the lover's embrace, and as compassion toward the poor and the suffering. But all of these are forms of one basic emotion related to sex—attraction or sexuality. That is why the *Brihadranayaka Upanishad* says, 'Man is sexual.' Sexuality is the semen of the mind.

1.1.24 Talismans, spells, and charms are an integral part of our civilization. They have been a part of Indian life from the *Rig Veda* and *Atharva Veda* down to our own times. That is why it was necessary for Vatsyayana to reflect on this subject. By describing these practices at the end of the text, Vatsyayana has paid respect to public sentiment, interest, and welfare. So that ordinary people should not get confused or upset on reading it, he has referred at various places in the text to the aims of non-violence, chastity, and empathy with the suffering of others.

1.3.16 Vatsyayana has not divided the arts into categories but merely enumerated them. The best-known number of the arts is sixty-four, which Shukraniti and Tantric texts also give, although some sources number the arts at sixteen, thirty-two, sixty-four, or even more. It is clear from Vatsyayana's list that in his view art is what enchants a woman. Any activity or skill that pleases a woman, seduces her, is art.

1.4.6 The servants of the man-about-town prepared, every week in advance, a mixture of scented substances for his use in brushing his teeth. The sticks used for brushing were soaked for seven days in cow's urine in which myrobalan powder was dissolved. After that, the stick was soaked in water containing cardamom, cinnamon, antimony, and honey. The stick prepared in this way was considered beneficent. The man-about-town of those times did not brush his teeth only for reasons of health or cleanliness but also considered it auspicious. Careful attention was given to the selection of the stick according to the type of tree and the phase of the moon. The man's servants and his priest took care that the selection of the stick was proper. After brushing his teeth, he rubbed his body with sandalwood paste or other substances, such as aloe and saffron mixed with cream. The *Ayurveda* tells us that anointing the body with these substances makes it supple and scented.

Then the hair was scented with the smoke of fragrant resin. This was done to prevent hair loss, to keep it from becoming grey, and to make it soft and glossy. Varahamihira warns, in his *Grihya Samhita*, 'You can wear the finest of clothes and scented garlands, and decorate your limbs with the most expensive ornaments, but if your hair becomes grey, all this decoration is useless.' After the hair was scented with camphor, saffron or musk, it was left loose until he took his bath.

After his hair was done, he put on a garland of flowers. The flowers used were champa, jasmine, and white ixora. At the time of making love, garlands of yellow amaranths were recommended, since they do not fall or fade in the course of embracing, kissing or hugging.

After discussing the garland, Vatsyayana talks of painting with lac-coloured dyes. There is no indication in ancient texts that men dyed their lips or feet red. Perhaps Vatsyayana is talking about colouring the nails. Afterwards, the man-about-town looked at himself in a mirror. Glass mirrors were not in use, but mirrors were made of highly polished square sheets of gold or silver.

Vatsyayana does not give a description of the bath because the right way of taking a bath was familiar to everyone. But the ordinary bath of those days seems like a special yogic exercise today. A description is provided in Bana's *Kadambari*:

Having finished his day's business a little before noon, the man-about-town was ready for his bath. Before the bath, he exercised a little with his friends. After resting for a while, he entered the bathroom. It had a marble seat and gold and silver vessels filled with herbal scented water. Female servants slowly rubbed scented myrobalan in his hair. Then they massaged his body with scented oil. The man then sat in a boat-shaped vessel filled with water for a little while and then on the marble seat for his bath. After the bath he went into the prayer room for worship.

1.4.35 Brahmins were not only reciters of the Vedas but became rich merchants by trading within and outside the country. This was also true of the Kshatriyas. They were not only kings and warriors but also high-quality merchants. The role of the jester in almost all the Sanskrit dramas was played by a Brahmin. This proves that in ancient times Brahmins were merchants as well as libertines, panders, and clowns.

2.1.38 In his work, *Nagarasarvasva*, Padmashri has described the preparations for intercourse. After dressing herself up according to the wishes of her husband, a woman should both expose and hide her limbs. Shy and smiling, she should approach her husband. If he tries to pull her near she should withdraw in feigned modesty. When he gets up and gathers her in his arms, she should behave like a startled doe and try to hide her limbs. But after a little while she should let herself go. She should first hide whichever part of her body her husband wants to touch, scratch, or bite, and then offer it passionately to his caress. If he hugs her tightly, bites her, or scratches her, she should make loud noises expressing pain. If he embraces and kisses her she should say such loving words as 'O heartless man, do not torture me so much!' According-ing to the occasion, the woman should respond to biting and scratching by using her own teeth and nails or by becoming helpless or saying, 'Go away, I won't talk to you', and turning over on her side. When the man tries to win her over she should turn back and engage in intercourse. After the intercourse is over, the woman should lie there exhausted with an infatuated expression on her face and close her eyes. This makes a man give his all for her.

2.1, *end* On reflection, one finds that the sprout of love grows first in a woman. Women are also more passionate than men. This kind of attraction, passion, and desire between men and women has a natural cause. The cause is a lack. A woman eagerly wishes to receive from a man what is missing in her, and vice versa. People generally believe that men get infatuated with women. But the fact is the opposite. A woman is more capable of infatuation than a man. Man and woman are two currents of electricity. One is a debt, the other a wealth. The two currents are oppos-ites. One attracts, the other repulses. When both meet, electricity appears. Indian science believes that a woman possesses the essence of the sun, and a man, that of the moon. The sun draws in the juice of the earth through its power, while the moon bathes the earth in dew. The sun-possessed woman draws the moon-possessed man's semen inside herself. This is the main cause of the attraction and love between man and woman.

2.2, *end* Padmashri is of the opinion that it is proper to sleep only with a girl and a young woman (*taruni*). Till the age of sixteen, a woman is called a girl, from sixteen to thirty a *taruni*, from thirty to fifty middle-aged, and after fifty she is called an old woman. To sleep with a girl in summer and autumn is beneficial. In early and late winter one should sleep with a young woman, and in spring and the rainy season, with a middle-aged woman. A man's energy increases if he enjoys a girl. A young woman saps his energy and a middle-aged woman makes him old.

From the new to the full moon, the god Kama first mounts the woman's thumb, then her feet, thighs, navel, breasts, nipple, throat, cheeks, lips, eyes, eyebrows, and forehead. That is why knowledgeable men awaken the god by holding the woman's hair, kissing her eyes and forehead, biting her lips, pressing her nipples, and stroking her breast and navel.

Sushruta says that just like the invisible presence of juice in the sugar-cane stalk, butter in milk, and oil in seasame seed, semen is present in all parts of a man's body. When a man thinks of a desired woman, sees, hears, or embraces her, he feels sexual pleasure, and semen is drawn from different parts of the body to enter the urinary canal. Sushruta's statement that semen is the material form of an individual soul is true and scientific. The seed (*bija*) inside the semen is the abode of the soul. Sexual desire is present in a human being right from birth. In childhood it is spread all over the body. As one gets older desire becomes concentrated in the genitals.

Padmashri says that there are twenty-four nerves in the vagina, which give rise to the desire for intercourse. The place where these nerves end is called 'Kama's umbrella' (the clitoris). It should be rubbed slowly with the fingers. Of the nerves which excite sexual desire, there are two in the face, two in the eyes, one in the throat, one at the base of the thumb. Pressing these nerves in an embrace soon excites desire. Scratching the ears, thighs, lower back, and forehead with the nails excites sexuality. *Sati, asati, subhaga, durbhaga, putri, duhitrini* are the six great nerves in the vulva, which give rise to an irresistible urge for intercourse when excited. Deep inside the vagina are the *putri* and *duhitrini* nerves. In the left part of the vulva is *sati*, in the right, the *asati*. At a little distance inside the vaginal canal are the *subhaga* and *durbhaga* nerves. Hugging excites the *sati* nerve; caressing both the armpits excites the *sati*. Kissing excites the *subhaga*; caressing the waist excites the *durbhaga*. Kissing the face excites the *putri* and caressing the buttocks produces agitation in the *duhitrini*, which leads to immediate orgasm.

2.3.4 Women are tender not only in body but also in character and mind. They should be handled as if they were flowers so that they neither fade nor lose their scent. If force is used in embracing or kissing them, a lifelong fear, suspicion, or hate can distort their minds.

The first three days [of marriage] demand utmost care. If within this period any kind of aversion arises toward the man, then it will always remain in the mind as hate. A woman's modesty should also be taken into account. Women prefer intercourse in the dark.

Generally, intercourse depends on the two mental inclinations of love and sexual hunger. Love makes one generous and sentimental, and sexual hunger makes one selfish.

2.3.32 Lips are considered the most important part of kissing because they are the tenderest parts of the body. Lips carry an electric charge which, when touched, excites those nerves and joints that carry an internal flow of this electric current. This electric current is responsible for the pleasure given by touch.

2.4, *end* Medical science is of the opinion that the upper part of a woman's skin has some areas which are connected to the womb. Exciting them slowly or rapidly in certain directions not only arouses desire but creates preliminary conditions for intercourse. Women are liable to become epileptic if these areas are not properly handled. That is why to preserve her mental and bodily health it is essential to use the nails and teeth on those parts of a woman's body that are recognized as erotic centres.

2.6, *end* It is quite acceptable for an authoritative treatise (*shastra*) to mention, describe, and reflect upon all kinds of sexual practices, whether good or bad, and to seek to understand their real import. But what can be the purpose of sculptures depicting intercourse and other sexual acts found in our ancient temples? If we study human behaviour closely, we find that in every human being a wish for salvation is born only after he is fully satisfied. Total satisfaction and salvation are the two goals of our existence. The sculptures of couples engaged in sexual intercourse found on the temples of Konarak, Puri, Khajuraho, and other places represent the first goal of life. That is why they are shown on the outside walls of the temple. Salvation is the second goal, which is represented by the image of the god in the inner sanctum. The sculptures of couples in intercourse on the outer door and walls remind the seeker that one who has not crossed the portals of sexual satisfaction has no right to take the second step toward god and salvation.

2.8.6 When the woman lies on top of the man and makes love, the flowers in her hair scatter. She begins to pant even as she laughs. When she brings her mouth close to her husband's for a kiss, her breasts press against his chest. At this time, the woman fully imitates the man. She scratches, bites, hits, kisses in the same way as the man. Then she laughs like a victor and says, 'First, you laid me low. Now I am taking revenge by laying you under me.' But when her sexual desire is satisfied, she becomes bashful and closes her eyes. She lies down on the cot because she is tired. Then she starts to show her love towards her husband like a man.

2.10, *end* All men and women have their own distinctive smells. Bodily smell is related to the surge of sexuality. With the onset of youth, a man or a woman gets a distinct smell. One sometimes hears about incidents in which a beautiful girl belonging to a good family surrenders completely to a low-born, ugly man. These surprising incidents can be attributed to the effect of smell. Saffron, musk, ambergris, and sandalwood are substances whose scent is similar to that of women and thus have a high sexual significance. That may be why women have traditionally used them. One thing is certain: bodily smell creates an atmosphere around itself which either attracts or repels.

3.1, *end* Vatsyayana says that it is the opinion of some teachers that one should marry a girl with whom one falls in love. The *Apastamba-dharmasutra* is of the same opinion. But before translating this scriptural injunction into practice, it is necessary to use one's own judgement. If a girl is physically handicapped or does not belong to an equal caste-group, then one should not marry her even if one is in love.

3.2, *end* The core of whatever Vatsyayana has to say in this useful exposition on how to relax a girl is that a man needs to be a specialist in the psychology of women. Without a knowledge of a woman's emotions, his marriage and married life will be failures.

3.5, *end* Love marriage has been common in India since ancient times and has enjoyed great popularity. The choosing of a husband in open assembly by a princess was a love marriage. Nala and Damayanti, Aja and Indumati, Rama and Sita, Udayana and Vasavadatta, Malati and Madhava were all married in this way. In Vatsyayana's view, even though love-marriage is not ritually the highest form of marriage, it is still pre-eminent. This is because the ultimate goal of marriage is to develop love between the couple, and a love-marriage has this from the beginning.

4.2.45 The unfortunate among these second-hand women are those who are harassed by the other co-wives. Such an unlucky woman should take the side of a co-wife who is favoured by the husband. She should show the arts that can be exhibited because a demonstration of proficiency often ends misfortune.

5.1, *end* In this section Vatsyayana has described ten sexual states of man which come to the fore at the time of separation from a woman. It is not necessary that these states become manifest only in relation to another man's wife. These ten states appear whenever desire is frustrated. Whether the object of desire is a man or woman, one's own wife or another man's, this section is concerned with the states when the object is unavailable. The ten states mentioned by Vatsyayana torment not only men but also women. Just as men sleep with other men's wives, women sleep with other women's husbands. The effort made by a man to sleep with the wife of another man is the same as made by a woman to sleep with the husband of another woman. It is a different matter that men have more courage and are less shy while women are more diffident in this particular enterprise. But one should not turn one's face away from the reality that, like men, women too desire other men. The conversation between Yama and Yami in the *Rig Veda* gives evidence of this. Commenting on the *Chandogya Upanishad*'s statement, 'Do not refuse any woman', Shankara says that one should not turn away a lustful woman who comes to one's bed, while Ramanuja writes in his commentary, 'To sleep with another man's wife when her longing for intercourse is intense is part of the worship of Shiva, and the adultery is not forbidden.' Besides, the Puranic legends of Ahalya and Indra, Kunti and the Sun, the stories of Dushyanta and Shakuntala, Malati and Madhava, and many other love stories testify to an unbroken chain of adultery since creation.

5.6, *end* Like Vatsyayana, other scholars of erotics have also inquired into the causes of women's sexual misconduct. Padmashri says that women should take care not to indulge in or listen to lewd talk when they go out to festivals, on pilgrimages, to temples, houses of neighbours or to the fields, because the intoxication of youth robs them of discrimination and they are apt to lose their chastity and virginity.

6.2, *end* The author of the *Kamasutra* has not asked why men frequent courtesans in spite of having young, beautiful, and accomplished wives at home. The answer to this question is given by the verses that speak of the courtesan's erotic accomplishments. Actually, courtesans are educated in sexual play since childhood. How to attract a man, how to make him a slave through sex, are arts which are uniquely those of the courtesan, not of a housewife.

6.3, *end* The essence of this section on the nature of a courtesan is found in the dialogue between the sage Maricha and the courtesan

Kamamanjari in Dandin's *Dashakumaracharita*. Kamamanjari says that there is an inborn tendency among courtesans to try to transform a girl into a celestial beauty. All the ways mentioned in the texts on erotics and beauty are employed to make her beautiful. From childhood, the girl eats a balanced diet so that bodily defects are corrected and her attractiveness increases. After she becomes five years old, she is hidden from men in such a way that even her father cannot meet her. From this age onwards, the girl is educated in the sixty-four arts and is taught different languages. All kinds of ways to cheat and deceive are taught to her. The arts of intercourse are imparted by a man who will not cause her much pain and will also remain discreet.

6.5, *end* The *Kamasutra* recommends to the courtesan that she determine her own fee according to the country, its state of affairs, the times she is living in, her qualities, beauty, etc. But Kautilya's *Arthashastra* gives the right of fixing her fees not to the courtesan but to the administration. Kautilya would appoint a Commissioner of Courtesans who keeps an eye on their security and their doings, keeps track of their visitors and income, and lays down the fee to be charged. The independence enjoyed by the courtesan at the time the *Kamasutra* was composed was absent at the time of the composition of the *Arthashastra*.

7.2, *end* A man cannot satisfy a woman through intercourse once his sexual power weakens. The woman then becomes detached and depressed. Women who suppress their strong wish for intercourse under such conditions often fall sick. They become epileptic, are subject to fainting fits, and become irritable by nature. Vatsyayana has said that a man who comes too soon should first excite the woman and make her wet by means other than intercourse. Such a way of proceeding satisfies both man and woman. At what time each part of a woman's body is erotically sensitive can be learned through a study of the principles of Moon-Art [a theory that links different parts of a woman's body to different phases of the moon]. Pressing the appropriate part of the woman's body at a particular time excites her and she soon becomes wet. The man who comes too soon, whose sexual power has weakened, but who still wants the pleasure of intercourse, should practise Yoga. The Yogashastras talk of the Ashvini-mudra. A person who attains proficiency in this particular *mudra* will remain sexually adequate.

EXPLANATORY NOTES

V = Vatsyayana   Y = Yashodhara

[Y] 1.1.1 The three aims of human life (*purusharthas*)—religion (*dharma*), power (*artha*), and pleasure (*kama*)—also known as the triple path (*trivarga*), are discussed in the Introduction. The metaphor of the bookworms is analogous to the odds against a monkey randomly typing out the works of Shakespeare. At 1.2.19 Y tells us that Vatsyayana is the author's family name; Mallanaga (literally, 'elephant among wrestlers') is the name given at his initiation. See O'Flaherty, *Dreams, Illusion*, for the bookworm metaphor.

1.1.2 The word that we have translated as 'text' is *shastra*, which sometimes also means a whole body of knowledge, what we would call a discipline or even a science, or sometimes a particular textbook. Pururavas, a mortal king, fell in love with the celestial nymph and courtesan Urvashi; when he broke his promise to her, she left him, though according to later versions of the myth, they were later reconciled. The story that Y tells here closely resembles the Greek myth of Paris, who, forced to choose between three goddesses, chose Aphrodite (= Kama) over Artemis and Athene (roughly = Dharma and Artha), and was cursed by Athene and Artemis. Kama functions as a god quite often in Hindu mythology; the god Shiva burns him to ashes, but he is revived, invisible. He is also invoked as the patron saint of adultery: One day Kama caught sight of the wife of a Brahmin and pricked his heart with his own flower arrow. She, too, was pierced by one of Kama's arrows and lusted for him. As Kama was wooing her, her husband caught them and cursed Kama to become a leper and the woman to become a broken stone *khanda-sila*, a pun on 'broken virtue'. Kama propitiated the sage and was freed from his disease, but the woman remained in the form of a stone. If a man worships her in this form on the thirteenth day (of the month), there will be no offence either for the man or for his lover when adultery occurs. And a woman who is being neglected by her husband should offer flowers to her (*Skanda Purana* 6.134.1–80). For Pururavas and Urvashi see *Rig Veda* 10.95 (*Rig Veda*, trans. O'Flaherty, 253–6); *Shatapatha Brahmana* 11.5.1.1–17; O'Flaherty, *Women, Androgynes*; and Doniger, *Splitting the Difference*. For Kama and Shiva, see O'Flaherty, *Siva*.

1.1.6 Manu, the son of the Creator, is the mythical author of the *Laws of Manu*.

1.1.7 Brihaspati is the guru of the gods, the planet Jupiter, and the putative author of a Machiavellian handbook of politics from which the extant text known as the *Arthashastra*, composed by Kautilya, is said to have been derived, just as Vatsyayana's *Kamasutra* is said to have been derived from that of the mythical Nandin. The human editions of these two texts, as well as Manu's text on *dharma*, are still in existence now, though perhaps not in the form in which V or even Y knew them. The texts cited in 1.1.9–13 no longer exist, but almost certainly existed at the time of V, since he and, later, Y often quote directly from them.

[Y] 1.1.8 Y is here making explicit the fact that the Nandin in question is actually a god, not merely a human named after a god (as a man, especially in Spanish-speaking countries, might be called Jesus). Nandin, a bull or a bull-headed deity, is the son of the Great God, Shiva, and is often stationed to guard the door to the bedroom door of his parents, Shiva and Uma (also named Parvati). A statue of Nandin often guards the door to a temple of Shiva. It is most appropriate for a bull, and for the god Shiva (whose phallus is worshipped throughout India, but who also controls his sexuality through his asceticism), to be associated with the textbook of sex and pleasure. A year as the gods count them is usually counted as ten thousand human years.

[Y] 1.1.9 The verses that Y cites contrast 'the guru's son', Manu, son of the Self-born (cited in the previous verse), who made the rules about wine, with Uddalaka's son, who made the rules about other men's wives.

Shvetaketu Auddalaki is cited often in the *Kamasutra*, henceforth just by his patronymic, Auddalaki. The story that Y tells is told at greater length in the great Sanskrit epic the *Mahabharata* (1.113.9–20): 'The great sage named Uddalaka had a son, named Shvetaketu, who became a hermit. Once, right before the eyes of Shvetaketu and his father, a Brahmin grasped his mother by the hand and said, "Let's go!" The sage's son became enraged and could not bear to see his mother being taken away by force like that. But when his father saw that Shvetaketu was angry he said, "Do not be angry, my little son. This is the eternal *dharma*. The women of all classes on earth are not fenced in; all creatures behave just like cows, my little son, each in its own class." The sage's son could not tolerate that *dharma*, and made this moral boundary for men and women on earth, for humans, but not for other creatures. And from then on this moral boundary has stood: A woman who is unfaithful to her husband commits a mortal sin that brings great misery, an evil equal to killing an embryo, and a man who seduces another man's wife, when she is a woman who keeps her vow to her husband and is thus a virgin obeying a vow of chastity, that man too commits a mortal sin on earth.' The epic keeps insisting that this is all hearsay, as if to make us doubt it; the primal scene that it imagines is a vivid, quasi-Freudian narrative, explaining a kind of sexual revulsion. Shvetaketu Auddalaki is well known as a hero of the Upanishads, the ancient Sanskrit philosophical texts that argue for renunciation; in those texts, his father teaches him the central doctrines of Indian philosophy. It is surprising to find Shvetaketu here in the *Kamasutra* cited as an expert sexologist, and this seeming incongruity may have inspired V to allude to, and Y to tell, this story here: it explains how a sage became simultaneously chaste, an enemy of male adultery, and an authority on sex.

A Brahmin's right to demand the sexual services of any woman he fancied evoked violent protest in ancient Indian texts; a notorious example is the story of Yavakri, who tried to exert this right on the wife of another Brahmin and died. For Shvetaketu, see *Brihadaranyaka Upanishad* 6.2.1; *Chandogya Upanishad* 5.3.1–6; 6.1–16; *Kaushitaki Upanishad* 1.1. For Yavakri, see O'Flaherty, *Tales of Sex and Violence*; Doniger, *The Bedtrick*.

1.1.10 Babhravya, like Auddalaki, is an authority with whom V will argue often in the course of the *Kamasutra*. We have translated *kanya* as 'virgin', in part to distinguish the term from *bala*, meaning 'a female child', which we translated as 'a young girl'. *Kanya* actually covers a range of meanings including maiden, virgin, unmarried girl, bride, and a girl who has not yet menstruated. In the context of this text, whose central concern is the sexual act, we felt that 'virgin' was usually the foregrounded meaning. What we have called 'erotic esoterica' is 'Upanishadic' (which might be translated as 'mystical'); it designates, in this text, aphrodisiac drugs, magic recipes, sex tools, and so forth.

1.1.11 The courtesans de luxe are said to be Pataliputrikas, 'Daughters of the Trumpet Flower'. To touch anyone, let alone a god, with your foot is an act of great disrespect and a common source of curses in India. Men are often turned into women, and back again, in Hindu and Buddhist mythology, as Teiresias was in Greek mythology; Narada, Bhangashvana, and Ila are the most famous of the serial androgynes. The difference between a courtesan and a courtesan de luxe is set forth in 1.3.17 and in Shastri's note on 1.5.3, cited in the Introduction. For Ila and Bhangashvana, see Doniger, *Splitting the Difference*; for Narada, see O'Flaherty, *Dreams, Illusion*.

1.1.15 The titles of books given here are repeated in the text at the beginning of each book; the chapters do not have titles. Instead, the text is divided into the sections listed here, and often (though not always) the title of the section is given at the end, set off by the word *iti* that also indicates the end of a direct quotation or a long list: 'That is . . .'. We have inserted all of the section headings at the appropriate places, in brackets, giving them the sixty-four numbers that Yashodhara gives them. There are also three unnumbered sections, at 1.5.1, 4.2.67, and 6.6.50.

1.1.16 The 'man-about-town' is literally the *nagaraka*, the man of the city (*nagara*), an urbane playboy.

1.1.20 Lists of the women with whom one can and cannot have intercourse are set-pieces in the *dharma* literature; cf. *Mahabharata* 13.107, *Laws of Manu* 3.4–50.

1.1.23 V says here that his text has 1,250 *sutras*, a nice, round number; the Shastri edition that we are using makes it 1492, also an easy number (date) to remember, and the Goswami edition numbers 1683.

1.2.1 A hundred years is the ideal lifespan, used as the benchmark in Vedic and Ayurvedic texts; but, as 1.2.5 indicates, it was understood that not everyone reached this ideal age.

1.2.2 V lists power rather than religion as the predominant goal of childhood, which Manu regards as a period of spiritual rather than worldly education. But V consistently regards knowledge (*vidya*, which may more specifically designate knowledge of the Veda) as a form of power, as, for instance, in 1.2.9. Moreover, V regards progeny both as an issue of religion, for the son must make the funeral offerings that free his dead father from limbo, and as an issue of power, probably because of the importance of inheritance. Compare Y's tabulation of the ages of men with Shastri's tabulation of the ages of women (at 2.2.23): until the age of sixteen, a woman is called a girl, from sixteen to thirty a young woman, from thirty to fifty middle-aged, and after fifty she is called an old woman. After the first age, when they are equal, the men are much older than the women with whom they are matched: a woman is old at fifty, a man at seventy.

1.2.4 Release (*moksha*) is the fourth human goal; see Introduction.

[Y] 1.2.4 The four classes are Brahmin, Kshatriya, Vaishya and Shudra, roughly priest, warrior/ruler, commoner, and servant. The four stages are the chaste student (*brahmacarin*), householder (*grihastha*), forest dweller (*vanaprastha*), and renouncer (*sannyasin*). Y, at 1.1.1, does not use the usual terms for the last two stages of life, but calls them a *vaikhanasa* (literally, 'digger', presumably for roots to eat) and a *bhikshu* (literally, one who begs for food to eat, more broadly designating a monk).

1.2.6 This passage seems to forbid pre-pubescent eroticism, which the previous passage (permitting the pursuit of pleasure in any stage of life) theoretically allowed. Y here also expands upon the previous passage's statement that the young student is concerned with power—here not merely knowledge, but land.

1.2.7 An alternative translation would be: 'Religion consists in engaging . . . in sacrifice and other such actions that people do not generally engage in . . . and in refraining . . . from . . . such actions that people generally do engage in.'

1.2.8 'Sacred scripture' is *shruti*, 'what is heard', the term for the most ancient Sanskrit texts, the Vedas, Brahmanas, and Upanishads, that are so named because they were 'heard' by the ancient sages (presumably from words uttered by the gods). *Shruti* was followed by *smriti*, 'what is remembered', man-made texts such as the textbooks referred to in 1.1.6–7 and the *Kamasutra*.

1.2.10 'The Tasks of the Superintendent' is the title of a chapter in the *Arthashastra*.

1.2.12 What we have translated, literally, as 'bearing fruit' Y interprets as 'culminating in a climax', but V may mean that the fruit is the production of a child. In the light of Babhravya's remarks cited at 2.1.18 about female orgasm, this passage may refer not only to the man's climax but also to the woman's, and to the ejaculation of seed by both of them that results in pregnancy. Y defines what V calls erotic arousal (*abhimana*) in terms of such things as kissing and caressing. The verb from which the noun *abhimana* is derived appears (with a direct object) at 1.2.35, where it seems to mean 'to desire', 'to be aroused (by)'. But it also means 'high self-esteem' (as well as 'arrogance'), perhaps combined in an erotic feeling that heightens the sense of self, a meaning which may also be relevant here; it suggests that there is some sort of self-definition involved in the sexual act.

1.2.15 It seems cynical of V to say that power and wealth (*artha*) are more important than religion (*dharma*) for a king; the *dharma* texts, not surprisingly, rank *dharma* above *artha* for a king, but, more surprisingly, so do the *artha* texts.

1.2.16 Now begins what Indian logic calls the 'other side' (literally, the 'former wing,' *purvapaksha*), the straw man, the arguments that imagined opponents might raise, followed by the author's rebuttals. In 1.2.16–20, V defends textbooks of sex against arguments that may in fact have been current in India in his time. In 1.2.21–5, he defends the pursuit of *dharma* against the materialists, then (in 1.2.26–31) the pursuit of *artha* against the fatalists, and finally (in 1.2.32–39) the pursuit of *kama* against the pragmatists.

[Y] 1.2.17 Y here alludes to the well-known Hindu belief that matter consists in three 'strands' (torpor, passion, and lucidity), and that different creatures are made up of different proportions of these strands. By omitting scholars of pleasure from his list, he implies that those who make the objections in 1.2.16–17 do not know what they are talking about.

[Y] 1.2.20 The fertile season is the time immediately after menstruation, according to Hindu medical theory. Here Y is quoting Manu 3.45.

1.2.21 Materialists (*Lokayatikas*) express doctrines that correspond, roughly, to what we call materialism; they are also sometimes called Charvakas and sometimes Nastikas ('Those who say [the gods] do not exist'), roughly, atheists. Their own texts, if they ever existed, have not survived; they are known only as the straw men in other texts such as this one.

1.2.26 *Kalakarinikas*, literally, 'People [who believe that] fate or time is the cause [of everything]', correspond to our 'fatalists'.

1.2.29 For Bali and Indra, see O'Flaherty, *The Origins of Evil*.

1.2.32 Pragmatists or utilitarians are *Arthachintakas*, literally people who are always thinking about success, power, and everything that *artha* implies. They have also been called 'opportunists' and 'Philistines'. The *Sarvadarshanasamgraha*, composed after the *Kamasutra*, describes the arguments of materialists called Charvakas in these terms.

1.2.35 Danda, the son of Manu, raped Ara (also called Araja), the daughter of the great sage Shukra (also called Ushanas or Bhargava), who was at that time Danda's royal chaplain and later became the royal chaplain of the demons. See the *Ramayana*.

[Y] 1.2.36 Unlike most other variants of this myth, Y's version does not mention that the king of the gods, Indra, took the form of Gautama to seduce Ahalya; also unique is its suggestion that Gautama had intended to make love to her himself. Other variants also attribute the form of the curse (to have the mark of vaginas all over his body) to the fact that Indra was caught in the 'womb' of Ahalya, not of the hermitage. Most famous of all, which is perhaps why Y does not bother to tell the story, is the abduction of Sita, wife of Rama, by the demon Ravana, whom Rama subsequently destroyed. All these seductions involved tricks: Indra pretended to be Ahalya's husband; Kichaka was foiled (and killed) when a man took the place of the woman he intended to seduce; and Ravana masqueraded as an ascetic to abduct Sita, while (in many tellings after the first Sanskrit version) a shadow Sita took the place of the Sita that Ravana thought he had abducted. All illusory seductions, they were all the more deadly for that. For Ahalya and Sita, see the *Ramayana* and Doniger, *Splitting the Difference*; for Kichaka, see the *Mahabharata* and Doniger, *The Bedtrick*.

1.2.38 The word for diseases, or 'flaws' (*doshas*), is also a technical term for the three 'humours' of the body, the basis of Hindu medical theory; they must be kept in proper balance through a careful diet. The implication is that aspects of sex, too, must be balanced or they will become pathological. The parable of the deer and barley appears in the *Shatapatha Brahmana* (*c.*900 BCE) as a metaphor for the seduction of other men's wives: 'When the deer eats the barley [the farmer] does not hope to nourish the animal; when the low-born woman becomes the lover of a noble man, [her husband] does not hope to get rich on that nourishment' (13.2.9.6–9). Cynically, V assumes that people are as unwilling to offer food to beggars as they are to offer up their crops to deer to browse.

1.3.4 The meaning of the techniques and the distinction between arts and techniques or practices are discussed in the note on 1.3.16.

1.3.7 V refers specifically to the *uha*, the technique of glossing a word.

1.3.14 'Girlfriend' is used through this text in the meaning of a friend who is a girl, not a female friend who is an erotic partner.

1.3.15 'The lute and the drum' are more precisely the *vina*, a stringed instrument, and the *damaru*, a small drum in the shape of an hour-glass. 'Languages made to seem foreign' (*mlecchita*, literally 'barbarianized') seem to be the antecedent of our Anguish Languish or tricks such as the French phrase 'Mots d'heures, faux cœurs', which has another meaning when pronounced in French but heard in English.

1.3.16 The distinction between fine arts (such as singing, described in Book One) and the arts of love (described in Book Two) is sometimes blurred in the *Kamasutra*. Often, but not always, the arts of love are called the sixty-four 'techniques'. Thus, at 1.3.22, V contrasts the (fine) arts in one line with the techniques in the next. But at 3.3.20, Y glosses the arts as 'cutting leaves into shapes, and so forth', and immediately, at 3.3.21, V refers to the sixty-four techniques. At 4.2.44 Y glosses the sixty-four arts as 'those beginning with embracing and ending with the sexual movements of a man', i.e. the arts of love, but at 4.2.45 he switches to the other definition ('cutting leaves into shapes, and so forth'). Wherever possible, we will specify 'fine' when non-sexual arts are intended, and 'of love' when sexual arts are intended, but where the usage of the term is ambiguous, perhaps intentionally ambiguous, we will just say 'arts', *tout court*. The term 'sixty-four techniques' is unambiguous in referring to the arts of love, not the fine arts.

1.3.17 Both *veshya* (courtesan) and *ganika* (courtesan de luxe) are words suggesting multiple sexual partners, *veshya* from *vish* (everyone, the people) and *ganika* from *gana* (a crowd or host). Other Sanskrit texts seem to use these terms interchangeably, but clearly the *Kamasutra* differentiates between them. See Sternbach, *Texts about Courtesans*.

1.3.22 'Luck in love', literally 'good luck' (*saubhagyam*), is a term used in the *Kamasutra* in the technical sense of the good luck of being loved, particularly of a woman's luck in being loved by her husband. When applied to a man, it means that he has the luck of being loved by many women, a significant asymmetry. The adjective *subhaga* also means handsome or beautiful, and the opposite term (*durbhaga*, for the prefixes *su* and *dur* are cognate with our *eu* and *dys/dis*) is used particularly for a woman whose husband hates her. (See 4.2.54). Oddly, since *bhaga* also designates the female sexual organ, *durbhaga* might also designate a woman with a bad vagina.

1.4.1 The man-about-town (*nagaraka*) is literally a man who lives in a city (a *nagara*), but the term designates a sophisticated connoisseur of the good life in general, of pleasure in particular, and of sex even more particularly. In our day, he would be called a playboy. He lives all by himself—which is very strange in India, where people are always connected to their families—and is rich. He has no caste, and V does not even refer to his class, though Y's gloss on this passage interprets the four sources of his wealth in terms of the four classes.

1.4.4 Betel (*tambula*, nowadays called *paan*) is a delicacy made of a betel leaf rolled up around a paste made of areca nuts (sometimes called betel nuts), cardamom, lime paste, catechu, and other flavours, sometimes including tobacco or other stimulants. The finished product, shaped rather like a stuffed grape-leaf, is eaten as a stimulant, digestive, and aphrodisiac, to redden the mouth (it produces a blood-red paste), and to freshen the breath.

1.4.8 The 'libertine', 'pander', and 'clown' are further defined at 1.4.31–4.

1.4.11 Both male and female messengers are mentioned in this text; we will specify the gender when it is not clear from the context.

1.4.15 Sarasvati, goddess of arts and letters, is the appropriate muse for a man-about-town, a connoisseur.

1.4.21 The phrase 'who love all men equally' is more literally 'for whom all men are alike when it comes to love' and might also be translated 'who are all the same for men to love' or 'who are the same as the men when it comes to love'.

1.4.28 The 'silk-cotton' tree (*shalmali*, *Bombax heptaphyllum* or *Salmalia malabarica*) is a great tree with massive thorns that are said to be used to torture people in hell. The 'morningstar' tree (*kadamba*, *Nauclea cadamba*) is said to put forth its fragrant buds at the roaring of thunderclouds.

1.4.31 The 'libertine' is the *pithamarda*, who appears in Indian drama as the hero's sidekick. The collapsible chair is a kind of shooting-stick, a portable seat.

1.4.32 The 'pander' is the *vita*, the usual messenger, a well-educated but parasitic courtier. In his commentary on 6.1.24, Y says that the *vita* is a man worn out by his former life as a man-about-town. *Vita* may also sometimes be better translated as 'voluptuary'.

1.4.33 The 'clown' is the *vidushaka*, a kind of jester in the drama, usually a Brahmin who teases the king.

1.4.34 These terms are satirically borrowed from the political players in the *Arthashastra*, as is Y's commentary on the next passage, in which he glosses the women's sophistication in the arts (presumably of love, not the fine arts) by punning on the words for a bawd (*kuttani*, literally 'crusher') and for crushing an enemy army (*kutt*).

1.4.35 The beggar women (*bhiksuki*) may be Buddhist nuns. Shaved heads are the sign of a particular kind of beggar, who, like the beggar women listed first, may belong to a religious order, particularly a renunciant order. Female renunciants, being cut off from normal social rules, have, in Sanskrit literature, a freedom denied to any other women except courtesans. But see note to 1.5.23.

1.4.37 This may also be translated, 'The man who speaks in society neither too elegantly nor too colloquially'.

1.5.2 The passage may also mean that pleasure under these circumstances is a means of getting illegitimate sons, a bad reputation, and social ostracism. Note the switch from the singular in the first passage, about a permitted woman, to the plural in the second passage, about forbidden women. The 'second-hand' woman is discussed at 4.2.31–44, and the wife unlucky in love at 4.2.45–54. Y here is quoting Manu 3.13.

1.5.3 'Women who may be lovers' are the *nayikas*. When they are the subjects of verbs, we generally translate *nayaka* and *nayika* as 'the man' and 'the woman', the male and female protagonists, designating a man or woman who may be a sexual partner. These terms should not be confused with 'a man', translating either the term *purusha*, a male, or the assumed male subject of most verbs with unstated subjects; and 'a woman', translating the term *stri* or one of its synonyms (such as *nari* or *yoshit*). In some contexts, *nayaka* or *nayika* is best translated as 'lover'. Where the context does not make clear, in English, the gender of the lover (which is unambiguously indicated by the ending of the Sanskrit word), we specify men or women. *Gamya*, the sexually accessible man or woman, may also be translated as 'lover' (also of both genders), but sometimes as 'eligible'; it means both permitted and available.

[Y] 1.5.11 Manu (8.350) says it is no violation of *dharma* to kill a man who has raised a weapon to kill you.

[Y] 1.5.12 Y here paraphrases Manu 8.389 and 10.99.

1.5.20 The verb *pra-kr*, which we have translated as 'seduce', more literally reproduces the English slang usage of 'make'.

1.5.23 The 'wandering ascetic' (*pravrajita*) is a woman who wanders about, presumably on a religious quest. It is a stunning indication of V's attitude to religious renunciation that he even considers here, without either approval or censure, a renunciant woman as a potential sexual partner. Yet at 1.5.29 he disqualifies wandering ascetic women as sexual partners.

1.5.26 'These women' are those mentioned in 1.5.22–5.

1.5.27 V simply gives this opinion without commenting on it as he comments on all the others; he appends it after his own statement of judgement. Here, as elsewhere, he refuses to commit himself to any absolute moral view of the third nature. V's attitude to the third nature is discussed in the Introduction.

[Y] 1.5.28 The context suggests, against Y, that 'both' may refer to both the open and the concealed lover.

[Y] 1.5.29 Manu 11.59. Defiling the guru's bed is the paradigmatic sin in ancient Hinduism, a crime regarded as a form of incest.

[Y] 1.5.30 Draupadi, the heroine of the Sanskrit epic the *Mahabharata*, had five husbands, the five sons of Pandu, under circumstances extenuated in various ways by various texts (both in the original Sanskrit version and in various retellings in Sanskrit and in vernacular languages) but never sufficiently to protect her from frequent slurs against her chastity.

1.5.34 It is important for V to define the boundaries of 'friend' in terms of both of the goals of this chapter: to make sure, first, that the lover does not sleep with the wife of his friend and, second, that he may use the friend as a messenger. The friends are just the sorts of people who appear on Manu's list of people to avoid at all costs.

1.5.37 Lee Siegel's inspired translation of these two final lines is: 'This man, if knowing when and where to make his passes, | Will surely captivate even the most obdurate of lasses' (Siegel, *Love in a Dead Language*, 74).

BOOK TWO · SEX

[Y] 2.1.1 The verse that Y cites is probably using the measurement of 'fingers', approximately ¾ in. each. The lengths therefore would be 4½, 6¾, and 9 in. Burton, in the *Anangaranga*, estimates lengths of 3, 4½, and 6 in., the latter 'of African or Negro dimensions'.

2.1.3 The couplings with the man larger than the woman are ideally better, though physically more difficult. The social category of hypergamy (in which the woman marries a man—a bridegroom, *gamos*—above—*hyper*—her) is what the Hindus call *anuloma* ('with the hair', or, as we would say, 'with the grain'), while hypogamy (in which the man is lower than she is) is called *pratiloma* or *viloma* ('against the hair', 'against the grain'). These two categories, and the favouring of hypergamy over hypogamy, may well have been derived from the more basic cultural assumption expressed in the animal metaphors: in terms of size, all of the couplings are 'against the grain', because the biggest man (the stallion) is hardly bigger than the smallest woman (doe), and grotesquely smaller than the largest woman (the elephant cow). The mare is regarded as sexually enormous, bigger than the bull, in Hindu mythology. Here Y uses the terms *anuloma* and *pratiloma* in another sense, meaning 'easily' or 'the hard way': the couplings with the man larger than the woman, though better (and hence *anuloma* in the sense of social value) are more difficult (and hence *pratiloma* in the sense of practicality). For the mare, see O'Flaherty, *Women, Androgynes*.

2.1.4 There are two different, conflicting agendas embedded in this passage: 'equal is best', but in fact the man has to be bigger.

2.1.10–30 These twenty passages follow the structure of a formal argument like that of 1.2.16; but this one is more complex. Auddalaki states his view (10–12) and imagines an objection (13–14*a*), to which he replies (14*b*); then another objection is stated (15) and answered (16–17). The followers of Babhravya then state their views (18); an objection is raised (19–20) and answered (21–2). V then states his views (23–6), imagines an objection (27*a*), and deflects it (27*b*); he imagines another objection (28) and answers it (29*a*); and he imagines a final objection (29*b*) and answers it (29*c*–30). The objections to Auddalaki and Babhravya are presumably V's; the objections to V's views may be those of the scholars that he cites or just the positions of straw men. In order to distinguish the views of the two scholars with whom V argues (Auddalaki or the Babhravyas) from those of their opponent (V), we have placed quotation marks around the views of those scholars, but not around V's objections to their views. By contrast, we have placed quotation marks around the objections to V's views, but not around his views. That is: V's opinions are never in quotation marks.

[Y] 2.1.11 The idea that worms inhabit women's sexual organs is also reflected in the belief held by Jains in ancient India, that the insects inside a woman are killed by the friction of intercourse, making every sexual act a mass murder.

2.1.12 The word *rasa*, which we have glossed as 'feeling', following Y, also means 'fluid'. The first meaning seems more relevant here because Auddalaki assumes that women do not emit any fluid at all, and in any case he has not mentioned semen or any fluid of the man from which the woman's could be said to differ. But the passage might nevertheless mean that the woman emits a different fluid.

[Y] 2.1.15 Y puns on the verb *snih* which means both 'to become oily or wet' and 'to be affectionate'.

[Y] 2.1.18 Y cites Charaka and Sushruta, authors of the most famous of the medical texts, which include a large section on embryology. Both of them assume that a woman has seed, as does Y (at 6.1.17). Manu, too, states (at 3.49) that a male child is born when the man's semen is greater, and a female child when the woman's semen is greater. Some Indian texts also assume that the woman must have an orgasm in order to conceive. Yet other embryologies assume that the woman's menstrual blood, rather than her semen, combines with the man's semen to form the embryo; this model gives women a much smaller role in the child, since it also assumed that semen was a much refined and concentrated form of blood. The story of the two women who make love and produce a boneless child is well known: A king died without an heir, and one of his two wives ate a special bowl of rice consecrated to make her pregnant, and the other 'acted the part of a man' with her, and she became pregnant; but the child had no bones, because that is the father's contribution to the embryo. The child lacked bones because the man contributes, from his semen, the white and hard parts of the embryo, bones and sinews, while the woman contributes, from her blood, the red and the soft parts, blood and flesh. There is also an example of the opposite case, in which the child (Shiva's son Bhringin) is cursed to be without flesh because he denies his mother. (These two embryologies correspond roughly to the European systems that follow Galen—in which the woman has seed like the man—and those that follow Aristotle—in which the man's semen alone forms the child, and a chicken is just an egg's way of making another egg.) Both of these models were available simultaneously at the time of the *Kamasutra*'s composition. The decision about gender, about whether women are or are not equal, may predetermine the choice of embryological mode, with two seeds or one.

Babhravya's assumption (in contrast with Auddalaki's) is that a woman, like a man, emits semen during orgasm; and that her seed, like his, is necessary for conception. V does not comment on this assumption but seems to share Babhravya's belief that women do have orgasms and not to share his belief that they have them continually. In focusing upon the issue of women's pleasure, and not only upon their ability to conceive, V differs dramatically from the medical and legal texts, all of which deal obsessively with the issue of conception. For the story of the two queens, in the *Padma Purana*, see O'Flaherty, *Textual Sources*; for the tale of Bhringin, see O'Flaherty, *Siva*; for menstrual blood and semen, see O'Flaherty, *Women, Androgynes*.

2.1.21 (and 2.1.35). There is an ambiguity here: whose fluids are used up, his or hers? The phrase could refer to the semen of either the man or the woman, or to the man's semen and the woman's lubricating juices, or to the man's semen and the woman's menstrual blood, or to both components of any of these options. The 'wish to stop' is similarly gender-neutral. Y's comment in 2.1.35 indicates his belief that both the man and the woman might wish to stop, but V in 2.1.36 tells us that the man runs out of fluid first, from which we might conclude that he is the one intended here too.

[Y] 2.1.24 The example chosen seemingly at random, the mating of a man and a mare, is actually attested in a number of Hindu myths. See O'Flaherty, *Women, Androgynes*.

2.1.27 'Species' (or 'form', *akriti*) is replaced, in 2.1.30, by 'genus', *jati*, a word, cognate with 'genus', that also, significantly, means 'caste', in contrast with 'class' (*varna*, as in 1.2.25 and 1.5.1).

[Y] 2.1.28 Devadatta is the ancient Sanskrit equivalent of John Doe, and the sentence about the rice is the standard sample sentence in Sanskrit, as 'See Dick and Jane run' used to be in English. Y uses grammatical terms such as noun and verb, subject and object, and glosses a grammatical sentence as an example, quoting the great Sanskrit grammarian Panini. In this gloss, the sexual act is a sentence in which the man is the subject, the object is sexual pleasure (for both of them), and the woman is the locative case. The double meaning is enhanced by the fact that 'object' and 'meaning' are the same word in Sanskrit—*artha*.

2.1.29 Wood apples, like croquet balls or lawn bowls, are used in a game in which they hit one another.

2.1.30 The conclusion that the woman must have her orgasm *first* results from an argument that Y, rather than V, spells out: since a woman can have an orgasm she should have an orgasm (or else she will not conceive a child, according to 2.1.18), and a man cannot satisfy a woman after he has had his orgasm. But cf. 2.1.36, which remarks without comment on the fact that men run out of fluids before women do—yet another submerged assumption that Y spells out: women are not easy to satisfy.

The Greek philosopher Hippocrates believed that women ejaculated, but in the modern era female ejaculation was first described by the German gynecologist Ernst Graefenberg. It occurs as a result of the stimulation of the 'Graefenberg Zone', popularly termed the G-spot. The G-spot is a particularly sensitive area within the vagina, about halfway between the pubic bone and the cervix adjacent to the rear of the urethra. It is constituted out of an erectile tissue and leads to a discharge of a clear, transparent liquid from the urethra during orgasm. This female ejaculation—distinct from the vaginal secretions—and the G-spot, controversial till the 1980s, are now accepted as facts in medical and reference literature. Renate Syed has persuasively demonstrated that besides Yashodhara's *Jayamangala*, other Indian erotic texts, such as the *Panchasayaka* (11th century), *Ratira-hasya* (13th century), and *Anangaranga* (16th century), describe both the G-spot and female ejaculation in convincing detail. Outside the scientific literature, female ejaculation is already mentioned in a seventh-century verse collection, the *Amarushataka*. See Ernst Graefenberg, 'The role of the urethra in female orgasm' (*International Journal of Sexology*, 3 (1950), 145–8).

2.1.32 *Rati*, *rata*, and *surata* are all derived from the same word, *rata*, the past passive participle from the verb *ram*, meaning, among other things, to enjoy sexual intercourse. The first set of words describes sexual feelings, the second set, sexual actions.

2.1.35 Y works out the various permutations for men and women of all twenty-seven types, but V realizes that the problem is general: at first, the man has fierce sexual energy and ejaculates quickly, while the woman at that time is slow to rouse and takes a long time to finish, not a satisfactory combination. After that, the man is slower to rouse and takes a long time to finish, while the woman is quick to rouse and does not last long, not so bad as the first coupling but not ideal either.

[Y] 2.1.36 So too the serial female-to-male bisexual Chudala says, when she is a woman, that a woman has eight times as much pleasure (*kama*) as a man, which could also be translated as eight times as much desire; but Bhangash-vana, the Indian Teiresias (male-to-female), just said women had more desire than men. Some Greek texts maintain that Teiresias, too, said that women have not just more pleasure, but *nine times* as much pleasure as men—thereby slightly upping the ante in comparison with the Hindu story of Chudala. For Chudala, see O'Flaherty, *Dreams, Illusion*. For Teiresias, see Apollodorus 3.6.7; Doniger, *Splitting the Difference*.

2.1.38 Cf. 1.1.24, where V speaks in more positive terms of wise people who want to have things spelt out in detail.

2.1.41 The implication is that, since these activities do not involve the sexual act itself, they generate love only through the erotic arousal of the imagination (*abhimana*), presumably the imagination of the sexual act. See note to 1.2.12.

2.1.43 When there is a comparison between a past and a present love, the present lover is loved for his resemblance to the past lover, in a kind of transposed love or *idée fixe*, as in 2.10.21.

2.2.1 In this passage and in 2.2.3, V uses the word 'part' (*anga*, literally 'limb'), perhaps referring to the original portions of the Ur-*Kamasutra* (which he calls 'parts' or 'limbs' in 1.1.14), but in fact designating the 'part' (of the total text) that we have called 'Book Two' (the second *adhikarana*).

2.2.2 V himself states at 1.1.23 that his text has sixty-four sections.

2.2.3 The *Rig Veda* is sometimes called (according to Monier-Williams's Sanskrit dictionary) 'the sixty-four', because there are sixty-four sections in it (eight parts, each actually called an *ashthaka*, 'eight'), or (according to Y) 'the ten', because there are ten 'circles', a separate enumeration, overlapping with that of the eight eights. The argument seems to be that the *Kamasutra* as a whole is named 'the sixty-four' because (1) it has sixty-four sections and (2) the term 'sixty-four' brings the text honour through the connection with the *Rig Veda*, for several reasons: (*a*) because both texts are called 'the sixty-four' and (*b*) because both one of the authors of the *Rig Veda* and one of the authors of the *Kamasutra* have names that connect them with Panchala, which is a name both of a place and of a family from that place. But Book Two alone is also named 'the sixty-four' because (1) that book is about the sixty-four sexual arts (1.3.16) and (2) like the *Rig Veda*, which is also called 'the sixty-four', it is divided into ten parts. In fact, though V does indeed count ten chapters in Book Two (at 1.1.17), they are not precisely the ten that Y cites here (for he omits the introductory and final chapters and compensates by numbering separately each of the two separate sections in chapters seven and eight). Finally, in 2.2.5 V dismisses all the contradictory numbers as mere manners of speaking. At 1.3.16, after listing the sixty-four fine arts (singing, etc.), V remarks that 'the sixty-four different techniques (*prayogas*) that come from Babhravya of Panchala are different'.

2.2.18 'Rice and sesame' has something of the meaning of our 'peas and carrots' or 'rizzy pizzy': a close mixture from which it is almost impossible to separate the component parts.

2.3.32 An inspired, if rather loose, translation of this verse by Lee Siegel ends: 'For love asks an eye for an eye, a tooth for a tooth; | while love gives a truth for a lie, a lie for a truth' (Siegel, *Love in a Dead Language*, 112).

2.4.7 V does not seem to care very much about the right or left hand; at 2.2.18, he says that the man and woman may lie on either side, freeing either hand, but here and at 2.4.7, 2.10.2, and 2.10.7 he specifies the left hand or arm. According to Hindu tradition, people use the left hand to cleanse themselves after emptying bladder or bowels, and their right hand to eat; sex would come in the former category, and require the left hand. Yet V's considerations here seem to be purely practical: nails on the right hand might become broken in the course of use, and hence unsuitable for the subtleties of scratching. See also the note on 2.6.18.

2.5.4 The actual order of the bites as they are described differs somewhat from the list of bites in this introductory passage.

2.5.27 The country where women rule is a mythical land in the far North; there have never been matriarchal dynasties in Indian history, though there are still matrilineal societies, especially in Northeast India and South India.

2.6.11 What we have called 'Junoesque' is literally 'of Indrani'. Indrani is the wife of Indra, the king of the gods (see 1.2.29 and 35), and resembles Juno, the wife of Jupiter, king of the Roman gods (or Hera, wife of the Greek Zeus), in many ways, including her own enormous sexual appetite and her jealousy about her husband's notorious adulteries.

[Y] 2.6.17 Y notes that the second variant of this position, the equivalent of our 'missionary position', is so easy, and presumably so common, that it needs no explanation.

2.6.18 According to this passage, the man, lying on his left side, has his right hand free. To avoid the implication that the man uses his right hand for sex (see note on 2.4.7), Y argues that V is talking about *sleeping*, not about *sex*, and that for sex the left hand is free to function, while the right is free only during sleep.

2.6.21 Hindu mythology uses the mare as the symbol of the hyper-sexualized woman. This position is called Carezza or Pompoir in Europe.

2.6.33 This is also known as the 'windmill'.

2.6.35 Manu forbids a man to emit his semen in water, which the commentator takes to mean 'when having intercourse with a woman in water' (11.174). See also 2.6.44.

2.6.48 The men are said to do this in the king's harem; see Section 38.

2.7.6 We have tried to find English equivalents for various Sanskrit terms for what are, after all, inarticulate sounds. The word we have translated as 'moaning' is literally 'making the sound "Seet!"', which means suddenly drawing in the breath between the teeth in an instinctive reaction to pain or intense pleasure. 'Screaming' (*viruta*) is the generic term, which includes the following: 'Whimpering' is making the sound 'hnnn', and 'groaning' is a sound like thunder. 'Babbling' (*kujita*) and 'crying' (*rudita*) are known from other contexts. 'Panting' is making the sound 'Soot!', 'shrieking' is making the sound 'Doot!', and sobbing, the sound 'Phoot!'

2.7.12 The climax in question here is presumably hers, though neither V nor Y says so specifically. This same ambiguity applies to this phrase in 2.7.20.

2.7.20 It is not clear whether the phrases 'in the throes of passion,' 'as passion nears its end', and 'until the climax' refer to him or to her, but their place-ment makes it more likely that he is intended, and this is what Y assumes. The passage simultaneously suggests that he is getting out of control and hitting her too hard and that she enjoys the slaps and is crying out in ecstasy. This sort of ambiguity is particularly disturbing to a contemporary reader, as it seems to lodge in the very heart of the philosophy of rape.

2.7.22 'Natural talent' (or 'glory' or 'vital power' [*tejas*]) is also, significantly, the word for semen.

2.7.24 The other forms of slapping were discussed at 2.7.2.

2.7.28–30 The kings who commit these excesses are all from South India, where V generally locates sexual excess. In contrast with such figures as Shakuntala and Ahalya, these kings are not well known to Sanskrit mythology.

2.8.6 The 'sexual strokes' (*upasriptani*, from the verb *upa-srip*, *srip* being related to the word for serpent in Sanskrit and in English), are, in particular, the snake-like movements that a man makes with his penis when he is inside the woman; often this term is supplemented by the word for 'man' (*puru-sha*), as in, 'a man's sexual strokes'. Another term for the woman 'playing the man's part' is the 'inverse' position (*viparita*), where the woman acts the man's part and the man acts the woman's part, or as we would say, the woman is on top. Significantly, V resists this value judgement and never uses this term. Yashodhara's commentary on this passage implies that the woman does not resume her 'natural talent' until the sexual act is over.

2.8.7 From the Sanskrit text, we might now expect a description of women doing things to men; but in fact we encounter a passage (2.8.8–31) where the man is the active party. The express subject of 2.8.8 is 'man' (*purusha*), and the express object is 'woman' (*yoshit*); there is no ambiguity at all in the text here. To account for this transition between subjects, Y makes explicit his interpretation of the connection between the two subjects—women acting like men and men acting like men—and points out that the author is now telling us what men do to women. At the end of this passage, at 2.8.32,

V reverts to the first sort of 'acting like a man', the reversed position with the woman on top.

2.8.16 This is what we would call the 'G' spot. Cf. note on 2.1.30 above.

2.8.30 See 2.6.16.

2.8.34 See 2.6.33.

2.8.36 See 2.8.22.

[Y] 2.8.41 The belief that a child with ambiguous sexual characteristics will result from incorrect forms of sexual union is a much-discussed topic in ancient Indian medical textbooks. See the Introduction.

2.9.3 V uses the pronoun 'she' for the third nature, the man who plays the sexual role of a woman. What we have translated as 'oral sex' literally means 'upper sex', a term that, like Freud's 'upward displacement', implies that the bottom line is the genitals.

[Y] 2.9.27 The passage that Y cites from Vasishtha is at 12.23, where the ancestors of the man who copulates in the mouth of his wife do not starve for fifteen years but, rather, are forced to eat nothing but his semen for a month; he adds that all unusual sexual practices are against the law. Cf. also Manu's injunction (at 11.174) against emitting semen 'in something other than a vagina'.

2.9.31 The word here translated as 'men of the city' is *nagaraka*, elsewhere translated as 'men-about-town', but in the present context it probably has a more specifically geographical meaning. Y says the city is Pataliputra, and it may well be.

2.9.33 The passage appears in this form, more or less, in the *Baudhayana Dharmasutra* (1.5.9). The verse also appears in Manu (5.130), where it is modified to desexualize it somewhat:

> A woman's mouth is always unpolluted,
> as is a bird that knocks down a fruit;
> a calf is unpolluted while the milk is flowing,
> and a dog is unpolluted when it catches a wild animal.

Manu has subtracted from the line about a woman's mouth the phrase, 'in the ecstasy of sex'. Cf. also *Baudhayana Dharmasutra* 1.5.49. The underlying assumption is that, normally, a dog, a calf's mouth, a bird's beak, and a woman's mouth would pollute anything they touched; but when they are needed, the pollution rules are nullified.

2.9.38 The crow is a symbol of doubling-up, in part because of the Indian folk belief that the crow has just one eye, which he switches to whatever side of his head you happen to be looking at.

[Y] 2.10.12 The incarnate god Krishna danced in a circle with the cow-herd women, and by his magic powers created doubles of himself so that each woman thought she was dancing with him and making love with him.

2.10.22 Monier-Williams's dictionary (citing older Sanskrit dictionaries) glosses 'coarse servant' (*pota*) as a female servant or a woman with masculine features such as a beard; Y says it is a 'non-male' (the term he uses as a synonym for someone of the third nature) who swings both ways. The passage itself makes no such allusions but merely designates unskilled female servants, presumably of unremarkable sexuality.

2.10.27 The lover's mistake in calling the woman with whom he is actively making love by the name of another woman, termed 'stumbling on the name' (*gotraskhalana*), is a classic trigger for lovers' quarrels. See Doniger, *The Bedtrick*.

[Y] 2.10.37 Y spells out what remains in V merely an implicit etymology, based on the equation of *puja* (which means to 'respect' or 'revere' or 'honour' or, stretching it a bit, 'delight in') with *nandana* ('delight').

[Y] 2.10.39 Y here is anxious to include all four kinds of eligible women in this list, and so argues that the fourth, the second-hand woman, is implied within the third, other men's wives.

BOOK THREE · VIRGINS

3.1.1 At 1.5.1, V gives a somewhat different set of criteria for the qualities of the ideal wife.

3.1.4 'Both sides' may refer to both parents, probably of the man (whose parents are mentioned earlier in this same passage) but also possibly of the girl; but it might simply refer to the man and the girl, as V specifies at 1.5.35.

3.1.6 Impersonating a fortune-teller is a minor blasphemy, but not as bad as the *Arthashastra*'s advice to the king, to have spies dress up as gods and praise the king.

3.1.8 It was a custom to take note of the first words overheard outside the family quarters, and regard them as an omen.

3.1.11 'Tawny' is an educated guess at the hapax word *ghona*, which Shastri translates as 'reddish-blond'. 'Promiscuous' (*samkariki*) is glossed by Monier-Williams, from lexicons, as, 'a girl said to be unfit for marriage (as having applied fire to her father's or other person's house)'; Upadhyaya makes this 'a girl who has lit her father's funeral pyre'. Y suggests that it means 'defiled by another man', and Shastri glosses it as 'promiscuous'. We relate the word to *samkaryam*, a promiscuous mixture. For *phalini*, literally, 'bearing fruit', which we have translated as 'pregnant', Monier-Williams cites the definition by Sushruta ('a girl whose vagina has been injured by violent intercourse'), while Y says, 'mute, excluded from communication'. Manu gives rather different criteria (3.8 and .10): 'A man should not marry a girl who is a redhead or has an extra limb or is sickly or has no body hair or too much body hair or talks too much or is sallow . . . He should marry a woman who does not lack any part of her body and who has a pleasant name, who walks like a goose or an elephant, whose body hair and hair on the head is fine, whose teeth are not big, and who has delicate limbs.'

3.1.12 Cf. Manu (3.9): 'A man should not marry a girl who is named after a constellation, a tree, or a river, or who has a low caste name, or is named after a mountain, a bird, a snake, or has a menial or frightening name.'

3.1.19 Manu (3.27–30) offers more details: 'It is said to be the law of Brahma when a man dresses his daughter and adorns her and he himself gives her as a gift to a man he has summoned, one who knows the revealed canon and is of good character. They call it the law of the gods when a man adorns his daughter and, in the course of a sacrifice, gives her as a gift to the officiating priest who is properly performing the ritual. It is called the Sages' law when he gives away his daughter by the rules, after receiving from the bridegroom a cow and a bull, or two cows and bulls, in accordance with the law. The tradition calls it the rule of the Lord of Creatures when a man gives away his daughter after adorning her and saying, "May the two of you together fulfil your *dharma*."' V lists only four official weddings, where Manu lists eight, and although V deals below (3.5.12–30) with the other four kinds of wedding that Manu lists (at 3.31–4), he never names them and seems to regard them all as variations on the form that dominates the *Kamasutra*, the love-match or Gandharva wedding.

3.1.20 'Completing verses' is one of the sixty-four arts listed in 1.3.15.

3.1.21 The 'upward alliance', in which the woman is higher than the man, goes against the grain; cf. 2.1.4 and the note.

3.2.3 There may be a double meaning in the man's silence, for 'conversation' is often a euphemism for sex in India. Referring to a man's desire for sex, women in the Hindi heartland often say, 'Admi bolna chahta hai' ('A man wants to speak'). See Sudhir Kakar, *Intimate Relations*.

3.2.6 'Gentle persuasion', *saman*, is also the term for negotiating a treaty with an enemy (especially when one does not have the force to win by an outright attack).

3.2.22 The 'gooseflesh' scratch is described at 2.4.12.

3.2.31 What we have translated as 'rub her the right way' is more precisely 'with the hair' or 'with the grain'. See the note to 2.1.3.

3.2.33 The beast (*pashu*) is either any animal, in contrast with a human, or more particularly a domesticated or farm animal, in contrast with a wild animal, or most particularly, an animal used for sacrifice (bull, horse, sheep, or goat) in contrast with an unconsecrated animal.

3.2.35 We have translated *vidvishta* as 'hated', presumably by the man (taking the last syllable as a passive suffix), but it might also be translated as 'full of hate', presumably for him (taking the last syllable as an agent-suffix or a periphrastic future). This is a significant ambiguity, but the sense of 'hated' is perhaps the more commonsense reading and recurs with this meaning, unambiguously, in 3.5.6; because he hates her, he refuses to sleep with her, and so she finds another man. A further ambiguity is raised by the possibility that, if she is 'full of hate', that hatred might be directed either at him or at pleasure in love-making; cf. 3.2.6, where she is said to hate sex itself if mistreated at the beginning of her experience. Y takes it to mean that she hates him, precisely because he has not given her pleasure, though this might just as likely drive her from sex altogether as into the arms of another man.

3.3.7–8 Games for grown-ups are described at 1.4.28. The game of the fist apparently consists in guessing what is held in the fist; 'eyes shut tight' is like our 'hide-and-seek'; and the game of six pebbles is very much like the game of jacks that American girls used to play.

3.3.10 The foster-sister, more precisely the nurse's child, is defined among the friends, at 1.5.32.

3.3.16 The word we have translated as 'little penis' (*medhraka*) also means 'little ram', which is the sense in which previous translators, and Y, have taken it, in conjunction with the next phrase, 'male and female' (ignoring the 'and', so that they render it, 'two sheep, male and female, joined together'). This overlooks the fact that sheep are listed separately in the very next item. But could one give a young girl a carving of entwined penises? Perhaps. Images of the *lingam*, the erect penis of the god Shiva, have been, for centuries, everyday items in any Hindu household; the yab-yum image of god and goddess in intercourse is widespread in Tibetan and Tibetan-influenced cultures; and right here in the *Kamasutra*, at 3.4.4, the man is said to give a virgin an image of a man and woman coupling, cut out of a leaf (though Y quickly bowdlerizes this as a couple of *geese*).

[Y] 3.3.20 Spring and summer in North India are too hot for outdoor sports (and, perhaps, for indoor sports). In traditional poetry, the rainy season (when travellers have to return home and/or remain at home), autumn, winter, and spring are the erotic seasons.

3.3.21 The sixty-four techniques, in contrast with the fine arts mentioned in the previous passage, are the sexual arts described in Book Two.

3.3.32 According to Padmashri, as quoted by Shastri on 2.2.31, a young girl (*bala*) is under sixteen years old; the woman in the prime of her youth (*yauvane sthita*) is between sixteen and thirty; and the mature woman is between thirty and fifty. The arts here are probably, as Y suggests, the fine arts, mentioned in 3.3.20, but they may be the arts of love, mentioned in 3.3.21. Shastri says that these are the sixty-four arts of the science of *kama*, surely the erotic techniques.

3.4.3 The 'touching' embrace is described at 2.2.8.

3.4.7 The game of 'new leaves' is among the group games mentioned at 1.4.28.

3.4.34 These gestures and signals (usually given by facial expressions, especially the eyes) are sometimes said to be involuntary, sometimes intentional. In the *Kamasutra*, they are usually, but not always, intentional.

3.4.36 Cf. the rather different qualifications for a man in this situation mentioned in 3.3.1.

3.4.40 Apparently she is treating him as if he were a young girl, a role reversal akin to that of the woman playing the man's part (in 2.8).

3.4.44 Who is touching whose hidden place(s)? The Sanskrit leaves it ambiguous, since the compound can allow for either an objective or a subjective relationship, and for either a singular or plural. (Y glosses 'hidden place' in the singular here but in the plural at 6.2.17.) Y says that she touches him. The text says that he merely wants her to understand his arousal, not necessarily to bring it about (as Y glosses it), though this purpose, too, might be served by having her touch him. On the other hand, the euphemism of 'hidden place', which also means 'a cave', in the singular sometimes designates the female rather than the male organ. Both his hidden place(s) and hers may well be understood in the context of the text, and perhaps V meant to imply that any of these possibilities would be difficult for her.

3.5.1 The verb here translated as 'insinuates himself into intimacy' is precisely the same (*upasrip*) as the verb denoting a man's sexual strokes inside a woman. See 2.8.6 and the note.

3.5.5 This story did not turn out so well as V implies; Shakuntala suffers greatly in the version of her story told in the *Mahabharata* and less, but still significantly, in the version told by Kalidasa a few centuries later.

3.5.13 Whose mother and father does he inform? The passage does not say, but we have specified hers because (1) the man tells his own people two passages later, so that here he is probably telling hers; and (2) the concern, throughout this section, is with her parents, never with his. Shastri says the statement refers to both his parents and hers, but the text clearly specifies one mother and one father.

3.5.18 The love-match wedding is called a Gandharva wedding, because it is consummated by a sexual act witnessed by no one but Gandharvas, demigods concerned with fertility (and horses; their name is cognate with 'centaurs'). V goes on (at 3.5.19–22) to describe variants of the Gandharva wedding. This is how Manu describes it (3.32): 'In the wedding in the manner of the Gandharvas, the girl and her lover join with one another in sexual union because they want to, out of desire.'

[Y] 3.5.19 Y assumes that the go-between's intimacy is with the man, but it might also be with the girl.

3.5.23 This corresponds only roughly to what Manu describes as the wedding in the manner of the Demons (*asuras*) (3.31): 'In a wedding in the manner of the Demons, a man takes the girl because he wants her himself, when he has given as much wealth as he can to her relatives and to the girl herself.' But Y (at 3.5.28) seems to assume that V has described the wedding of Demons after the Gandharva wedding (3.5.18–22) and before the Ghouls (3.5.25–60), which narrows it down to this passage.

3.5.25–6 These two passages regard as two separate types of weddings two of the three methods appropriate to the wedding in the manner of the Ghouls (*pishacas*), which Manu describes like this (3.34): 'In the lowest and most evil of marriages, known as that of the Ghouls, a man secretly has sex with a girl who is asleep, drunk, or out of her mind.'

3.5.27 This is the wedding of the Ogres (*rakshasas*) (Manu 3.33): 'In the manner of the Ogres, a man forcibly carries off a girl out of her house, screaming and weeping, after he has killed, wounded, and broken.' V uses the word *yoga* here in the sense of a trick or an underhanded device.

3.5.28 V lists them in this descending order: Brahma (3.1.19), Gandharva (3.5.18), Demons (3.5.23), Ghouls (3.5.25–6), and Ogres (3.5.27). He differs here from the rankings according to Manu, who, after the Brahma wedding, regards the wedding of Demons as superior to that of the Gandharvas, and that of the Ogres, and the Ghouls as worst of all. It is natural for V to have a higher opinion of the Gandharva wedding than Manu has.

BOOK FOUR · WIVES

4.1.4 At 1.1.12, V names Gonardiya as the author of the section of the primal *Kamasutra* that deals with wives.

[Y] 4.1.14 'Wrongly' may mean that he pays too little, or pays for shoddy merchandise, or buys from disreputable merchants. Y seems to take it in the second sense.

4.1.19 The word we have translated as 'infidelities' can also mean, more rarely, 'misdeeds' of a more general nature, but the counter-measure rejected in 4.1.20 strongly suggests that it means 'infidelities' here.

4.1.20 Love-sorcery worked with roots is black magic, making use of roots like mandrake, to get a lover back or to destroy an erotic rival. It is alluded to in the *Rig Veda* and described at some length in the *Atharva Veda* and in Book Seven of the *Kamasutra*.

4.2.1 Manu offers different justifications for supplanting a wife (9.80–1): 'A wife who drinks wine, behaves dishonestly, or is rebellious, ill, violent, or wasteful of money may be supplanted at any time. A barren wife may be superseded in the eighth year; one whose children have died, in the tenth; one who bears [only] daughters, in the eleventh; but one who says unpleasant things (may be superseded) immediately.' Manu focuses on rules for the inheritance of the sons of the various wives, distinguishing the wives by their seniority and their class (which Vatsyayana, as usual, does not mention) rather than by their sexual past, as V does.

4.2.7 The passage seems to imply that the senior wife treats the co-wife's children just as she treats her own, but Y assumes that the senior wife has no children, in which case the passage would mean that she treats them just as she treats other children, perhaps the children of the other wives.

4.2.31 We have translated *punarbhu* (literally, 'coming into existence again') as 'second-hand', following the inspiration of Laura Desmond (who points out that it has the same connotation of 'damaged goods' in both English and Sanskrit). Yashodhara says that these women, who have been owned by men before, are widows; Monier-Williams says they were widowed as virgins; and Shastri (citing the lawbook of Yajnavalkya and the commentary of Mitakshara) says that they are not widows at all, but women who lost their maidenheads before marriage or had a relationship with another man after marriage. The fact that widows are listed separately, in 1.5.22, suggests that the women in this passage are not widows. Manu (9.175–6) groups together, as second-hand women (*punarbhu*), a woman who remarries after her husband has deserted her, or a widow, or a woman who still has her maidenhead intact (when she remarries), or who returns to a man she had left. In the *Kamasutra*, the term seems to mean simply that the woman has previously been with a man, not necessarily her husband. The woman with whom she is contrasted is the *ananyapurva*, the woman who has not been with another man before—the permitted woman (1.5.1); this term covers not just a virgin but a married woman who remains faithful to her husband. The variation in interpretation doubtless reflects the wide swings of the law concerning the rights of women, and of widows, to remarry, in different times and places. This passage invokes the word 'again' [*punar*] to explain the name of the second-hand woman [*punarbhu*]; the Babhravyas make yet another point about 'again' in the next passage.

4.2.34 The implication is that she will not leave a well-endowed lover.

4.2.42 The arts here are presumably the fine arts, mentioned again in passage 45, in contrast with the arts of love mentioned in passage 44. Y says her knowledge is greater than that of the man, but it may be greater than that of the other women or simply greater than average.

4.2.45 The last half of this passage is doubly ambiguous. There are, first of all, two different readings in the Sanskrit text: Shastri has arts 'that give pleasure' (*prakamya*) while Goswami (whom we follow, along with Y) has arts 'that can be revealed' (*prakashya*). And the last sentence can mean either that the unlucky wife has no way of keeping secrets, since she must use what she knows to make alliances with the other wives, or that she has no erotic secrets and therefore has to get the other woman to tell her the tricks that she lacks, since, ironically, not knowing them has kept her out of her husband's bed, where she might have learned some. Shastri seems to take it in the first sense, of 'the arts that can be exhibited', because 'a demonstration of proficiency often ends misfortune.'

4.2.54 For the women lucky or unlucky in love (*subhaga* or *durbhaga*), see note to 1.3.22.

4.2.56 The chamberlain and bodyguard are called the Kanchukiya and Mahattarika.

4.2.57 The word used here for these leftovers is *nirmalyam*, literally 'leftover garlands', more precisely designating the leftovers from flower offerings to a god (or, by extension, to a king), returned to the worshippers (or subjects) as a kind of grace (hence the other term for them, *prasad*, literally, 'grace').

BOOK FIVE · OTHER MEN'S WIVES

5.1.30 Here both V and Y conflate size ('doe' vs. 'stallion') with sexual energy ('fierce' vs. 'dull').

5.1.31 Presumably the fine arts are intended here, but the arts of love are not out of the question. Y does not specify. The lifestyle of the man-about-town is described at 1.4.

5.1.42 Religion clearly is an afterthought, but even so this passage contradicts 5.1.10, which insists that women never think about religion at all. The phrase may be a common saying; at the end of the story of the clever and virtuous wife of Muladeva, the author remarks, 'So you see, your majesty, there really are in this world some women of good family who love their husbands; not all women misbehave always' (*Ocean of Story* 124 (18.5).131– 237).

[Y] 5.1.44 Y links each of these remedies with an abbreviated version of a problem stated above; he finds a place for all causes except for her fear that 'He will soon go away. There is no future in it; his mind is attached to someone else' (5.1.24). Is this because there is no remedy for this problem? Because the fear of the future is the one thing that you cannot talk someone out of? Is this a philosophical moment in the *Kamasutra* (or in the commentary)?

5.1.50 Vulnerable spots are literally chinks in the armour.

5.1.51 This passage, and its intersection with the next, is different in Goswami's edition, and Y does not recognize it at all.

5.1.52 Schmidt and Mylius follow Y in assuming a singular rather than plural form for 'who can be had merely by making advances', applying it only to the first woman on the list, rather than to all of them.

5.1.53 Manu says that it is no crime to commit adultery with the wife of an actor, 'for these men have their women embrace other men, concealing themselves while they have them do the act' (8.362).

5.1.55 The longing here is the desire of a woman for the man.

5.2.7 The friend of a man is always, unless indicated, a man, and of a woman, a woman, whom we have referred to as a girlfriend.

5.2.18 Perhaps he says 'How amazing!' in order to avoid saying 'You must be wrong.'

5.2.19 These methods are described in Book Three.

5.3.5 Burton calls this woman a trifler in love, Schmidt, a coquette. Cf. the teasing male wooer, at 5.1.28.

5.3.13 Y says she is just pretending to be asleep, but V elsewhere (3.5.26) acknowledges that a man may in fact rape a sleeping girl.

5.3.18 What we have translated as 'rub her the wrong way' is more precisely 'go against the hair', or 'go against the grain'. See the note to 2.1.4.

5.4.9 This is the very opposite of the opinion given as a 'common saying' at 5.2.3.

5.4.10–25 Throughout this section, the subject of each sentence is the messenger, and the other woman is the intended woman. Then, in 5.4.26–9, the woman is the subject, until the messenger is explicitly named as the subject again in 5.4.30.

[Y] 5.4.14 Y tells the same story of Ahalya in a negative mode at 1.2.36, and in much more detail, as a warning to a man about the trouble that desire can cause him. And the story of Shakuntala, which Y does not tell here at all, he tells in a curiously truncated version at 3.5.5. Both of these are, as V says, famous stories. Avimaraka is the hero of a play by Bhasa. The Shabaras are a wild, savage tribe of mountaineers.

[Y] 5.4.15 Here Y goes on to give definitions of both kinds of arts, fine arts and arts of love.

5.4.42 The absolute single-mindedness of the true lover has never been demonstrated more powerfully than here, where a fire, robbery or invasion does not deter him from trying to arrange an adulterous rendezvous.

5.4.54 The unfaithful lover who 'stumbles on the name', calling the woman he is in bed with by the name of another woman he is thinking of, is a set piece in Sanskrit erotic poetry and narrative. See Doniger, *The Bedtrick*.

5.4.58 The naïve wife is a stereotype, the wife who is so innocent of sexual technique, and perhaps has been so unresponsive to her husband's initial attempts to arouse her, that her husband has stopped sleeping with her. The woman who intends to sleep with this wife's husband helps the wife to 'send a message' to her husband, not in words but in her actions; the wife thinks that the message is that she herself desires him, but the husband knows that the actual message is that the other woman desires him. The title can be glossed either as 'the messenger of a foolish person' or as 'the foolish messenger'. Y's gloss explicitly makes the title fit the second description by making the wife herself the foolish messenger, even though this interpretation requires a sudden shift of subject at the end of this paragraph, and back again in the next, which is awkward, though not impossible. The wife is explicitly the messenger in the next passage, but she differs from the foolish (wife) messenger in that the husband manipulates the wife as messenger, whereas the other woman manipulates the foolish (wife) messenger.

5.4.64 This verse can be read in two ways. What it seems to say, literally, is that in order to make the intended woman hate her own husband, the messenger praises his sexual charms and makes her jealous by reminding her that many other women have enjoyed them. But Y reads an implicit shift from the husband, in the first quarter of the verse, to the would-be lover, in the rest of the verse, contrasting the husband's ugliness (alluded to in Y's commentary on the first passage that he quotes here, 5.4.3) with the lover's sexual charms. And Y therefore says that the 'other women' in the last line merely hear about the lover's sexual accomplishments, where we take the Sanskrit to imply that these women have themselves experienced the husband's sexual accomplishments.

5.5.2 The three worlds are sometimes said to be sky, air, and the earth, or heaven, earth, and hell. In either case, the phrase refers to all the living creatures in the universe. This is the only chapter that Vatsyayana *begins* with a verse, perhaps to emphasize his moral ambivalence about its contents.

5.5.8 The man in charge of threads superintended the women who had no families and therefore made their living by spinning and weaving.

5.5.27 The word for 'secret methods' is in the plural, not the dual, but Y wants to restrict the term to the last two rather extreme methods.

5.5.36 At 1.1.9 Y tells another myth about the origin of adultery. The story of Ahalya, as told in the *Ramayana*, also contains a statement that it was on this occasion that Indra, the king of the gods, invented adultery.

5.5.37 Surely significantly, the word here used for the king's pleasure (*rata*) in the welfare of his people is the word used elsewhere (as in 2.1.32) for the sexual act. The *Shatapatha Brahmana*, in the 8th century BCE, already tells a parable about the king violating the people sexually. See O'Flaherty, *Textual Sources*.

5.6.3 Schmidt notes that a manuscript of this text in the Indian Institute in Oxford reads 'distinct' rather than 'indistinct' sexual characteristics, and this is the reading that makes sense to us. Y, however, reads 'indistinct' and glosses that reading.

[Y] 5.6.5 Manu says this about wet-dreams (2.181): 'A twice-born chaste student of the Veda who has spilled his semen in his sleep, not out of lust, should bathe, worship the sun, and chant, three times, the Vedic verse that begins, "Let my sensual power return to me again".' As for sex 'in things other than the vagina, in things other than the human species', Manu says (11.174): 'If a man has shed his semen in non-human females, in a man, in a menstruating woman, in something other than a vagina, or in water, he should carry out the Painful Heating vow.' (Manu tells us (11.213) that the 'Painful Heating' vow is traditionally said to consist of drinking cow's urine, cow-dung, milk, yogurt, melted butter, and water infused with sacrificial grass, and then fasting for one night.)

5.6.24–5 Hindu mythology tells stories of people who disappeared, leaving behind a shadow or reflection, a kind of after-image, which other people mistook for the person who had disappeared. (See Doniger, *Splitting the Difference*.) Evidently there are magic spells that enable one to do this, and those are *not* the spells that should be used in this situation. See also the spells at 7.1.34.

5.6.38 This section begins with the women taking the initiative (1–9), then alternates between male agency (10–28, 36–7) and female agency (29–35), ending with bi-gendered agency (38).

5.6.41 The *Arthashastra*, the textbook of power and politics, describes (at

1.10.1–20) the trinity (*trivarga*) of trials that the king is to set for the ministers in charge of the uprooting of dissidents (the trial of religion, *dharma*), the treasury (the trial of power or money, *artha*), and the harem (the trial of pleasure or desire, *kama*), with a fourth test (not *moksha*, but fear) for his bodyguards. A man who passes all four may become the prime minister, and a man who fails all four may still be used in some distant mines. V quotes as the opinion of 'scholars' the part of this traditional quartet that applies to the harem, but he does *not* recommend applying the traditional test of *kama* to the harem guards (nor, as the Babhravyas recommend, to the women themselves). Instead, he recommends for harem guards the trial that the *Arthashastra* thought appropriate for bodyguards (fear) and the uprooters of dissidents (religion).

5.6.45 The word we have translated as 'restraint' literally means 'elephant goad'. The meaning is that the women are out of control, like elephants in rut.

BOOK SIX · COURTESANS

6.1.9, 13, 31 The arts here could refer either to the fine arts or to the arts of love, or to both. Y does not specify.

6.1.10 These fatalists are called *Daivapramana* ('those for whom fate, or the gods, are the authority); the fatalists mentioned at 1.2.26 are *Kalakarinikas* ('those who invoke fate, or time, as the cause').

6.1.13 Y glosses what we have translated as 'true to one type' (*ekajatiya*) as meaning that the woman does not keep changing her appearance (losing and gaining weight, one might suppose, changing her hairdo, etc.)

6.1.14 These qualities are apparently appreciated in all women, in contrast with the qualities enumerated in 6.1.13, which are appreciated only, or specially, in courtesans.

[Y] 6.1.15 Y takes his examples from each of the three groups of qualities: bad family (the inverse of a great family, the first quality in 6.1.12), ugliness (in contrast with beauty, 6.1.13), and stupidity (in contrast with intelligence, 6.1.14). This means that the faults apply to both men (6.1.12) and women (6.1.13–14).

6.1.16 'Worms in the faeces' may offer a speculative explanation for some venereal disease.

[Y] 6.1.17 Y assumes that women have semen, a belief that he and the Babhravyas express in the discussion of female orgasm (at 2.1.18). Ravana raped Rambha by threatening to kill her, but she cursed him so that he could never rape another woman again. This story is told in the *Ramayana*; see Doniger, *Splitting the Difference*. Devadatta and Anangasena are two courtesans, and Muladeva is a master-thief, in Somadeva's tenth-century *Ocean of Story* and Kshemendra's eleventh-century work the *Kalavilasa*.

6.1.20 'And so forth' may refer to the twenty reasons for a courtesan to take a lover, listed in 6.1.17; though why 'fear' should come first and stand for the group in this case is puzzling; one would expect 'passion', the first reason listed there.

6.2.11 The word for leftover garlands also means the flowers left over from an offering to the gods, whose leftover food (called *prasada*) is distributed to worshippers together with the leftover flowers, or to a king, as described at 4.2.57.

6.2.13 These techniques are discussed at 2.2.3.

6.2.26 This can mean either that she expresses her passion for him by faking drunkenness and so forth and then blames them on her sexual deprivation, or that she uses those feigned conditions that strip away pretences as an excuse to tell him how she feels. Y takes the first two (drunkenness and sleep) in the first sense and the third (disease) in the second sense.

6.2.31 She says, 'Live!' in the spirit of our 'God bless you', or 'Gesundheit', and for a similar reason: the widespread folk belief that the soul temporarily leaves the body during a sneeze (when the heart does in fact stop for a split second).

6.2.36 The word *vrittha*, that we have translated as 'false', can also mean 'casual' or 'in vain', and the compound as a whole can apply either to him or to her. Y takes it in the sense of 'false', and applies it to the woman's infidelity; but it could also apply to him in this sense, or be taken in the sense of 'casual', and applied to either him or her: 'When s/he has been accused of a casual infidelity . . .' Her fasting in the context of his infidelity is well attested in Sanskrit literature, which makes it more likely that it is the man's infidelity that V intended. The word *vyasana*, that we have rendered as 'misfortune', may also mean 'addiction, evil passion, vice', presumably his, but, again, possibly hers.

6.2.47 Or, if this quarrel is between them, and about the vow mentioned in the previous passage, she may be arguing that it is too demanding even for him to carry out.

6.2.54 She asks that when she is reborn, he be reborn as her husband.

6.2.69 A pot full of presents is distributed to anyone who brings good news.

6.2.70 Crows are said to be auspicious omens with the power to make wishes come true.

6.2.72 To follow him beyond death means to die a natural death after his death and wait to be joined with him in heaven or in the next rebirth. Only later, and very rarely, did it come to mean mounting his funeral pyre alive to burn to death with his corpse.

6.3.4 She gets the money ostensibly to pay for the things but actually buys them on credit and keeps the money; he sees the things and thinks she has bought them with the money he gave her.

6.3.36 This may also mean that she does this before he realizes that she is going to take the money and run.

6.3.44 The word 'release' (*moksha*) more generally refers to a person's spiritual release from the world of transmigration (as in 1.2.4); there may be an intended irony in its use here to designate the release of a man from a courtesan's thrall.

6.4.12 The idea seems to be that there is no more reason to take him now than there was when the other woman got rid of him, since he still has no money.

6.4.16 'As fickle in his affections as turmeric is in its colour' puns on the word *raga*, which can mean either 'colour' or 'passion', and on the fact that turmeric cannot hold its colour for long.

6.4.28 There is some confusion in the editions of this passage about the person who is the object of contempt. According to Shastri's reading, it is the courtesan; according to Goswami's, it is the man (treated with contempt by his wife). And according to Y, it is the man's wife (treated with contempt by the courtesan). We have followed Shastri here.

6.4.40 The attitude to the man who is 'attached', according to this verse and, even more sharply, in the commentary on it, is far more cynical than the one expressed in earlier discussions of the attached man, as at 6.2.73. There, he was a willing devotee; here, he seems to be either entirely besotted or simply the man with her at the moment, or both. There, he was cherished; here he is taken for granted and scorned, explicitly contrasted with the man she does love. This may be an example of a different origin for the prose and verse passages of the text.

6.5.5 A series of choices is made here between paired alternatives, and there is a running disagreement about them between V and earlier scholars. In passage 5 the scholars rank at the top the man who gives her what she seeks or needs, a general category that will be broken down, in passage 8, into those who fulfil temporary and future needs and that V, in passage 6, epitomizes in the man who gives gold. Passage 8 offers another set of categories, which are debated in the passages that follow, together with yet other criteria. In passage 9, the scholars rank the generous man over the man in love, and V disagrees in 10–11. In passage 12 (and again in 14, 19 and 22), the scholars rank the man who does what she needs to have done over the generous man, and V disagrees in 13. In 15 the scholars rank the generous man over the grateful man, and V disagrees in 16–18. In 20 the scholars rank the general category of getting money over a friend's advice, and V disagrees in 21. In 24 the scholars rank getting money over counteracting losses, and V disagrees in 25–7.

6.5.18 The text allows the reading that the man himself cannot be slandered, which is a more logical conclusion from his own good character, but Y links it to passage 16 and takes it to mean that he does not believe slander against her.

6.6.5 This triad may well be a satirical twist on the famous triad of the three aims of human life (1.1.1), which here are reduced to three aspects of one of them: money or power—which (in Sanskrit, *artha*) itself also means 'gain'.

6.6.12 This triad is, theoretically, that of losses connected with money, religious merit, and pleasure, though V spells these out neither for gains (which he has discussed at 2.1.1) nor for losses. Significantly, V here reverses the usual order, putting *artha* first. One might also see a triad in situations that result in positive gain (6.6.13–14), mixed gain and loss (6.6.15–16), and loss (6.6.17–18).

BOOK SEVEN · EROTIC ESOTERICA

7.1.20 'Oriental practices' is a euphemism that V uses (at 5.6.2–3) for the lesbian activities of the women in the harem.

7.1.26 Y specifies both a male and a female object of this magic, assuming both a male subject (as V does) to put the spell on a woman and, presumably, either a female subject or a person of the third nature to put the spell on a man. Shastri assumes a male subject, instructing the reader to smear the powder on his own penis when he makes love to the woman he wants, as V specified in the previous passage. The bird that Y says is *not* a peacock he calls *jivanjivaka*, a bird whose call sounds like 'Jiva! Jiva!'—'Live! Live!'

7.1.27 Presumably this powder is used in the same way as the one in 7.1.26.

7.1.32 There is a pun here: the demigods are Gandharvas (fertility deities that validate love-marriages; see 3.5.18) who like an ointment made with a special perfume (*gandha*, in Sanskrit).

7.1.33 Another pun: the acacia tree is called the Naga tree, and the semi-serpents are *nagas* (a word that also means 'cobra' and 'elephant'), serpents from the waist down and human-like from the waist up. The panic-seed plant (*priyangu*) is said to put forth blossoms at a woman's touch, a play on the word *priya*, which means 'love' or 'pleasure'.

7.1.34 The marigold plant is the *bhringaraja*, literally 'king of the bees'. These eye-salves (which are also described at 5.6.24–5) work by projection: you put them on your own eyes, like eyeshadow or eyeliner, and they distort the vision of the people that you look at or that look at you.

7.1.43–4 The 'and so forth, as above', is in the text.

7.1.45 The exact amounts of the measurements given in the text are uncertain, though their relative size is generally agreed upon: 1 *prastha* = 32 *palas*, and 1 *pala* = 4 *karshas*. If we accept one educated guess that a *karsha* weighs 11 grams, or approximately half an ounce (and, therefore, that a *pala* = 44 grams, or 2 ounces, and a *prastha* = 64 ounces, or 4 lb.), this mixture consists of 4 ounces each of butter, honey, sugar, and licorice, half an ounce of wine-palm hemp, and 64 ounces of milk.

7.1.46–7 Spring is the season that begins when the moon is in the constellation of Paushya.

7.1.48 Here we are guessing that the two *palas* that the text prescribes weigh 2 ounces apiece.

7.1.49 The Veda of Long Life is the *Ayurveda*, the general science of medicine that is expounded in several texts; and the Veda is the *Atharva Veda*, the fourth Veda, a specific text, which deals with magic.

7.2.2 This passage, like most of this section with the exception of 7.2.3, seems to refer to the kindling of the woman's passion when the man cannot satisfy her.

7.2.4 Sex tools include dildos (used instead of a penis), bracelets or rings (put on a penis), sheaths (put over and around a penis), and objects inserted through a hole pierced in the penis. Dildos are described in 5.6.2 and elsewhere in the *Kamasutra* where women use them with other women. Passages 7.2.4–7 may apply to either dildos or bracelets; passages 7.2.8–11 describe bracelets; 7.2.12 describes a sheath; 7.2.13 describes dildos; and passages 7.2.14–24 describe the piercing and its accoutrements.

7.2.6 The adjective used here for 'violent', *dhrishnu*, is derived from the verb connoting sexual violence or rape.

7.2.9 The word for 'wraparound' is also used for the robe of a Buddhist monk, perhaps one of V's jokes about religion.

[Y] 7.2.12 Y assumes that the size of the penis is what determines the force with which this sheath is employed, but V might have had in mind the size of the vagina, as Y does in 7.2.24. Y also assumes that the 'balls' are tiny bumps that provide friction, as in 7.2.8; but here the 'balls' appear to be the testicles.

7.2.16–17 N. N. Bhattacharya's comment on these two passages is telling: 'A man with some commonsense must admit that by keeping the perforated organ under water the wound can only be made poisonous in which pus will be formed and that it is impossible to make sexual intercourse in such a condition on the very day when the perforation is made. There is no reason to believe that the ancient peoples did not know such simple things.' (*History of Indian Erotic Literature*, 91).

7.2.24 The devices may be soft or hard, and they may be rough or smooth.

7.2.25 In his translation of the *Anangaranga*, Burton remarks on 'the application of insects, as it is practised by some savage races; and all Orientalists will remember the tale of the old Brahman, whose young wife insisted upon his pudendum being again stung by a wasp' (p. 47).

7.2.33 Who smears these substances on the woman? The woman herself? Her lover who wants to destroy a rival lover? Or the man who wants to break out of her thrall? In the first two cases, though not in the last, the woman must acquiesce in this project. In 7.2.34, however, the woman must surely be the one who knowingly bathes in the magic substances and so must be the one who wants to destroy the man's passion for her.

7.2.36–7 Presumably these ointments, like the one in 7.2.33, are smeared on the woman's vagina, to make it contract or expand, as in 2.6.1–2.

7.2.38–40 Presumably you put this mixture on your own hair; but it might be used in some other way to affect the hair on someone else's head. The same applies to the lip in 7.2.41–2.

7.2.54 Here V makes starkly explicit what he has in fact done at the end of most of the other books, too: rescinded the apparent licence given by the rest of the book.

BIBLIOGRAPHY

Editions of the Kamasutra *(in chronological order)*

1891   Edited by Pandit Durgaprasad. Bombay.

1912   *Kamasutra* of Vatsyayana, with the commentary of Yashodhara. Edited by Sri Damodar Lal Goswami, Varanasi: Kashi Sanskrit Series, 29.

1934   *Kamasutra* of Vatsyayana, with the commentary of Yashodhara. Edited with the Hindi 'Purushartha' commentary by Madhavacharya, Bombay: Lakshmivenkateshvara Steam Press.

1964   *Kamasutra* of Vatsyayana, with the commentary of Yashodhara. Edited with the Hindi 'Jaya' commentary by Devadatta Shastri. Kashi Sanskrit Series, 29. Varanasi: Chaukhambha Sanskrit Sansthan.

1997   *Kamasutra* of Vatsyayana, with the commentary of Yashodhara. Edited with the Hindi 'Jaya' commentary by Ramanand Sharma, Bitthaldas Sanskrit Series, 4, Varanasi: Krishnadas Academy.

Translations of the Kamasutra *(in chronological order within each language)*

Into English

[1883] *The Kama Sutra of Vatsyayana.* Translated by Sir Richard Burton and F. F. Arbuthnot. Foreword by Santha Rama Rau, Introduction by John W. Spellman, New York: E. P. Dutton & Co., 1962.

——— ed., with a preface, W. G. Archer, London: George Allen and Unwin, 1963.

——— ed. John Muirhead-Gould, Introduction by Dom Moraes, London: Panther Books, 1963.

——— ed., with a preface, W. G. Archer, Introduction by K. M. Panikkar, New York: Berkeley Books, 1966.

1921   K. Rangaswami Iyengar, Lahore: Punjab Sanskrit Book Depot.

1943   B. N. Basu, *The Hindu Art of Love*, rev. S. L. Ghosh, Calcutta: Medical Book Company.

1946   Santosh Kumar Mukherji, Calcutta.

1946   Umendra Verma, *Complete and Unexpurgated: The Most Comprehensive Manual ever written on the Hindu Art and Techniques of Love*, special illustrated edition, Lahore.

1961   S. C. Upadhyaya, Bombay: Taraporevala's Treasure House of Books. Illustrated.

1963   Vipin Shastri, Delhi.

1982   M. R. Anand and L. Dane, Delhi.
1994   From the [1992] French edition. Alain Daniélou, *The Complete Kama Sutra*, Rochester, Vt.: Park Street Press.

Into French, German, Italian, and Russian

1883   Isidore Liseux. *Kama Sutra de Vatsyayana. Manuel d'Érotologie Hindoue*, Paris: Georges-Anquetil, 1925 (Varanasi, 1883).
1891   Pierre Eugène Lemairesse, Paris (repr. 1952).
1992   Alain Daniélou, *Kama Sutra. Le Bréviaire de l'Amour. Traité d'érotisme de Vatsyayana*. Commentaire *Jayamangala* en sanskrit de Yashodhara. Extraits d'un commentaire en hindi de Devadatta Shastri, Paris: Éditions du Rocher.
1897   Richard Schmidt. *Das Kamasutram des Vatsyayana. Die indische ars amatoria, nebst dem vollständigen Kommentare (Jayamangala) des Yasodhara. Aus dem Sanskrit übersetzt und herausgegeben von Richard Schmidt*, Leipzig; 2nd edition Leipzig, 1900; rev. Berlin, 1907, 1912, 1920, 1922 ... 1956.
1987   Klaus Mylius. *Mallanaga Vatsyayana: Das Kamasutra, übersetzt von Klaus Mylius*, Verlag Philipp Reclam jun., Leipzig, 1987.
1945   Antonio Velini. *I kamasutra, codice indiano dell'amore; nella traduzione integrale di Antonio Velini*. Rome: De Carlo, 1945.
1993   Alexander Y. Syrkin. *Vatsyayana Mallanaga Kamasutra, perevod s sanskrita, vstypitelnaya statya i kommentarii*, Moscow: Nauka.

Other Sanskrit Texts Cited

Amarushataka, with the commentary of Arjunavarmadeva, Bombay: Nirnayasagara Press, 1954.
Anangaranga of Kalyanamalla, Delhi: Chowkhamba Sanskrit Pratishthana, 1988.
Arthashastra of Kautilya, critical edition, ed. R. P. Kangle, Bombay: University of Bombay, 1960.
Baudhayana Dharmasutra, in *Dharmasutras*, trans. Patrick Olivelle.
Dharmasutras: The Law Codes of Apastamba, Gautama, Baudhayana, and Vasistha, trans. Patrick Olivelle, World's Classics, Oxford: Oxford University Press, 1999.
Kathasaritsagara, Bombay: Nirnara Sagara Press, 1930. English translation: *The Ocean of Story*, ed. N. M. Penzer, trans. C. W. Tawney, 10 vols, London: Chas. J. Sawyer, 1924.
Kumarasambhava of Kalidasa, in *The Complete Works of Kalidasa*, ed. V. P. Joshi, Leiden: E. J. Brill, 1976.
Laws of Manu (Manusmrti), ed. Harikrishna Jayantakrishna Dave, Bombay: Bharatiya Vidya Series, 29 ff., 1972–91.

Laws of Manu, trans. Wendy Doniger, with Brian K. Smith, Harmondsworth: Penguin Books, 1991.

Manu. See *The Laws of Manu*.

Natyashastra of Bharata Muni, ed. M. M. Batuk Nath Sharma and M. M.
Baldeva Upadhyaya, Varanasi: Chaukhamba, Kashi Sanskrit Series, 60,
1929.

Ocean of Story. See *Kathasaritsagara*.

Rig Veda, with the commentary of Sayana, 6 vols. London: Oxford
University Press, 1890–92. See also Griffith.

—— trans. Wendy Doniger O'Flaherty, *The Rig Veda: An Anthology, 108
Hymns Translated from the Sanskrit*, Harmondsworth: Penguin Classics,
1981.

Shiva Purana, Varanasi: Pandita Pushtakalaya, 1964.

Shakuntala (Abhijnanashakuntalam) of Kalidasa, in *The Complete Works
of Kalidasa*, ed. V. P. Joshi, Leiden: E. J. Brill, 1976.

Shatapatha Brahmana, Varanasi: Chowkhamba Sanskrit Series, 1964.

Skanda Purana, Bombay: Shree Venkateshvara Steam Press, 1867.

Upanishads. In *Upaniṣads*, trans. Patrick Olivelle, World's Classics, Oxford:
Oxford University Press, 1996.

Vasishtha Dharmasutra, in *Dharmasutras*, trans. Olivelle.

Secondary Sources

1. About Sir Richard Burton

Archer, W. G., Preface to *The Kamasutra of Vatsysyana*, trans. Sir Richard
Burton and F. F. Arbuthnot, ed. with a preface, W. G. Archer, London:
George Allen and Unwin, 1963.

Brodie, Fawn M., *The Devil Drives: A Life of Sir Richard Burton*, New
York: Ballantine, 1967.

Casada, James A., *Sir Richard F. Burton: A Biobibliographical Study*,
Boston: G. K. Hall, 1990.

Dearden, Seton, *The Arabian Knight: A Study of Sir Richard Burton*,
London: Arthur Barker, 1936; 1953.

Lovell, Mary S., *A Rage to Live: A Biography of Richard and Isabel
Burton*, New York and London: W. W. Norton, 1998.

McLynn, Frank, *Snow upon the Desert*, London: Murray, 1993.

Rice, Edward, *Captain Sir Richard Francis Burton: The Secret Agent who
Made the Pilgrimage to Mecca, Discovered the Kama Sutra, and Brought
the Arabian Nights to the West*, New York: Charles Scribner's Sons, 1990.

2. Other Secondary Sources

Bhattacharya, Narendra Nath, *History of Indian Erotic Literature*, New
Delhi: Munshiram Manoharlal, 1975.

Biggs, Jonathan, *The Pop-Up Kama Sutra*, New York: Bonanza, 1984.

Burton, Sir Richard Francis, [*Anangaranga*] *The Hindu Art of Love (Ars Amoris Indica) or Ananga-Ranga (Stage of the Bodiless One)*, translated from the Sanskrit of Kalyana Malla and annotated by A. F. F. and B. F. R., privately issued by the British Bibliophiles' Society, 1907 [1885].

Burton, Sir Richard Francis, *The Illustrated KamaSutra, Ananga-Ranga, Perfumed Garden: The Classic Eastern Love Texts*, the Sir Richard Burton and F. F. Arbuthnot translations, edited and introduced by Charles Fowkes, Rochester, Vt.: Park Street Press, 1991.

Chakladar, H. C., *Social Life in Ancient India: A Study in Vatsyayana's Kamasutra*. Calcutta: Susil Gupta, 1954 [1929].

Comfort, Alex, trans. *The Koka Shashtra*, with a preface by W. G. Archer, New York: Ballantine Books, 1964.

Conte, Gian Biagio, 'The Inventory of the World: Form of Nature and Encyclopedic Project in the Work of Pliny the Elder', in Conte, *Genres and Readers* [1991], trans. Glenn W. Most, with a foreword by Charles Segal, Baltimore/London: Johns Hopkins University Press, 1994, 67–104.

De, Sushil Kumar, *Ancient Indian Erotics and Erotic Literature*, Calcutta: Firma K. L. Mukhopadhyay, 1959.

Desmond, Laura, 'Love and Marriage: The Gandharva marriage form in ancient India', autumn 2000, unpublished MS.

Doniger, Wendy, 'Echoes of the *Mahabharata*: Why is a Parrot the Narrator of the *Bhagavata Purana* and the *Devibhagavata Purana*?', in Wendy Doniger (ed.), *Purana Perennis*, Albany: State University of New York Press, 1993, 31–57.

—— 'Three (or More) Forms of the Three (or More)-Fold Path in Hinduism', in Andrew D. Weiner and Leonard V. Kaplan (eds.), *Graven Images: Studies in Culture, Law and the Sacred*, 3, Madison: University of Wisconsin Law School, 1996, 201–12.

—— *The Implied Spider: Politics and Theology in Myth*, The 1996–7 ACLS–AAR Lectures, New York: Columbia University Press, 1998.

—— *Splitting the Difference: Gender and Myth in Ancient Greece and India*, Chicago: University of Chicago Press, 1999.

—— 'Presidential Address: "I Have Scinde": Flogging a Dead (White Male Orientalist) Horse', *Journal of Asian Studies*, 58/4 (November 1999), 940–60.

—— *The Bedtrick: Tales of Sex and Masquerade*, Chicago: University of Chicago Press, 2000.

—— See also: O'Flaherty, Wendy Doniger.

Douglas, Nik, and Slinger, Penny, *The Pillow Book: The Erotic Sentiment and the Paintings of India, Nepal, China and Japan*, New York: Destiny Books, 1981.

Foucault, Michel, *The History of Sexuality*, i. *An Introduction*, trans. Robert Hurley, New York: Vintage Books, 1990.

Ganguly, Anil Baran, *Sixty-four Arts in Ancient India*, New Delhi: English Book Store, 1962.

Griffith, Ralph T. H., *The Hymns of the RgVeda*, Delhi: Motilal Banarsidass, 1973 [1889].

Hampiholi, Viswanath K., *Kamashastra in Classical Sanskrit Literature*, Delhi: Ajanta Publications, 1988.

Hunt, William Bradford, 'Sex for Dharma: Framing the *Kamasutra* in Manu's World', autumn 1999, unpublished MS.

Jamison, Stephanie W., *Sacrificed Wife, Sacrificer's Wife: Women, Ritual, and Hospitality in Ancient India*, New York: Oxford University Press, 1996.

Jolly, J., *Arthasastra of Kautilya*, i, Lahore: Moti Lal Banarsi Das, 1923.

Jong, Erica, *Fear of Flying: A Novel*, New York: New American Library, 1974.

Kakar, Sudhir, and Munder Ross, John, *Tales of Love, Sex and Danger*, New York: Basil Blackwell, 1987.

Kakar, Sudhir, *Intimate Relations: Exploring Indian Sexuality*, Chicago: University of Chicago Press, 1989.

Keith, A. B., *History of Sanskrit Literature*, Oxford: Oxford University Press, 1928.

Lane, Harriet, 'A Book at Bedtime', *The Observer*, 21 January, 2001.

Levinas, Emmanuel, *Totality and Infinity: An Essay on Exteriority*, trans. Alphonso Lingis, The Hague: Martinus Nijhoff, 1979 [*Totalité et Infini*, 1961].

Lutz, Catherine A., and Collins, Jane L., *Reading National Geographic*, Chicago: University of Chicago Press, 1993.

Manara, Milo, *Manara's Kama Sutra*, trans. Joe Johnson, New York: Eurotica: Mantier, Beall, Minoustchine, 1998.

Meyer, Johan Jakob, *Sexual Life in Ancient India*, New York: Barnes and Noble, 1953.

Monier-Williams, Sir Monier, *Sanskrit–English Dictionary*, Oxford: Clarendon Press, 1899.

O'Flaherty, Wendy Doniger, *Asceticism and Eroticism in the Mythology of Siva*, Oxford: Oxford University Press, 1973; retitled *Siva: The Erotic Ascetic*. New York: Galaxy, 1981.

—— *Hindu Myths: A Sourcebook, translated from the Sanskrit*, Harmondsworth: Penguin Classics, 1975.

—— *The Origins of Evil in Hindu Mythology*, Berkeley: University of California Press, 1976.

—— *Women, Androgynes, and Other Mythical Beasts*, Chicago: University of Chicago Press, 1980.

—— *Dreams, Illusion, and Other Realities*, Chicago: University of Chicago Press, 1984.

—— *Tales of Sex and Violence: Folklore, Sacrifice and Danger in the Jaiminiya Brahmana*, Chicago: University of Chicago Press, 1985.

—— *Textual Sources for the Study of Hinduism*, Chicago: University of Chicago Press, 1990.

—— See also: *Rig Veda*, *Laws of Manu*, and Doniger, Wendy.

Oldenberg, Herman, 'Widerruf der Angabe, dass die anonyme englische Übersetzung von Shankar Pandit stammt', in *Deutsche Literaturzeitung*, 19 (1898), 454.

—— 'Zur englischen Übersetzung des Kamasutra', *Zeitschrift der Deutschen Morgenländischen Gesellschaft*, 56 (1902), 26–128.

Olivelle, Patrick, trans. See *Dharmasutras* and *Upanishads*.

Panniker, K. M., *Studies in Indian History*, Bombay: Asia Publishing House, 1963.

Penzer, Norman, *An Annotated Bibliography of Sir Richard Burton*, London, 1923.

Pichard, Georges, *The Illustrated Kama Sutra*, New York: Eurotica—Mantier, Beall, Minoustchine, 1991.

The Pillow Book Kama Sutra, San Francisco: Harper, 1991.

Pollock, Sheldon, 'The Theory of Practice and the Practice of Theory in Indian Intellectual History', *Journal of the American Oriental Society*, 105 (1985), 499–519.

Rai, Ram Kumar, *Encyclopedia of Indian Erotics*, Varanasi: Prachya Prakasan, Chowkhamba Sanskrit Series Office, 1981.

Rawson, Philip, *Erotic Art of the East*, New York: G. P. Putnam's Sons, 1968.

Rocher, Ludo, 'The *Kamasutra*: Vatsyayana's Attitude toward Dharma and Dharmasastra', *Journal of the American Oriental Society*, 105/3 (1985), 521–9.

Schmidt, Richard, *Beiträge zur Indischen Erotik. Das Liebesleben des Sanskrit Volkes*. Berlin: Verlag von H. Barsdorf, 1911.

—— *Liebe und Ehe im alten und modernen Indien*, Berlin: Verlag von H. Barsdorf, 1904.

Sen, Amartya, 'East and West: The Reach of Reason', *New York Review of Books*, 20 July, 2000, 33–8.

Siegel, Lee, *Love in a Dead Language*, Chicago: University of Chicago Press, 1999.

Spayde, Jon, 'The Politically Correct *Kama Sutra*', *The Utne Reader* (November–December 1996), 56–7.

Spencer, Colin, *The Gay Kamasutra*, New York: St Martin's Press, 1996.

Sternbach, Ludwik, *Texts on Courtezans in Classical Sanskrit*, Hoshiarpur: Vishveshvaranand Institute Publications, 1953.

Sweet, Michael J., and Zwilling, Leonard, 'The First Medicalization: The Taxonomy and Etiology of Queerness in Classical Indian Medicine', in *Journal of History of Sexuality*, 3/4 (1993).

Syrkin, A. Y., 'Notes on the *Kama Sutra*', first published in *Trudy po znakovym sistemam*, 3 (1967), 71–80; reprinted in *Semiotica* 11 (1974), 33–42.

Tolputt, Sherry, *The Cartoon Kama Sutra*, London: Knockabout Comics, 1998.

Warren, Henry Clarke, *Buddhism in Translation*, New York: Atheneum, 1969.

Watson, Francis, 'Must We Burn Vatsyayana?', *Encounter* 22/3 (March 1964), 67–73.

Werbe, Chlodwig H., 'Frauen sind den Blumen gleich, gar zärtlich zu behandeln, oder, Auch Lust bedarf der Methode', Austro-Indian Association, Vienna, *Newsletter*, 7, May 2000, 7–18.

Wezler, Albrecht, 'Zum Verständnis des Kamasutra', *Zeitschrift der Deutschen Morgenländischen Gesellschaft*, 121 (1971), 269–83.

Winternitz, Maurice, trans. Subhadra Jha., *History of Indian Literature*, iii, *part 2*: *Scientific Literature*, Delhi: Motilal Banarsidass, 1967.

GLOSSARY AND INDEX

ivory tree, *kutaja* *Wrightia antidysenterica* (palay tree) 167, 170
ixora, white, *juhi* 174

jalashuka *see* leech
jambu *see* plum, Java
jasmine, wild, *nipa* *Nauclea cadamba, Ixora badhucca* 94, 170
Jayasena king of Varanasi 124
jihvika *see* ant

kadamba *see* 'morningstar' tree
Kalakarinikas *see* fatalists
Kalidasa great poet of the Gupta age xxx, xli, liii, 200
Kalinga an ancient country in East India between the Godavari and
    Mahanadi rivers, the present Orissa 129
Kama the incarnation of *kama*, the Indian Eros/Cupid 3, 14, 20, 59,
    141, 161, 176, 181
Kamasutra xi–lxviii, 4–5, 8–9, 13–15, 37, 39–40, 73–4, 107, 111, 134,
    161–2, 171–3, 179–187, 191, 193, 198–9, 201–3, 210
Kanchukiya a woman servant in the harem, so-called because she
    covered her breasts with a cloth called the Kanchuki 202
Karnataka an ancient country and present state in South India, just
    north of the Chola country 50
karsha a measure of weight, about 11 grams 209
kaseruka *see* kysoor root
Kathasaritsagara (**Ocean of Story**) 10th-cent. CE Kashmiri Sanskrit
    text xxii, xxvi–xxvii, 203, 206
Katyayana author of an ancient *dharma* text 53
khadira *see* cashew
Kichaka a lecherous general in the *Mahabharata* 12, 186
kidney bean, *uccata* *Abrus precatorius, Flacourtia cataphracta* (shrubby
    kidney bean of India, also bead tree, coral-bead plant, a species of
    cyperus) 164
kings 3, 9, 11–12, 14, 16–17, 22–6, 56, 59, 69, 102, 116–17, 122–9, 175,
    184, 188, 195, 202, 207
kinka oil-plant, *avalguja* *Vernonia anthelminthica* (khatzum oil-plant)
    169–70
kliba a non-functional male xxxiii
'**kohl-black' flower,** *anjanika* 170
kokilaksha *see* cuckoo's-eye
Kosala ancient Indian country, northeast of the central Ganges 49
Kotta ancient country in the present Gujarat 124
Krishna a god, incarnation of the god Vishnu 71, 196

Bhagavad Gita

The Bible Authorized King James Version
  With Apocrypha

Dhammapada

Dharmasūtras

The Koran

The Pañcatantra

The Sauptikaparvan (from the
  Mahabharata)

The Tale of Sinuhe and Other Ancient
  Egyptian Poems

Upaniṣads

ANSELM OF CANTERBURY   The Major Works

THOMAS AQUINAS   Selected Philosophical Writings

AUGUSTINE   The Confessions
  On Christian Teaching

BEDE   The Ecclesiastical History

HEMACANDRA   The Lives of the Jain Elders

KĀLIDĀSA   The Recognition of Śakuntalā

MANJHAN   Madhumalati

ŚĀNTIDEVA   The Bodhicaryāvatāra

The Oxford World's Classics Website

www.worldsclassics.co.uk

- Information about new titles
- Explore the full range of Oxford World's Classics
- Links to other literary sites and the main OUP webpage
- Imaginative competitions, with bookish prizes
- Peruse the Oxford World's Classics Magazine
- Articles by editors
- Extracts from Introductions
- A forum for discussion and feedback on the series
- Special information for teachers and lecturers

www.worldsclassics.co.uk

American Literature

British and Irish Literature

Children's Literature

Classics and Ancient Literature

Colonial Literature

Eastern Literature

European Literature

History

Medieval Literature

Oxford English Drama

Poetry

Philosophy

Politics

Religion

The Oxford Shakespeare

A complete list of Oxford Paperbacks, including Oxford World's Classics, Oxford Shakespeare, Oxford Drama, and Oxford Paperback Reference, is available in the UK from the Academic Division Publicity Department, Oxford University Press, Great Clarendon Street, Oxford OX2 6DP.

In the USA, complete lists are available from the Paperbacks Marketing Manager, Oxford University Press, 198 Madison Avenue, New York, NY 10016.

Oxford Paperbacks are available from all good bookshops. In case of difficulty, customers in the UK can order direct from Oxford University Press Bookshop, Freepost, 116 High Street, Oxford OX1 4BR, enclosing full payment. Please add 10 per cent of published price for postage and packing.